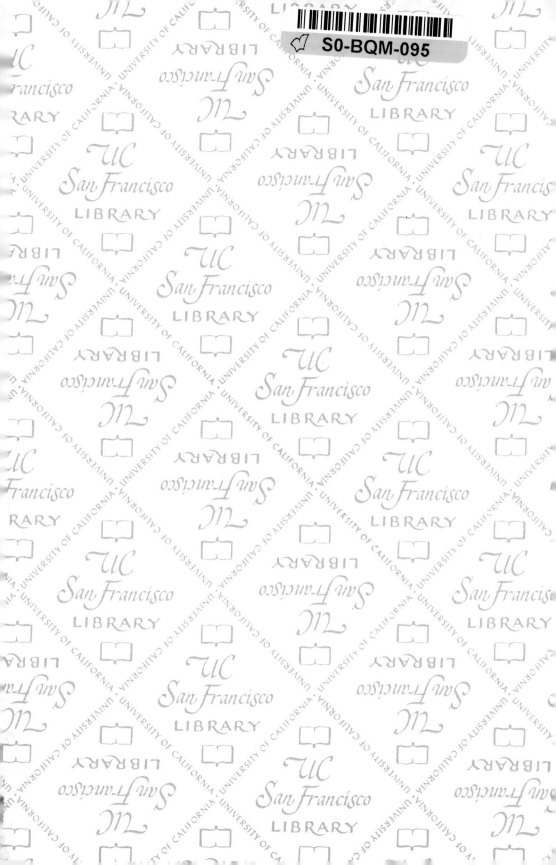

CARCINOGENESIS—
A COMPREHENSIVE SURVEY
VOLUME 5

Modifiers of Chemical Carcinogenesis

Carcinogenesis—A Comprehensive Survey

Carcinogenesis—
A Comprehensive Survey
Volume 5

Modifiers of Chemical Carcinogenesis:
An Approach to the Biochemical Mechanism and Cancer Prevention

Editor

Thomas J. Slaga, Ph.D.
Cancer and Toxicology Program
Biology Division
Oak Ridge National Laboratory
Oak Ridge, Tennessee

Raven Press ■ New York

Raven Press, 1140 Avenue of the Americas, New York, New York 10036

Made in the United States of America

Library of Congress Cataloging in Publication Data
Main entry under title:

Modifiers of chemical carcinogenesis.

(Carcinogenesis—a comprehensive survey; v. 5)
Includes index.
1. Carcinogens. 2. Cancer—Prevention.
3. Antineoplastic agents. 4. Carcinogenesis.
I. Slaga, Thomas J. II. Series.
RC268.5.C36 vol. 5 [RC268.6] 616.9′94′07108s
ISBN 0-89004-232-2   [616.9′94′071]   77-75652

Preface

Epidemiological studies suggest that 60 to 90% of all human cancer is caused by environmental factors. In addition to the epidemiological data, studies using experimental animals provide evidence that exposure to environmental chemicals plays a significant role in the etiology of cancer in man. Man is exposed daily to low-level amounts of a variety of cancer-causing chemicals, few of which are carcinogenic at such low levels. In all probability, such subthreshold amounts become carcinogenic only through an additive effect, cocarcinogenesis, or by expression through natural tumor promoters. A number of environmental chemicals, diet, radiation, and viruses may well be important modifying factors that increase cancer incidence by carcinogenic chemicals. It is with such factors that this book is concerned. Current information suggests that smoking, alcohol, asbestos, high-caloric and high-fat diets, an imbalance of endogenous hormones, to name only a few, are important cofactors in a large percentage of cancers in humans.

Although preventing exposure of the population to carcinogens is theoretically the best way to reduce the incidence of cancer, such an approach is obviously not practical. Therefore, alternative means of modifying the process of carcinogenesis in man must be found. Since carcinogenesis is a prolonged, multistage process, a variety of approaches may be considered, directed toward the inhibition of either the initiation or the promotion phase of carcinogenesis.

This volume discusses not only the above-mentioned modifying agents but also the potent inhibitory effects of certain vitamin A derivatives, antioxidants, protease inhibitors, antiinflammatory steroids, and modifiers of the mixed-function oxidases on chemical carcinogenesis. Some of these agents specifically inhibit the tumor initiation phase, whereas others inhibit primarily the promotion phase. It is the general aim of the contributing scientists to examine the role these modifiers have played in providing a better understanding of the mechanism of chemical carcinogens. In addition, scientific research may determine that some of these modifiers either singularly or in combination may also become important agents in the prevention of cancer in man.

Directed to all scientists and concerned laymen, this book should provide a better understanding of the induction of cancer as well as its possible prevention.

Contents

Contributors

D. L. Berry: *Biology Division, Oak Ridge National Laboratory, Oak Ridge, Tennessee 37830*

T. Colin Campbell: *Division of Nutritional Sciences, Cornell University, Ithaca, New York 14853*

Nancy H. Colburn: *Laboratory of Viral Carcinogenesis, National Cancer Institute, Bethesda, Maryland 20205*

John DiGiovanni: *The McArdle Laboratory for Cancer Research, University of Wisconsin Medical Center, Madison, Wisconsin 53706*

Johnnie R. Hayes: *Division of Nutritional Sciences, Cornell University, Ithaca, New York 14853*

M. R. Juchau: *Department of Pharmacology, School of Medicine, University of Washington, Seattle, Washington 98195*

Ralph J. Rascati: *Biology Division, Oak Ridge National Laboratory, Oak Ridge, Tennessee 37830*

Toby G. Rossman: *New York University Medical Center, Department of Environmental Medicine, New York, New York 10016*

James K. Selkirk: *Biology Division, Oak Ridge National Laboratory, Oak Ridge, Tennessee 37830*

Thomas J. Slaga: *Cancer and Toxicology Program, Biology Division, Oak Ridge National Laboratory, Oak Ridge, Tennessee 37830*

Michael B. Sporn: *National Cancer Institute, Bethesda, Maryland 20205*

Raymond W. Tennant: *Biology Division, Oak Ridge National Laboratory, Oak Ridge, Tennessee 37830*

Walter Troll: *New York University Medical Center, Department of Environmental Medicine, New York, New York 10016*

Robert L. Ullrich: *Biology Division, Oak Ridge National Laboratory, Oak Ridge, Tennessee 37830*

Lee W. Wattenberg: *Department of Laboratory Medicine and Pathology, University of Minnesota, Minneapolis, Minnesota 55455*

Friedrich J. Wiebel: *Gesellschaft für Strahlen- und Umweltforschung, Institute of Toxicology and Biochemistry, München-Neuherberg, Germany*

Carcinogenesis, Vol. 5: Modifiers of Chemical
Carcinogenesis, edited by T. J. Slaga.
Raven Press, New York, 1980.

1

Chemical Carcinogenesis: A Brief Overview of the Mechanism of Action of Polycyclic Hydrocarbons, Aromatic Amines, Nitrosamines, and Aflatoxins

James K. Selkirk

Biology Division, Oak Ridge National Laboratory, Oak Ridge, Tennessee 37830

Cancer is an ancient enemy. It was the same insidious disease eighteen million years ago. The fossil record shows a clear track of osteomas and hemangiomas in dinosaur remains (88,89). In addition, the appearance of plant tumors significantly predates that of animal tumors, pushing back the appearance of cancer fifty million years (87). Although the skeletal parts of ancient forms comprise the fossil record, it is not unrealistic to assume that these early creatures also developed cancer in the soft tissues. More recently, the history of man shows evidence of schistosomiasis in Egyptian mummies of the fifth dynasty (about 3,000 B.C.) suggesting that this civilization probably suffered from an inordinate degree of bladder cancer with no indication that the people ever recognized the relationship between bladder disease and the intermediate snail host (79). Attempts to overcome cancer also date back to civilizations' earliest periods. In India and Egypt, a salve consisting of vinegar and arsenic was applied to lesions with hot irons directly or after cautery. Although it is true that these methods were often directed more to exorcising evil spirits rather than killing malignant cells, our current approach to cancer chemotherapy, although philosophically oriented and scientifically grounded, is not altogether unrelated to that of the ancient physicians. Chemotherapy tries to exploit some more sensitive aspects within the tumor cell's biochemical or genetic apparatus that is more labile than normal cells. Most often, antimetabolites or alkylating agents depend upon the more rapid mitotic index of cancer cells to interrupt its programmed pattern of development to the point that the tumor cell is blocked from further development and can no longer divide. Since complete understanding of the biology and chemistry of the living cell has not been reached, our attempts at blocking cancer growth are all too often ineffective. Clinical data clearly show dramatic differences in how patients are affected by chemotherapeutic drugs: one patient will respond readily, whereas another will not respond at all. In

1

addition, leukemia therapy exhibits the phenomenon of overcoming the effectiveness of a given drug after a prolonged remission. It would appear that the surviving tumor cells had developed the capacity to bypass the biochemical block imposed by the drug. It is, therefore, increasingly important that we begin to understand the biochemical schemes within the growing cell that lead to the malignant state. Obviously this requires knowledge at the level of the gene and a thorough description of the critical steps involved in the transcription of this information to daughter cells as well as the translation into enzymes and structural elements that maintain the cell's own metabolic homeostasis. Concurrently, we must gain an understanding of the subtle interactions between chemicals that can cause permanent perturbation within a cell that in some manner invokes a signal to begin malignant transformation. There are now in the hands of researchers several families of carcinogenic chemicals that have become important probes into the cell's biochemistry. These compounds are, in some cases, structurally related as in polyaromatic hydrocarbons, aromatic amines, and aflatoxins, all of which possess benzenoid moieties as well as unrelated nonaromatic structures such as nitrosamines and carcinogenic metals. Studying structurally divergent carcinogens, especially where there are definite species or tissue preferences as target sites, tends to single out the critical steps necessary to transform that chemical into its carcinogenically active form. As the data base grows and we begin to understand the activation pathways for these divergent types of chemicals, we may eventually begin a general description of the mechanisms of action for all chemical carcinogens. To date, the only generalization that can be attempted, with a good degree of certainty, is the electrophilic nature of all chemical carcinogens (86). It appears that activated forms of carcinogens, irrespective of the parent molecular structure, become electron deficient. They readily attack nucleophilic sites on nucleic acid and protein. Although the actual chemical interaction may follow random kinetics, probability predicts that a finite number of interactions should occur at critical target sites for initiation of tumorigenesis.

Since human exposure to carcinogenic chemicals is, in most cases, a continuous bombardment of subthreshold doses (e.g., cigarettes, automobile exhaust), other noncarcinogenic vectors in our environment can enhance the effect of the relatively low doses of carcinogen (4).

The following sections comprise a summary of the current state of knowledge of several important naturally occurring and industrial carcinogens that have been studied in depth.

POLYCYCLIC AROMATIC HYDROCARBONS

Benzo(a)pyrenes (BP) as all PAH (polycyclic aromatic hydrocarbons) are prevalent contaminants of air, water, and soil. They are products of alkene free-radical conjugation during the incomplete combustion of fossil fuels (Fig. 1) and are, therefore, major exhaust components of transportation, industrial

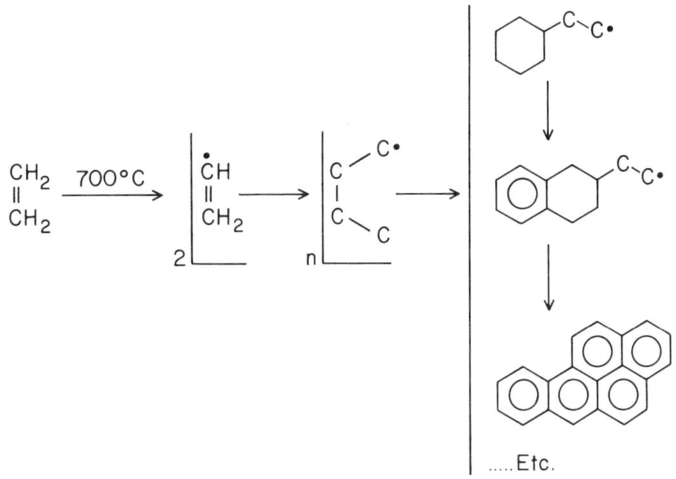

FIG. 1. Pyrolytic formation of polycyclic hydrocarbons by free-radical polymerization.

energy sources, and refuse burning (26). The observation by Percival Pott in 1775 that scrotal cancer in chimney sweeps in Britain was, in some manner, related to the tar and soot left in the chimneys after coal burning, proclaimed for the first time that the environment could be a factor in human cancer (97). Yamagiwa and Ichikawa confirmed this hypothesis when they produced the first laboratory tumor by chemicals using multiple treatments of coal tar extracts on rabbit ear (133). This demonstrated the presence of a tumorigenic substance in coal tar. This finding stimulated a British group to isolate a few grams of pure BP (Fig. 2) following a laborious extraction of two tons of pitch (29). This polyaromatic compound was an effective carcinogen and joined another polycyclic compound, dibenz*(a,h)*anthracene (Fig. 2), also a carcinogen that had been synthesized by the same group just previous to the isolation of the coal tar product (60).

During the next few decades, the majority of the work on polycyclic hydrocarbons was directed toward synthesis and *in vivo* testing of new derivatives (98). The recognition that these compounds were major environmental contaminants led to a burgeoning of research for elucidating the species and tissue susceptibilities for these compounds, including the biochemical pathways for activation and detoxification and their role in human carcinogenesis.

One of the most intriguing problems confronting these studies concerns the intracellular target site(s) with which the carcinogen reacts to induce malignant transformation. The working hypothesis has been centered around the fact that polycyclic aromatic hydrocarbons convalently bind to cellular macromolecules such as DNA (deoxyribonucleic acid), RNA (ribonucleic acid) and protein (9, 14,44,47,64,80,99,110). The amount of hydrocarbon bound is proportional to the concentration of macromolecule in the tissue, with cellular protein binding

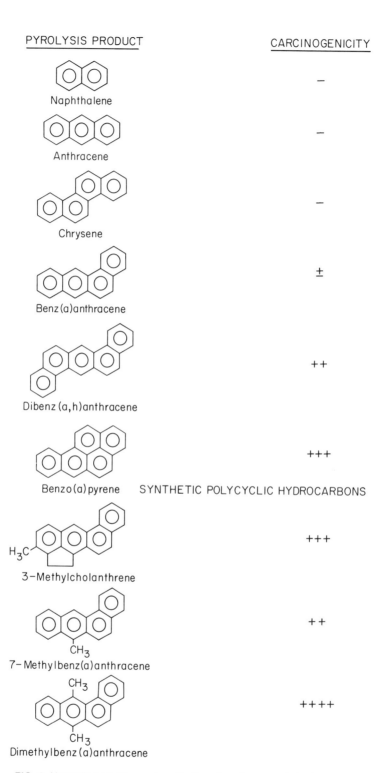

PYROLYSIS PRODUCT   CARCINOGENICITY

Naphthalene   −

Anthracene   −

Chrysene   −

Benz(a)anthracene   ±

Dibenz(a,h)anthracene   ++

Benzo(a)pyrene   SYNTHETIC POLYCYCLIC HYDROCARBONS

                                        +++

3-Methylcholanthrene   +++

7-Methylbenz(a)anthracene   ++

Dimethylbenz(a)anthracene   ++++

FIG. 2. Naturally occurring and synthetic polycyclic aromatic hydrocarbons.

most of the hydrocarbon, followed by RNA and then DNA. Although there is no unequivocal evidence that carcinogenesis is a mutagenic event, and epigenetic mechanisms are theoretically feasible (95), much of the current search for the critical target site(s) is with DNA.

Major emphasis in this area lies in determining which polycyclic derivatives are most efficiently bound to DNA, including what type of chemical bond is formed and which DNA bases are involved. Benzo*(a)*pyrene has become the prototype PAH carcinogen. It is a major environmental pollutant and potent laboratory carcinogen probe. Early studies showed that the hydrocarbon was probably bound covalently since rigorous solvent extraction failed to remove all the hydrocarbon from the macromolecules (14,45). Currently, there is much activity in comparative binding of hydrocarbons to macromolecules to ascertain which compounds are more relevant to carcinogenesis (8–10,58). Polycyclic hydrocarbons are metabolized by the microsomal mixed-function oxidase, arylhydrocarbon hydroxylase (AHH) (Fig. 3), which is predominantly found in liver. This enzyme has been extensively studied and has been the subject of several reviews (27,43,91). This enzyme complex is apparently involved with detoxification of xenobiotics and is also directly involved with the activation process whereby the molecule forms its active epoxide species (111,113). A second microsomal enzyme, epoxide hydrase, converts epoxides into vicinal glycols (93), and since epoxides are more active carcinogens than the parent hydrocarbon, this enzyme may play a critical role in carcinogenesis for rapid removal of the reactive intermediate epoxides (52,128) before interaction with a target site. However, it is now apparent that in some cases diols of aromatic hydrocar-

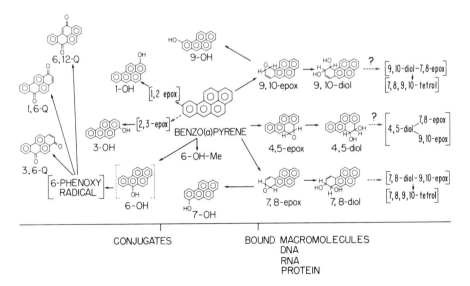

FIG. 3. BP metabolism: Known and suspected *(bracketed)* in vivo and *in vitro* metabolites.

bons can undergo another cycle of metabolic activation and become even more carcinogenic as diol epoxides than the epoxide by itself (53,112,114,115,131). This has been demonstrated for BP (Fig. 3) where the 7,8-diol is readily transformed by the microsomal oxidases into the 7,8-diol-9,10-epoxide (134). This labile intermediate is a major binding species of BP to nucleic acid from the 10-carbon of BP to the N-2 position of guanine (124). There is also some interaction with adenine but no significant pyrimidine binding has been reported.

The diol epoxide has proved to be an active mutagen (7,18,19,78,132) and is tumorigenic to mouse skin (68,116,117). Other intermediates currently under investigation in several laboratories, primarily using BP, are transient free radicals. This type of intermediate is known to be generated chemically and enzymatically (90,122). However, its instability has precluded its comprehensive testing and placement in the scheme of carcinogenesis by PAH. It is apparent that the biochemical steps are complex and the active intermediates are transient. The balance between carcinogen activation and detoxification and the relative physicochemical binding of reactive intermediates to the critical receptors are important determinants for transformation in the cell.

The carcinogenic species of PAH apparently occurs when the cellular biochemistry raises the molecule to a higher level of lability in order to metabolize it to a less toxic compound for removal from the cell (48).

The known metabolites of BP, as well as bracketed compounds not yet unequivocally identified or only hypothesized (shown by question marks), are seen in Fig. 3. The 7,8-epoxide and 9,10-epoxide have not been isolated intact, but their presence has been confirmed by enzymatic formation and inhibition studies of their respective dihydrodiols (50,108). The metabolite profile appears to be qualitatively identical in both susceptible and resistant species and tissues (111). Therefore, the susceptibility to tumorigenesis by these compounds may lie in the kinetic description of metabolite formation and removal. If one or two active intermediates are the primary carcinogenic species of polyaromatic hydrocarbons, then the rate of formation and disappearance of these particular intermediates affects the probability of the active compound reacting at a target site and subsequently dictates the susceptibility or resistance to tumorigenesis of any given species or tissue. Figures 4 to 8 show the metabolite profile variation of BP metabolized by rat liver microsomes in contrast to hamster liver microsomes, hamster embryo cell-tissue culture incubations, and microsomes prepared from hamster embryo cells. The metabolites shown have been separated by high-pressure liquid chromatography (107,109,111). The marked difference in the amounts of the various hydroxylated products formed between rodent liver microsomes and intact or lysed cells shows great range in the attack of the respective monooxygenases. Clearly, different regions of the BP molecule are favored. Rat (Fig. 4) and hamster liver (Fig. 5) microsomes show metabolite patterns containing three diols 8,10-, 4,5-, 7,8-dihydrodihydroxy-BP; three quinones, 1,6-, 3,6-, 6,12-BP quinone; and two phenols, 9-OH, 3-OH-BP. Liver

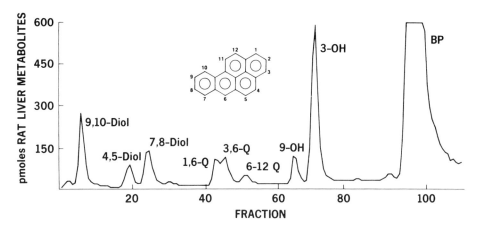

FIG. 4. Rat liver metabolism of BP. High-pressure liquid chromatographic separation of organic solvent extractable material after incubation of BP with tissue containing arylhydrocarbon hydroxylase and epoxide hydrase.

contains the highest level of drug-metabolizing enzymes but is not a major target site for polycyclic carcinogenesis.

Hamster liver produces almost exclusively 4,5-diol, although this metabolite forms a lesser component in rat liver metabolism. In contrast, microsomes from hamster cells (Fig. 6) either produce insignificant amounts or further metabolize

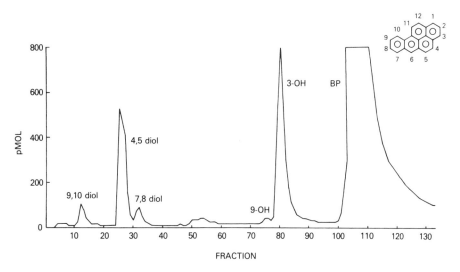

FIG. 5. Hamster liver metabolism of BP.

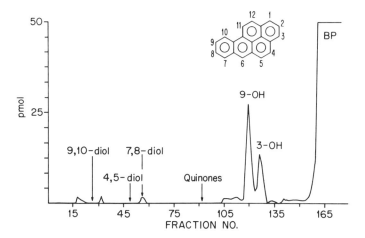

FIG. 6. Metabolism of BP by microsomes prepared from hamster embryonic fibroblasts grown in tissue culture.

diols and quinones while forming 9-hydroxy as the major metabolite with lesser amounts of 3-hydroxy. Conversely, BP metabolism in intact hamster cells (Fig. 7) reverses the metabolite pattern. The 9,10- and 7,8-diols are the major components with only trace amounts of phenols. It would appear that intact cells produce predominantly precursor diols for formation of the highly reactive diol epoxides. Disruption of the cells clearly alters metabolite ratios suggesting a requirement for spatial orientation of the enzyme complexes within the microsomal membranes. In addition, intact cells contain the cytoplasmic conjugates that are important for conversion of reactive tumorigenic and toxic intermediates

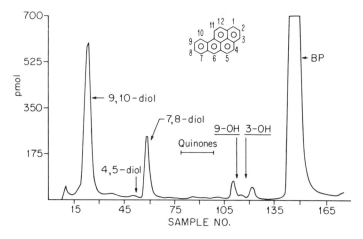

FIG. 7. Metabolism of BP by intact hamster embryo cells during 24-hr incubation period.

to water-soluble products for excretion. The conjugating enzymes become diluted or lost during cell disruption and microsome preparation. Species resistance and susceptibility may, indeed, be determined by the rate of the activation and detoxification steps, and therefore, the kinetics of formation and disappearance of the activated carcinogenic molecular species may dictate whether that given species is a significant risk to polycyclic hydrocarbon induced tumorigenesis.

Further developments in technology have allowed greater resolution of metabolite peaks to enable discovery of even larger numbers of potentially important metabolites. Since BP contains a number of possible isomeric phenols, it is important to know how many are metabolic products. This knowledge would help us to understand which regions are most susceptible to the microsomal enzymes.

In order to do this, multiple chromatography was needed without exposing the labile intermediates to air and light. In addition, more than a few columns in succession would cause the pressure head to reach the practical limits of the instrumentation. The problem was solved by recycling the partially resolved peaks through only two columns (110). Figure 8 shows a schematic representation of the recycle system and incorporates the same alternate pumping design with a 6-port, 2-position valve (Model CV-G-HPAX; Valco, Inc., Houston, Texas).

When the valve is set to position 1, compounds injected into the system pass first through ports 1 and 2 and into column 1. After eluting from column 1, they pass through the UV cell and back through ports 5 to 3 and enter column 2. At this point, the valve is changed to position 2, so the eluting compounds from column 2 pass through ports 4 to 2 and reenter column 1. As the compounds elute from column 1 and pass through the UV flow cell,

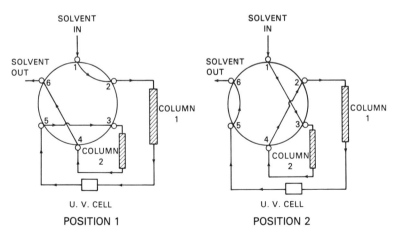

FIG. 8. Valve assembly for high-pressure liquid chromatography (HPLC) recycling between two microparticulate columns.

they may either be collected at port 6 after passing through three columns or recycled again through another two columns by changing the valve back to position 1 and allowing the compounds to enter column 2 via ports 5 to 3. Once the compounds are transferred onto column 2, which is complete after the final peak has passed through the UV cell, the valve is changed to position 2. The compounds can be collected after five columns at port 6 or the valve can be changed once again to position 1 to transfer the compounds once again onto column 2 repeating the recycle procedure.

Compounds that separate adequately without recycling can be injected into the system with the valve in position 2 and collected after passing through two columns.

Figure 9 shows the elution of 10 synthetic BP phenols, separated after one, three, and five passages through the column. After a single pass through one column, six peaks are observed; four of these peaks each contain two phenols, and two peaks each contain one phenol. After the first passage the 5-phenol is cleanly resolved as a single peak and the 7-phenol is partially resolved. The 4-phenol and 6-phenol, 10-phenol and 12-phenol, 1-phenol and 3-phenol, and 8-phenol and 9-phenol migrate in the indicated pairs in four different peaks. A structural basis for the separation seems to relate to the relative position of the hydroxy group since each of the latter four peaks contains pairs of phenols

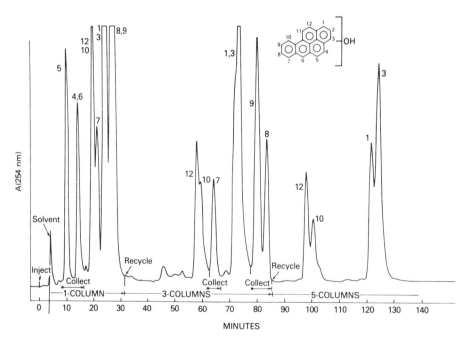

FIG. 9. HPLC separation of BP phenols using recycling with hexane:dioxane (9:1) as the elution solvent.

in which the hydroxyl groups are either adjacent or two carbon atoms apart. After passage through three columns, five peaks were clearly resolved. The 7-phenol, 8-phenol, and 9-phenol were completely separated as single peaks; the 12-phenol and 10-phenol migrated in one peak with the 10-phenol as a sharp shoulder on the 12-phenol and the 1-phenol a slight shoulder on the 3-phenol peak. The single 5-phenol peak and the peak containing the 4-phenol and 6-phenol were collected after a single pass through the column, since they elute first and pass through the UV cell and out of the system before the last peaks (8-phenol and 9-phenol) appear. This prevented recycling them further in the same system.

The two remaining doublets, the 12-phenol and 10-phenol and the 1-phenol and 3-phenol, were passed through two additional columns producing four separate peaks, the 12-phenol, 10-phenol, 1-phenol, and 3-phenol, respectively. Additional recycling resulted in some broadening of the peak bases.

Figure 10 shows the separation in an identical system of phenolic metabolites formed when BP was incubated with liver microsomes from methylcholanthrene-induced rats. The first two unidentified peaks are not metabolites but rather material absorbing at 254 nm which, when collected, show no UV spectrum related to BP. These peaks are derived from microsomal extracts. Three metabolite peaks are observed after passage through a single column. After passage through the entire five-column recycling system, four distinct peaks are resolved.

Each of the metabolites was isolated and characterized by cochromatography and UV spectra and compared to the 10 synthetic phenols. These correspond

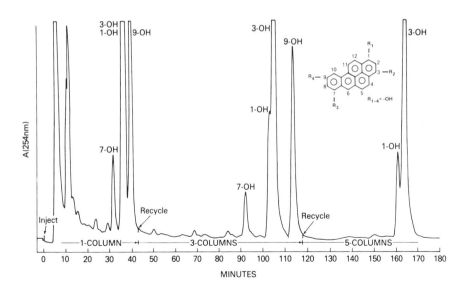

FIG. 10. HPLC separation of BP phenol metabolites formed by rat liver microsomes.

to the 3-phenol and 9-phenol previously identified as metabolites and two newly identified metabolites, the 1-phenol and the 7-phenol. The absorption maxima of the authentic compounds and the compounds formed by rat liver microsomes were identical.

Interestingly, all twelve BP phenols have now been tested as tumor initiator in mouse skin and whereas 1-OH and 7-OH have proved negative 2-OH and 11-OH are positive (129). Neither derivative has yet been isolated as a metabolite.

As the case for the metabolic diol epoxide becomes stronger, it may be possible that polyfunctional intermediates can be found with the active groups not necessarily in the same benzene ring.

AROMATIC AMINES

Aromatic amines comprise a large family of compounds, both industrial, and medicinal and consumer products. These compounds are related to polyaromatic structures because of the presence of benzene moieties. However, they differ since they possess reactive primary or secondary amine groups that play an active role in determining the carcinogenicity of the compound. Aromatic amines became suspect as human carcinogens in the late 19th century with an observation by Rehn that bladder cancer was more prevalent in workers in the chemical dye industry (102). The compound assumed to be carcinogenic was aniline (see Structure 1) which was the starting material for most synthetic azo dyes. However, Case and co-workers (23) showed by means of epidemiological studies that 2-naphthylamine and benzidine (see Structure 1) were more directly related to the incidence of bladder cancer. Epidemiologically, it appeared that only 6 months exposure to 2-napthylamine was equivalent to 5 years exposure to 1-naphthylamine with regard to the number of cases of bladder cancers reported. Workers outside the dye industry who were exposed to the same chemicals also presented higher than expected incidence of bladder cancer. This supported the argument that some aromatic amines were human carcinogens. Rubber workers (22), exterminators (6), and patients treated for polycythemia vera (120) were all exposed to naphthylamine and all were above the expected incidence. Population studies were followed in the laboratory by Hueper who

Aniline   2−naphthylamine   Benzidine

Structure 1.

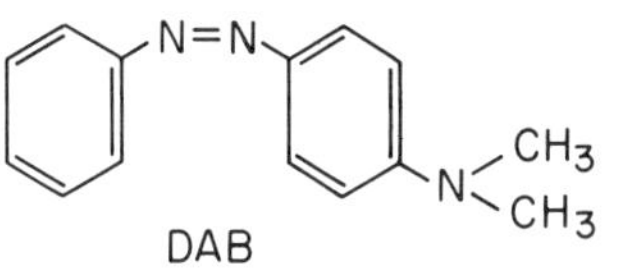

Structure 2.

DAB

showed 2-naphthylamine to be an effective bladder tumor agent in the dog (54).

In order to be tumorigenic, aromatic amines must be introduced parenterally, which is indicative of a requirement for metabolic activation (85). They do not produce tumors at injection sites, as do the polycyclic hydrocarbons; aromatic amines require a labile functional group that reacts readily with nucleophilic sites. However, carcinogenic polycyclic hydrocarbons are tumorigenic at the site of injection and largely ineffective systemically which suggests that the species and tissue specificity for many chemical carcinogens along with biochemical requirements include physical and chemical characteristics such as relative solubility, rate of hydrolysis, alkylating ability, etc. Polycyclic hydrocarbons are probably more hydrophobic and are more likely to remain locally in the tissue when injected than a less hydrophobic aromatic amine which would be more rapidly transported to the liver where the highest level of drug metabolizing enzymes are present and where they are very active tumor agents. The two most representative aromatic amines used in elucidating the metabolic pathways for activation and detoxification are *N,N*-dimethyl-4-phenylazoaniline (DAB or *p*-dimethylaminoazobenzene, Structure 2) and *N*-2-fluorenylacetamide (2-FAA, Structure 3) (Figs. 11 and 12). DAB, originally termed "butter yellow," was used to color margarine but was quickly removed from commerce when it was found to be a potent liver carcinogen (85) in rodents.

2-Fluorenylacetamide was patented as an insecticide but extensive tests previous to its marketing showed this compound also to be an effective liver and bladder tumor agent in rodents (126,127). A number of reviews extensively discuss many aromatic amine derivatives and compare their relative tissue range of susceptibility and metabolic products. The reader is referred to reviews by Clayson and Garner (25), Miller and Miller (82), and Weisburger and Weisburger (125).

Metabolic studies show a number of ring hydroxylation products. However, these compounds are extremely weak carcinogens or noncarcinogens and strongly

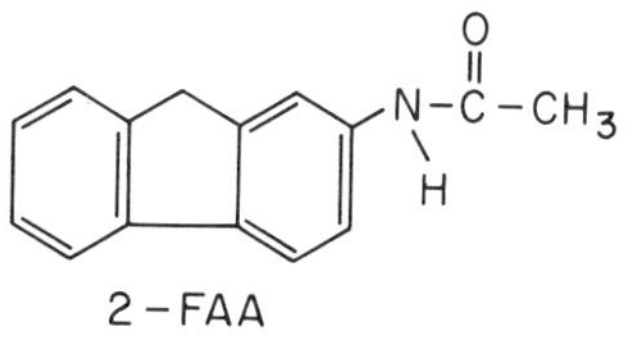

Structure 3.

2 – FAA

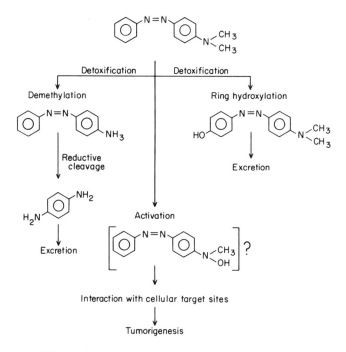

FIG. 11. Aromatic amine activation: metabolism of DAB.

suggest that hydroxylation of the aromatic rings is a detoxification pathway (125). Long-term treatment did produce a new urinary product that was not a ring-hydroxyl and was conjugated to glucuronic acid (81). This conjugate, when digested, yielded the side-chain metabolite, N-hydroxy-2-FAA.

Unlike the inactive ring hydroxylation metabolites, N-hydroxy-2-FAA (Structure 4) was even more tumorigenic than the parent 2-FAA molecule and would produce tumors at the site of injection (62). The expression "proximate carcinogen" was adopted with isolation of this metabolite since the N-hydroxy product was clearly metabolically closer to the actual reactive carcinogenic species than the parent 2-FAA. Although it appears all aromatic amines require N-hydroxylation for metabolic activation, not all N-hydroxy amines are carcinogenic (82).

Following hydroxylation, the next metabolic step in the pathway of aromatic amines is esterification, which was first discovered using methylaminoazobenzene (MAB) which, unlike 2-FAA, would not be readily N-hydroxylated and required some additional chemistry to achieve the next step. The benzoyloxy ester was prepared (Fig. 13) with the assumption that tissue esterases would rapidly release the free N-hydroxy-MAB (51,81,95).

When the ester was tested it proved to be a potent skin carcinogen at the site of injection (96). In addition, DNA-bound derivatives using *in vitro* incubations were similar to those found in DNA extracted from tissue treated

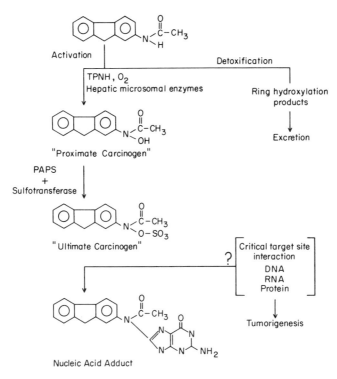

FIG. 12. Aromatic amine activation: metabolism of 2-FAA.

with MAB (83). Furthermore, the benzoyloxy ester rapidly formed a methylthio ether (Fig. 13) when mixed with methionine alone to form 3-methylmercapto-MAB indicative of a natural chemical equilibrium strongly in the direction of ortho addition.

This sulfation mechanism was also suspected for esterification of *N*-hydroxy-2-FAA since several types of synthetic esters were found to be tumorigenic, although none were isolated as metabolic products. Subsequently, a hepatic sulfotransferase activity utilizing 3′-phosphoadenosine-5′-phosphosulfate (PAPS) as the donor which formed *N*-sulfate-2-FAA (Structure 5) was demonstrated (30,61).

In species comparisons, the level of hepatic sulfotransferase activity and sus-

Structure 4.

N−hydroxy−2−FAA

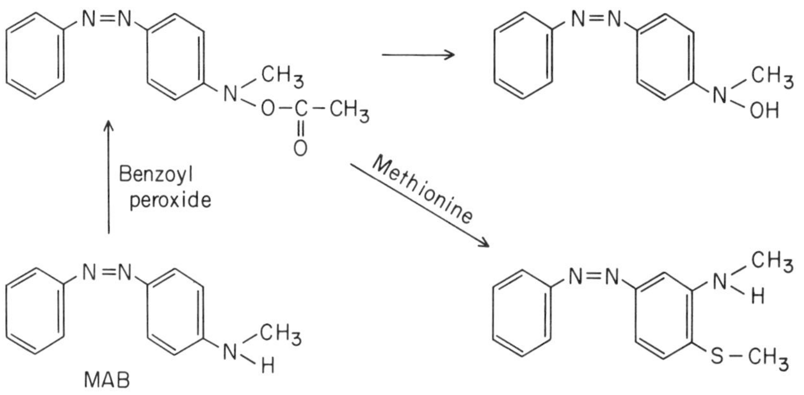

FIG. 13. Formation of 3-methylmercapto-MAB.

ceptibility to hepatocarcinogenesis from 2-FAA was found to be directly proportional (31), and it would appear that a similar mechanism occurs for DAB in addition to its known 3-mercapto derivative although sulfate esters of this compound have not been isolated. This supposition is circumstantially derived from the ease of reaction to form methionyl, tyrsoinyl, and guanyl derivatives (70, 71,84).

Activation to an *N*-hydroxylated alkylating species mediated through an ester intermediate is metabolically correct. However, there is sufficient variation in species susceptibility to assume there may be other types of active intermediates (55). Sulfotransferase activity has not been observed in subcutaneous, mammary, or in sebaceous ear duct, all of which are target sites for aromatic amines (32,57,61). Furthermore, 2-naphthylamine is carcinogenic in the dog, whereas acetylation of aromatic amines has not been shown in canines (28).

There are additional enzymatic mechanisms acting at the hydroxy ester stage which may have special carcinogenic or detoxification activity in certain instances. Stable glucuronides are formed as urinary metabolites which possess some covalent reactivity toward nucleic acids (56). Peroxidase activity produces nitroxide free radicals that can interact with 2-nitrosofluorene (11), and transacetylation can occur between *N*-hydroxy-2-FAA to form *N*-hydroxy-2-fluorenamine. These metabolic processes have not been clearly placed in the biochemical activation of the class of carcinogens. Aromatic amines represent an important class of man-made compounds that are used in a number of industrial applica-

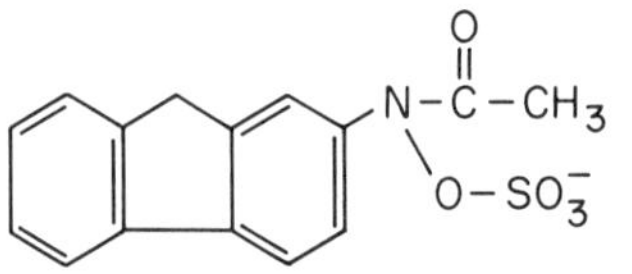

Structure 5. *N*-sulfate-2-FAA.

tions. It is therefore critically important to determine the chemical and physical characteristics that cause some of them to be carcinogenic. Mechanistically, they offer a different type of activated intermediate than epoxide-forming poly-cyclic hydrocarbons, and comparing the physical-chemical characteristics of these two classes may aid in forming a more unified concept of chemical carcino-genesis.

NITROSAMINES AND NITROSAMIDES

In 1937, Freund reported (39) two cases of severe liver toxicity in chemists preparing dimethylnitrosamine (DMN) (see Structure 6). Magee and Barnes subsequently discovered DMN to be a powerful hepatocarcinogen in rats that were being studied for chronic DMN toxicity. All the animals under study developed liver tumors between 26 and 40 weeks (74). This observation opened up an entirely new class of chemical carcinogens, the *N*-nitroso compounds.

The *N*-nitroso class of chemicals can be divided into two major categories, nitrosamines and nitrosamides. Nitrosamines fall into three subcategories, de-pending upon the nature of the R groups attached to the *N*-nitroso moiety (Fig. 14).

At present, over 100 *N*-nitroso derivatives have been synthesized in the labora-tory and tested for their carcinogenic potency and specificity (34,75,76). As increasing numbers of these *N*-nitroso compounds are tested for carcinogenicity, it is becoming apparent that there are wide variations in their carcinogenic specificity in terms of species and tissue susceptibility and the degree of carcino-genic activity. Part of the reason for this variance most likely lies in the relative chemical stability of the compounds under physiological conditions (87) and the constitutive level and inducibility of the drug-metabolizing enzymes in the tissue being tested.

Nitrosamines also require metabolic activation by the hepatic microsomal mixed-function oxidases and require oxygen and reduced pyridine nucleotides as cofactors. Unlike polycyclic hydrocarbons, nitrosamines require only the first activation step which forms a hydroxylated intermediate that is sufficiently unsta-ble to spontaneously decompose and generate a reactive carbonium which can rapidly alkylate target macromolecules in the cell. The activation pathway (Fig. 15) begins with the hydroxylation occurring at the α-carbon to form a labile hydroxyl whose proton is attracted by the nitroso oxygen. This most likely results in a concerted shift that produces an unstable diazohydroxide and elimi-nates an aldehyde. The diazo intermediate, in turn, forms an alkyldiazo salt

$$CH_3 \diagdown N-N=O$$
$$CH_3 \diagup$$

Dimethylnitrosamine

$$CH_3 \diagdown N-N=O$$
$$H_2N-C \diagup$$

N—methylnitrosourea

Structure 6.

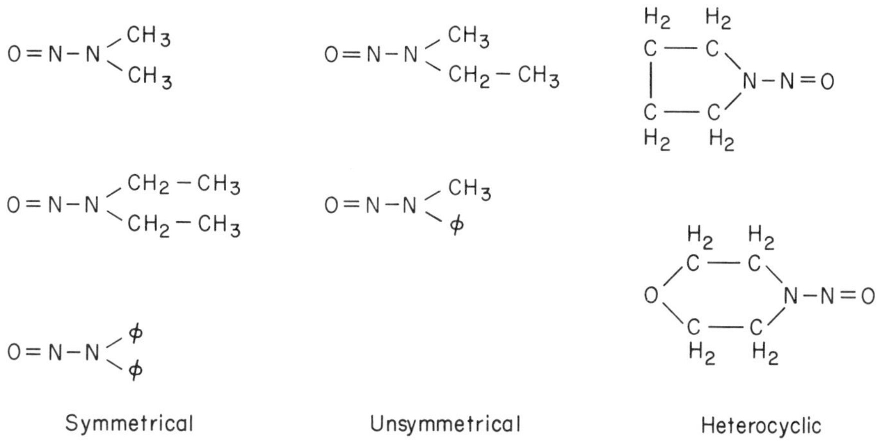

$$O=N-N\overset{CH_3}{\underset{CH_3}{\diagdown}}$$

$$O=N-N\overset{CH_3}{\underset{CH_2-CH_3}{\diagdown}}$$

$$\begin{array}{c}H_2\quad H_2\\ C-C\\ |\qquad\quad \diagdown \\ \qquad\qquad N-N=O \\ C-C\diagup \\ H_2\quad H_2\end{array}$$

$$O=N-N\overset{CH_2-CH_3}{\underset{CH_2-CH_3}{\diagdown}}$$

$$O=N-N\overset{CH_3}{\underset{\phi}{\diagdown}}$$

$$\begin{array}{c}H_2\quad H_2\\ \diagup C-C\diagdown\\ O\qquad\qquad N-N=O \\ \diagdown C-C\diagup \\ H_2\quad H_2\end{array}$$

$$O=N-N\overset{\phi}{\underset{\phi}{\diagdown}}$$

Symmetrical   Unsymmetrical   Heterocyclic

FIG. 14. Representative nitrosamines containing several forms of alkyl and aryl functional groups on the *N*-nitroso moiety.

that decomposes to molecular nitrogen and the carbonium ion which serves as the active alkylating moiety (35).

In contrast, nitrosamides (e.g., nitrosomethylurea, NMU) do not require metabolic activation because of inherent chemical instability in aqueous solution. Nitrosamides decompose at physiological pH nonenzymatically to produce the same class of reactive electrophiles as the nitrosamines. Alkyl urea is one example where the introduction of a proton from the solution to the nitrogen results in cleavage of the amide to produce the same intermediate diazohydroxide followed by rapid decomposition to the reactive electrophile. This marked difference in chemical stability between nitrosamines and nitrosamides clearly parallels the *in vivo* activity of these compounds. Since nitrosamines require metabolic

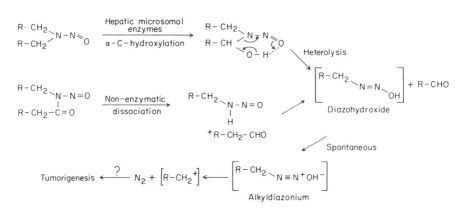

FIG. 15. Schematic representation of nitrosamine and nitrosamide activation.

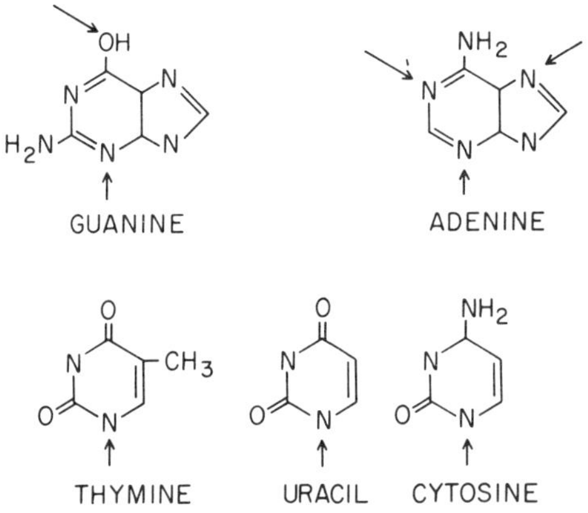

FIG. 16. Sites of nitrosamine and nitrosamide alkylation on purines and pyrimidines. Arrows represent known sites of alkylation, with N-2 position of guanine comprising 80% of nucleic acid alkylation.

GUANINE

ADENINE

THYMINE

URACIL CYTOSINE

activation, they persist in the body for relatively long periods where they are carried by the circulation to the liver yielding severe hepatotoxicity and tumorigenicity with relatively little pathology at the injection site. However, nitrosamides cause severe toxicity at the application site because of their almost immediate decomposition to the reactive carbonium ion. Interaction occurs in the immediately adjacent tissue with relatively little hepatotoxicity (67,82,87,105). The high degree of organ specificity of many *N*-nitroso compounds suggests the relative susceptibility of a given tissue is most likely a function of the ability of the cellular enzymes to activate the compound for decomposition in the proximity of the target site for malignant transformation. Although the actual target site for nitroso carcinogens is not yet elucidated, a number of alkylation sites in nucleic acids (66,118) are known (Fig. 16).

Studies have shown the main alkylation site to be the N-2 position of guanine which comprises 80% of the nucleic acid binding. However, at the present time it is not certain that alkylation in the N-2 position of guanine correlates with tumor induction (69).

Since the synthesis of *N*-nitroso compounds is accomplished through reaction of secondary amines and nitrous acid (Structure 7), it was suggested by Druckrey that nitrosamines could be produced biochemically by the naturally acidic conditions in the stomach with ingestion of secondary amines (34). The nitrosating agent would be formed by the reaction of gastric juice with nitrite compounds that are widely used as food preservatives and for food color enhancement (36,103).

$$NaNO_2 + \text{gastric juice} \rightarrow HNO_2$$

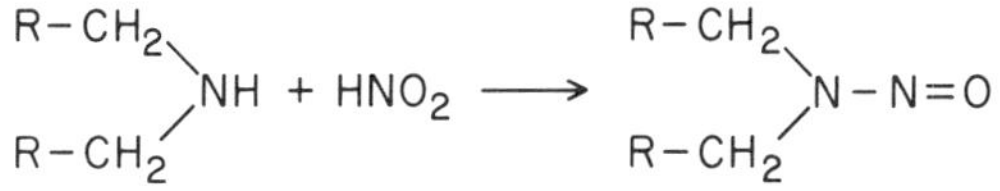

Structure 7.

In addition, nitrates that are high in certain vegetables such as spinach, beets, and egg plant may be reduced to nitrites under conditions of low acidity or during storage by nitroso reductase-containing bacteria. The highest incidences of gastric cancer are found in Japan, Chile, and Austria where cured meat and fish containing sodium nitrite preservative comprise a major part of the diet.

AFLATOXIN

In the early 1960s there were several large outbreaks in Great Britain of an unexplained toxicosis that resulted in heavy losses of young turkeys (2,12). Within a short time similar toxicity syndromes were seen in ducklings, chickens (7), pigs (46), and calves (73). The outbreaks appeared related to commercial feeds that contained both peanut meal and fish meal and the toxicity could be removed by replacing these ingredients with soybean meal or dried milk (3). Investigation disclosed that all the commercial feeds in question contained a particular shipment of Brazilian peanut meal from which the toxic principle could be extracted (104). It was shown that 6-day-old ducklings were killed in 13 days with only 6.5% of the suspected peanut meal in the diet (19,21). Sargeant et al. (104) first associated the toxicity with heavy mold infestation by several strains of *Aspergillus flavus* and gave the generic name aflatoxin to the toxic principle (12). Acute toxicity symptoms included liver necrosis, hemorrhage, fibrosis, and enlarged hepatic cells. In subacute toxicity studies, there was moderate damage to the liver as seen during acute toxicity studies, with the additional development of biliary hyperplasia as the most commonly observed lesion for all domestic animals studied with the exception of sheep (4).

As with nitrosamines, the carcinogenicity of aflatoxins became apparent during chronic toxicity studies using sublethal doses. Feeding contaminated peanut meal to rats for 6 months produced multiple liver tumors in almost all rats tested (65). However, tumor susceptibility to aflatoxins appears to have a narrower range than its toxicity. Tumor formation has been reported in rainbow trout (131), ferret (18), and mice (92,123), although not as extensive as that found in the rat. Chronic feeding of contaminated peanut meal to ducks beginning at 7 days of age at the 30-ppb level for 14 months produced hepatocellular carcinomas and cholangiocarcinomas (100). Ferrets fed a peanut meal diet containing 2.0 ppm aflatoxin produced similar liver tumors between 27 and 38 months. There appears to be variation in strain susceptibility in mice.

Mycotoxin metabolites as a factor in human liver cancer became suspect when it was shown that certain regions of Africa possessed favorable climate for mycotoxin growth (5). It was also discovered that these areas represented an inordinately high incidence of liver disease. In addition, coincident was the fact that the population indigenous to those areas ingested cereal grains and ground nuts which are the major substrates for growth of this fungus. The climate of the country and the microenvironment, namely the food storage areas, contribute greatly to the favorable conditions in which the mold proliferates. Furthermore, economic conditions in certain geographic areas may dictate a necessity for not rejecting partially spoiled foods for consumption.

Variance in species susceptibility to this carcinogen which confines its carcinogenic activity to liver also indicates that this compound requires metabolic activation to bring it to a higher level of chromatin reactivity. Once this active intermediate is formed, the probability that it will interact with the target site for tumor formation will most likely be dictated by the biochemical activation and the toxification rate inherent in the liver of that given species.

Aflatoxins were readily isolated from contaminated peanut meal by thin-layer chromatography (121). Extraction with methanol followed by chromatography in a number of solvent systems separated several heterocyclic five-ring structures (Fig. 17). Details of the structural analysis of these compounds have been reviewed (15).

The compound of major importance in terms of toxicity and carcinogenicity is aflatoxin B_1 (AFB_1) (Fig. 18) (130). This compound possesses an exposed double bond in the 2,3-position, which when compared to the microsomal activation of polycyclic hydrocarbons via an active epoxide intermediate, appeared to be a likely region of the molecule for similar activation (106). The other known aflatoxin metabolites appear to be secondary products derived from AFB_1. Aflatoxin B_{2a} containing the hydroxy group in the 2-position strengthens the argument for 2–3 epoxide as an intermediate since nonenzymatic epoxide ring opening to phenols is routinely seen for polycyclic hydrocarbons (113). In addition, aflatoxin B_{2a} is essentially nontoxic (1).

Aflatoxin M_1, which was named because of its presence in milk, yields acute toxicity symptoms analogous to AFB_1. This compound appears to have the same relative acute toxicity as aflatoxin B_1 (100), but its carcinogenicity and mutagenicity are considerably less (101). Although the toxicity may be due to

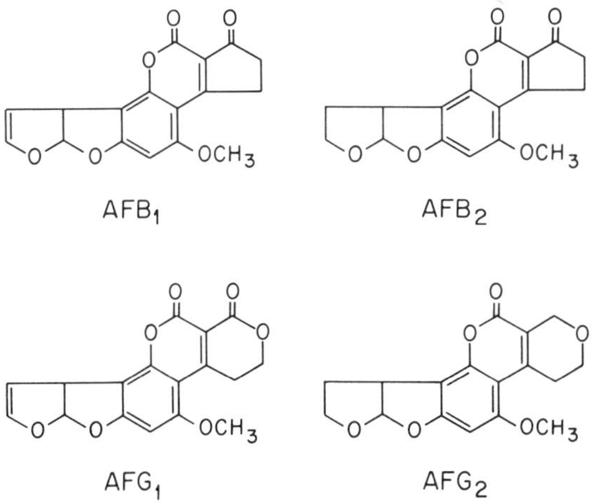

FIG. 17. Aflatoxins isolated from contaminated peanut meal.

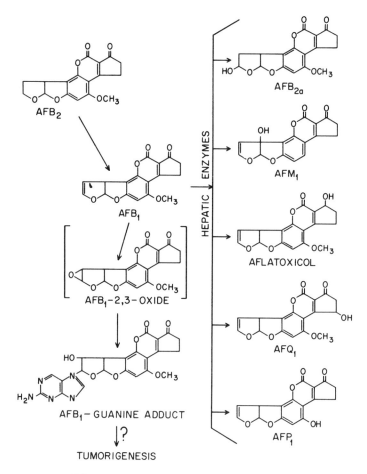

FIG. 18. Metabolites of AFB$_1$ isolated from liver.

one or more oxygenated portions of the molecule, the metabolic activation and the presence of the 4-position hydroxyl may also make aflatoxin M$_1$ less attractive to the microsomal activation system. In addition, its greater polarity would increase its water solubility and may facilitate rapid removal from the cell. Aflatoxicol is a nonmicrosomal reduction product formed by an enzyme in the soluble cytoplasmic fraction of the cell (33). The activity appears to arise from 17-hydroxy steroid dehydrogenase and is a reversible process that may act to maintain a pool of AFB$_1$ within the cell (94). The toxicity of aflatoxicol is very low when compared to AFB$_1$ but greater than aflatoxin M$_1$ (16,42) which indicates that this derivative is more readily converted to AFB$_1$ than the hydroxylated aflatoxin M$_1$ intermediate.

Aflatoxin P$_1$ is a microsomally mediated demethylation product of AFB$_1$ and shows extremely weak toxicity in newborn mice with an LD$_{50}$ of 150 mg/kg compared to 9.5 mg/kg for aflatoxin B$_1$ (17). Aflatoxin P$_1$ is nontoxic in both the chicken embryo and the *Salmonella typhimurium* assay system. Aflatoxin Q_1 which possesses a hydroxyl group in the cyclopetanone ring has been observed as a major metabolite produced by microsomes of monkey and human liver, although appearing as a minor metabolite with rat and chicken liver microsomes (77). As with the other aflatoxin metabolites, aflatoxin Q_1 is far less toxic than AFB_1 (51). It is not yet known whether this metabolite plays a special role in the activation and detoxification pathway of AFB_1 in primates.

The other three aflatoxins extracted from contaminated peanut meal (Fig. 15) are significantly less toxic than AFB_1 and therefore have not been studied in the same depth as AFB_1. Carnaghan measured the relatively lethal potency of the four aflatoxins in 1-day-old ducklings and showed the LD_{50} values at 7 days to be for aflatoxins B_1, 18.2 μg; B_2, 84.8 μg; G_1, 39.2 μg; and G_2, 172.5 μg per 50 g body weight (20).

In reviewing the toxicity of the AFB_1 derivative and the three other aflatoxins extractable from contaminated feed, we find that although AFB_1 far outreaches all the other metabolic products, many of the compounds still maintain some lethal potency. It is interesting to note that all compounds showing activity possess a double bond at the 2,3-position. The isolation of the 2,3-diol-AFB_1 from the hydrolysis of a microsome-mediated binding of AFB_1 to RNA strongly suggested an epoxide at the 2,3-position as an intermediate. Failure to isolate the 2,3-oxide itself from microsomal incubation and its inability to be synthesized chemically in the laboratory pointed to the high reactivity of this intermediate. In response to this, the AFB_1-2,3-dichloride which would decompose in water to yield a transient electrophilic site at carbon 2 should act as a model compound for the 2,3-oxide (119) (Fig. 19). This compound, as expected, showed high

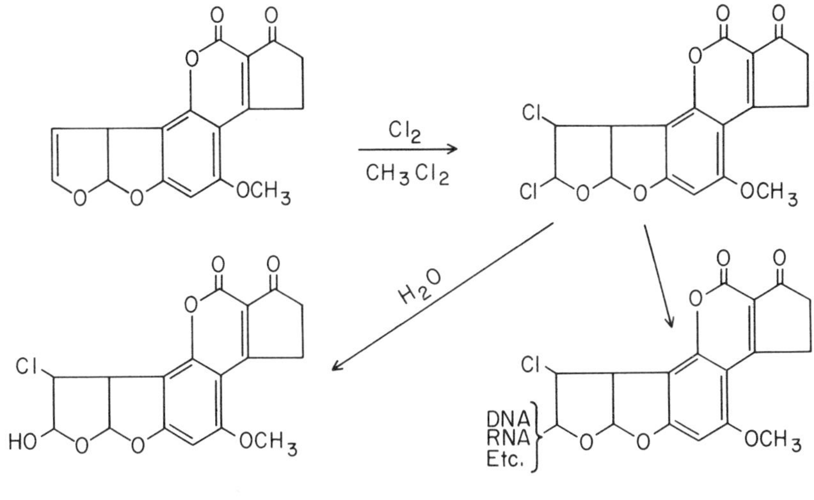

FIG. 19. Synthesis of AFB_1-2,3-dichloro intermediate.

affinity toward forming covalent adducts with DNA and RNA, and proved to be more active than AFB_1 in inducing sarcomas subcutaneously in rats in the formation of papillomas and by skin painting, and yielded strong evidence that the 2,3-oxide was probably a final carcinogenic form of this molecule.

Large-scale incubation of DNA with AFB_1 and isolation of the hydrolysis product has shown the major binding of AFB_1 to be from the 2-position to the N-7 position of guanine (37). The final role of this important covalent binding in the induction of tumor induction remains to be clarified.

Several other areas of growing concern require a larger data base before they can be comprehensively understood, namely the pesticides, food additives, and metals. Many of these chemicals induce the hepatic microsomal oxidases and are currently being tested by the National Cancer Institute. Their degree of carcinogenicity may be clarified during the next few years. Cancer as a result of drug treatment is another area of uncertain significance. During puberty, vaginal cancer in offspring of women treated with diethylstilbestrol to prevent spontaneous abortion is a classic example of iatrogenic cancer (49). The mechanism of action of this form of chemical carcinogenesis is unknown. Steroids in some cases are potent potentiators and at the same time used to treat cancer of the prostate. Although the cyclopentaphenanthrene structure strongly resembles the polyaromatic hydrocarbon, their potent multifocal physiological actions at ppm concentrations makes them difficult to study. Tumorigenesis by pituitary and steroid hormones has recently been reviewed (24,41,59).

A number of metals are known carcinogens and although their toxicity and tumorigenicity have been tested, the mechanism of action of these substances remains obscure (38,40). Recent work shows a number of the carcinogenic metals cause infidelity in polymerase activity during DNA synthesis, whereas noncarcinogenic metals are refractory (72). The same uncertainty surrounds solid-state carcinogenesis, that is, tumor formation from implanted plastics or glass (13). Table 1 lists synthetic chemicals, food additives, or drugs that are known or suspected carcinogens (63). In several cases the carcinogenic activity has been demonstrated in only a few species under special laboratory conditions and may not represent a significant hazard to the general population.

The final outcome of all of these diverse chemical entities, either discussed in detail or briefly mentioned, results in malignant transformation and suggests that the underlying perturbation of all of these seemingly unrelated substances is possibly or even probably the same. As the data base grows and the mechanism of activation and detoxification pathways become apparent, the rationale for organ, tissue, and species specificity should become clarified. Eventually it may become possible to develop a unifying concept of the metabolic steps required to bypass the host defense mechanism, whether immunological or catabolic, and result in a high-risk situation that the cell will become malignantly transformed. It is also probable that success of a formulated cancer mechanism will require a clear concept of the regulation of the genetic apparatus and intracellular events taking place during cell replication.

TABLE 1. *Compounds of known and suspected carcinogenic activity*

Ergot	Nickel	Carboxymethyl-cellulose
Luteoskyrin	Thorotrast	Polyoxyethyl-enemonostearate
Cyclochlorotine	X-rays	
Aflatoxins	Arsenic	Oil orange E
Sterigmatocystin	Chlornaphazin	Oil yellow HA
Ethionine	Coal tar products	Oil orange TX
Nitrosamines	INH (isonicotinic acid hydrazide)	Orange I
Polycyclic aromatic hydrocarbons		Yellow AB and OB
	Iron dextran	Light green SF
Pyrrolizodine alkaloids	Penicillin	Brilliant blue FCF
Safrole (from sassafras)	Griseofulvin	Fast green FCF
Oil of calamus	Mitomycin C	Butter yellow
Cycasin	Actinomycin D	8-Hydroxyquinoline
Bracken fern	Niridazole	FC&C red no. 32
Thiourea	Flagyl	Diethylpyrocarbonate
Tannins (tannic acid)	Diethylstilbestrol	Diethylstilbestrol
Carrageenan	L-dopa	Ponceaux MX
Beryllium	Dulcin	Citrus red no. 2
Chromium (hexavalent)	Cyclamates	
Cobalt	Tween 60	

ACKNOWLEDGMENTS

Oak Ridge National Laboratory is operated by Union Carbide Corporation under contract W-7405-eng-26 with the U.S. Department of Energy.

The author would like to thank Ms Nancy Trent for her most able secretarial skills during preparation of this manuscript.

REFERENCES

1. Abedi, Z. H., and Scott, P. M. (1969): Detection of toxicity of aflatoxins, sterigmatocystin and other fungal toxins by lethal action on Zebra fish larvae. *J. Assoc. Off. Anal. Chem.,* 52:963–969.
2. Allcroft, R., and Carnaghan, R. B. A. (1963): Toxic products in ground nuts. Biological effects. *Chem. Ind. (Lond.),* 50–53.
3. Allcroft, R., Carnaghan, R. B. A., Sargeant, K., and O'Kelley, J. (1961): A toxic factor in Brazilian ground nut meal. *Vet. Rec.,* 73:428–429.
4. Allcroft, R. (1966): In: *Mycotoxins in Foodstuffs,* edited by G. N. Wogan, p. 153. MIT Press, Cambridge, Mass.
5. Alpert, M. E., Hutt, M. S. R., Wogan, G. N., and Davidson, C. S. (1971): Association between aflatoxin content of food and hepatoma frequency in Uganda. *Cancer,* 28:253–260.
6. Annotation (1966): A dangerous rodenticide. *Lancet,* 11–26:1183.
7. Asplin, F. D., and Carnaghan, R. B. A. (1961): The toxicity of certain ground nut meals for poultry with special reference to their effect on ducklings and chickens. *Vet. Rec.,* 73:1215–1219.
8. Baird, W. M., Dipple, A., Grover, P. L., Sims, P., and Brookes, P. (1973): Studies on the binding of 7-methylbenz(a)anthracene to DNA: The hydrocarbon–deoxyribonucleoside products formed by the binding of derivatives of 7-methylbenz(a)anthracene to DNA in aqueous solution and in mouse embryo cells in culture. *Cancer Res.,* 33:2386–2392.
9. Baird, W. M., and Brookes, P. (1973): Isolation of the hydrocarbon-deoxyribonucleoside products from DNA of mouse embryo cells treated in culture with 7-methylbenz(a)anthracene-^{3}H. *Cancer Res.,* 33:2378–2385.

10. Baird, W. M., Harvey, R. G., and Brookes, P. (1975): Comparison of the cellular DNA-bound products of benzo(a)pyrene with the products formed by the reaction of benzo(a)pyrene-4-5-oxide with DNA. *Cancer Res.,* 34:54–57.

11. Bartsch, H., and Hecker, E. (1971): On the metabolic activation of the carcinogen N-hydroxy-N-2-acetylamino fluorene. *Biochem. Biophys. Acta,* 237:567–578.

12. Blount, W. P. (1961): Turkey "X" disease. *J. Br. Turkey Fed.,* 9:55–58.

13. Brand, K. G. (1975): In: *Cancer,* Vol. 1, edited by F. E. Becker, p. 485. Plenum Press, New York.

14. Brookes, P., and Lawley, P. D. (1964): Evidence for the binding of polynuclear aromatic hydrocarbons to the nucleic acids of mouse skin: Relation between carcinogenic power of hydrocarbons and their binding to DNA. *Nature,* 202:781–784.

15. Büchi, G., and Rae, I. D. (1969): In *Aflatoxin-Scientific Background, Control and Implications,* edited by L. A. Goldblatt, p. 55. Academic Press, New York.

16. Büchi, G., Spitzner, D., Paglialunga, S., and Wogan, G. N. (1973): Synthesis and toxicity evaluation of aflatoxin P_1. *Life Sci.,* 13:1143–1149.

17. Büchi, G., Muller, P. M., Roebuck, B. D., and Wogan, G. N. (1974): Aflatoxin Q: A major metabolite of aflatoxin B_1 produced by human liver. *Res. Commun. Chem. Pathol. Pharmacol.,* 8:585–592.

18. Butler, W. H. (1969): In: *Aflatoxin-Scientific Background, Control and Implications,* edited by L. A. Goldblatt, p. 223. Academic Press, New York.

19. Carnaghan, R. B. A., and Sargeant, K. (1961): The toxicity of certain ground nut meals to poultry. *Vet. Rec.,* 73:726–767.

20. Carnaghan, R. B. A., Hartley, R. D., and O'Kelly, J. (1963): Toxicity and fluorescence properties of the aflatoxins. *Nature,* 200:1101.

21. Carnaghan, R. B. A. (1965): Hepatic tumours in ducks fed a low level of toxic ground nut meal. *Nature,* 208:308.

22. Case, R. A. M., and Hosker, M. E. (1954): Tumour of the urinary bladder as an occupational disease in the rubber industry in England and Wales. *Br. J. Prev. Soc. Med.,* 8:39–50.

23. Case, R. A. M., Hosker, M. E., McDonald, D. B., and Pearson, J. T. (1954): Tumours of the urinary bladder in workmen engaged in the manufacture and use of certain dye stuff intermediates in the British Chemical Industry. *Br. J. Ind. Med.,* 11:75–88.

24. Clayson, D. B. (1962): *Chemical Carcinogenesis,* p. 315. Little, Brown and Company, Boston.

25. Clayson, D. B., and Garner, R. C. (1976): In *Chemical Carcinogens,* edited by C. E. Searle, p. 366. American Chemical Society, Washington, D.C.

26. Committee on Biologic Effects of Atmospheric Pollutants. (1972): Particulate Polycyclic Organic Matter. National Academy of Sciences, Washington, D.C.

27. Conney, A. H. (1967): Pharmacological implications of microsomal enzyme induction. *Pharmacol. Rev.,* 19:317–366.

28. Conzelman, G. M., Flanders, L. E., and Moulton, J. E. (1972): Dose-response relationship of the bladder tumorigen 2-naphthylamine: A study in beagle dogs. *J. Natl. Cancer Inst.,* 49:193–200.

29. Cook, J. W., and Hewett, C. L. (1933): Synthesis of 1:2 and 4:5-benzpyrenes. *J. Chem. Soc.,* 398–405.

30. DeBaun, J. R., Rowley, J. Y., Miller, E. C., and Miller, J. A. (1968): Sulfotransferase activation of N-hydroxy-2-acetylaminofluorene in rodent livers susceptible and resistant to this carcinogen. *Proc. Soc. Exp. Biol. Med.,* 129:268.

31. DeBaun, J. R., Miller, E. C., and Miller, J. A. (1970): N-hydroxy-2-acetylaminofluorene sulfotransferase: Its possible role in carcinogenesis and protein-(metheon-S-yl)-binding in rat liver. *Cancer Res.,* 30:577–595.

32. DeBaun, J. R., Smith, J. Y., Miller, E. C., and Miller, J. A. (1970): Reactivity in vivo of the carcinogen N-hydroxy-2-acetylaminofluorene: Increase by sulfate ion. *Science,* 167:184–186.

33. DeTroy, R. W., and Hesseltine, C. W. (1968): Isolation and biological activity of a microbial conversion product of aflatoxin B_1. *Nature,* 219:967.

34. Druckrey, H., Preussman, R., Ivankovic, S., and Schmähl, D. (1967): Organotrope carcinogene Wirkung bei 65 verschieden N-nitroso Verbindugen und BD-Ratten. *Z. Krebsforsch.,* 69:103–201.

35. Druckrey, H. (1972): In: *Topics in Chemical Carcinogenesis,* edited by W. Nakara, S. Takayama, T. Sugimura, and S. Odashima, p. 73. University Park Press, Baltimore.

36. Endo, H., Takahashi, K., Kinoshita, N., Utsunomiia, T., and Baba, T. (1975): An approach to the detection of possible idiologic factors in human gastric cancer. *Gann. Mono. Cancer Res.,* 17:17–29.
37. Essignmann, J. M., Croy, R. G., Nadzan, A. M., Busby, W. F. Jr., Reinhold, V. N., Büchi, G., and Wogan, G. N. (1977): Structural identification of the major DNA adduct formed by aflatoxin B_1 in vitro. *Proc. Natl. Acad. Sci. (USA),* 74:1870.
38. Fishbein, L. (1976): Environmental metallic carcinogens: An overview of exposure levels. *J. Toxicol. Environ. Health,* 2:77–109.
39. Freund, H. A. (1937): Clinical manifestations and studies in parenchymatous hepatitis. *Ann. Intern. Med.,* 10:1144–1155.
40. Furst, A., and Haro, R. T. (1969): A survey of metal carcinogenesis. *Prog. Exp. Tumor Res.,* 12:102.
41. Furth, J. (1975): In: *Cancer,* Vol. 1, edited by F. E. Becker, p. 75. Plenum Press, New York.
42. Garner, C. R., Miller, E. C., and Miller, J. A. (1972): Liver microsomal metabolism of aflatoxin B_1 to a reactive derivative toxic to Salmonella typhimurium TA 1530. *Cancer Res.,* 32:2058–2066.
43. Gelboin, H. V. (1967): Carcinogens, enzyme induction and gene action. *Adv. Cancer Res.,* 10:1–81.
44. Gelboin, H. V. (1969): A microsome-dependent binding of benzo(a)pyrene to DNA. *Cancer Res.,* 29:1272–1276.
45. Goshman, L. M., and Heidelberger, C. (1967): Binding of tritium-labeled polycyclic hydrocarbons to DNA of mouse skin. *Cancer Res.,* 27:1678–1688.
46. Harding, J. D. J., Done, J. T., Lewis, G., and Allcroft, R. (1963): Experimental ground nut poisoning in pigs. *Res. Vet. Sci.,* 4:217–229.
47. Heidelberger, C., and Moldenhauer, M. G. (1956): The interaction of carcinogenic hydrocarbons with tissue constituents: IV. A quantitative study of the binding to skin proteins of several C^{14}-labeled hydrocarbons. *Cancer Res.,* 16:442–449.
48. Heidelberger, C. (1973): Chemical oncogenesis in cultures. *Adv. Cancer Res.,* 18:317–366.
49. Herbst, A. L., Ulfelder, H., and Poskanzen, D. C. (1971): Adenocarcinoma of the vagina: Association of Maternal Stilbestrol Therapy with Tumor Appearance in Young Women. *N. Engl. J. Med.,* 284:878–881.
50. Holder, G., Yagi, H., Dansette, P., Jerina, D. M., Levin, W., Lu, A. Y. H., and Conney, A. H. (1974): Effects of inducers and epoxide hydrase on the metabolism of benzo*(a)*pyrene by liver microsomes and a reconstituted system: Analysis by high pressure liquid chromatography. *Proc. Natl. Acad. Sci. USA,* 71:4356–4360.
51. Hsieh, D. P. H., Salhab, A. S., Wong, J. T., and Yang, S. L. (1974): Toxicity of aflatoxin Q_1 as evaluated with the chick embryo and bacterial auxotrophs. *Toxicol. Appl. Pharmacol.,* 30:237–242.
52. Huberman, E., Kuroki, T., Marquardt, H., Selkirk, J. K., Heidelberger, C., Grover, P. L., and Sims, P. (1972): Transformation of hamster cells by epoxides and other derivatives of polycyclic hydrocarbons. *Cancer Res.,* 32:1391–1396.
53. Huberman, E., Sachs, L., Yang, S. K., and Gelboin, H. V. (1976): Identification of mutagenic metabolites of benzo(a)pyrene in mammalian cells. *Proc. Natl. Acad. Sci. USA,* 73:607–611.
54. Hueper, W. C., Wiley, F. H., and Wolfe, H. D. (1938): Experimental production of bladder tumors in dogs by the administration of beta-naphthylamine. *J. Ind. Hyg.,* 20:46.
55. Irving, C. C. (1962): N-Hydroxylation of the carcinogen 2-acetylaminofluorene by rabbit-liver microsomes. *Biochim. Biophys. Acta,* 65:564–566.
56. Irving, C. C., Veazey, R. A., and Hill, J. T. (1969): Reaction of the glucuronide of the carcinogen N-hydroxy-2-acetylaminofluorene. *Biochim. Biophys. Acta,* 179:189–198.
57. Irving, C. C., Janss, D. H., and Russell, L. T. (1971): Lack of N-hydroxy-2-acetylaminofluorene sulfotransferase activity in the mammary gland and Zymbal's gland of the rat. *Cancer Res.,* 31:387–391.
58. Irving, C. C. (1973): Interaction of chemical carcinogens with DNA. *Methods Cancer Res.,* 7:189–244.
59. Jull, J. W. (1976): Endocrine aspects of carcinogenesis. In: *Chemical Carcinogenesis,* edited by C. E. Searle, p. 52. American Chemical Society, Washington, D.C.
60. Kenneway, E. L., and Heiger, I. (1930): Carcinogenic substances and their fluorescence spectra. *Br. Med. J.,* 1:1044–1046.

61. King, C. M., and Phillips, B. (1968): Enzyme-catalyzed reactions of the carcinogen N-hydroxy-2-fluorenylacetamide with nucleic acid. *Science,* 159:1351–1358.
62. Kramer, J. W., Miller, J. A., and Miller, E. C. (1960): The hydroxylation of the carcinogen 2-acetylamine fluorene by rat liver: Stimulation by pretreatment *in vivo* by 3-methylcholanthrene. *J. Biol. Chem.,* 235:885–888.
63. Kraybill, H. F. (1977): In: *Environmental Cancer,* edited by H. F. Kraybill and M. A. Mehlman, p. 27. Halsten Press, New York.
64. Kuroki, T., Huberman, E., Harquardt, H., Selkirk, J. K., Heidelberger, C., Grover, P. L., and Sims, P. (1971): Binding of K-region epoxides and other derivatives of benz(a)anthracene and dibenz(a,h)anthracene to DNA, RNA and proteins of transformable cells. *Chem. Biol. Interact.,* 4:389–397.
65. Lancaster, M. C., Jenkins, F. P., and Philip, J. Mcl. (1961): Toxicity associated with certain samples of ground nuts. *Nature,* 192:1095–1096.
66. Lawley, P. D. (1966): Effects of some chemical mutagens and carcinogens on nucleic acids. *Prog. Nucleic Acid Res. Mol. Biol.,* 5:89–131.
67. Leaver, D. D., Swann, P. F., and Magee, P. N. (1969): Induction of tumours in the rat by a single oral dose of N-nitrosomethyl urea. *Br. J. Cancer,* 23:177–187.
68. Levin, W., Wood, A. W., Yagi, H., Dansette, P. M., Jerina, D. M., and Conney, A. H. (1976): Carcinogenicity of benzo(a)pyrene 4,5–7,8- and 9,10-oxides on mouse skin. *Proc. Natl. Acad. Sci. USA,* 73:243–247.
69. Lijinsky, W., Loo, I., and Ross, A. E. (1968): Mechanism of alkylation of nucleic acids by nitrosodimethylamine. *Nature,* 218:1174–1175.
70. Lin, J. K., Miller, J. A., and Miller, E. C. (1969): Studies on structures of polar dyes derived from the liver protein of rats fed N-methyl-4-amino-azobenzene. II. Identity of synthetic 3-(homocystein-S-yl)-N-methyl-4-*O*-aminoazobenzene with the major polar dye p26. *Biochemistry,* 7:1889–1895.
71. Lin, J. K., Miller, J. A., and Miller, E. C. (1969): Studies on structures of polar dyes derived from the liver protein of rats fed N-methyl-4-aminoazobenzene. III. Tyrosine and homocysteine sulfoxide polar dyes. *Biochemistry,* 8:1573–1582.
72. Loeb, L. A., Sirover, M. A., Weymouth, L. A., Dube, D. K., Agarwah, S. S., and Katz, E. E. (1977): Infidelity of DNA synthesis as related to mutagenesis and carcinogenesis. *J. Toxicol. Environ. Health,* 2:1297–1304.
73. Loosmore, R. M., and Markson, L. M. (1961): Poisoning of cattle by Brazilian ground nut meal. *Vet. Res.,* 73:813–814.
74. Magee, P. N., and Barnes, J. M. (1956): The production of malignant primary hepatic tumors in the rat by feeding dimethylnitrosamine. *Br. J. Cancer,* 10:114.
75. Magee, P. N., and Schoental, R. (1964): Carcinogenesis by nitroso compounds. *Br. Med. Bull.,* 20:102–106.
76. Magee, P. N., and Barnes, J. M. (1967): Carcinogenic nitroso compounds. *Adv. Cancer Res.,* 10:163–246.
77. Masri, M., Booth, N., and Hsieh, D. P. H. (1974): Comparative metabolic conversion of aflatoxin B_1 to M_1 and Q_1 by monkey, rat and chicken liver. *Life Sci.,* 15:203–212.
78. Malaveille, C., Kuroki, T., Sims, P., Grover, P. L., and Bartsch, H. (1977): Mutagenicity of isomeric diol-epoxides of benzo(a)pyrene and benz(a)anthracene in S. typhimurium TA98 and TA100 and in V79 Chinese hamster cells. *Mutat. Res.,* 44:313–326.
79. Mettle, R., and Cecilia, M. (1947): *History of Medicine,* Blakiston, Philadelphia.
80. Miller, E. C. (1951): Studies on the formation of protein bound derivatives of 3,4-benzpyrene in the epidermal fraction of mouse skin. *Cancer Res.,* 11:100–108.
81. Miller, E. C., Miller, J. A., and Hartman, H. A. (1961): N-hydroxy-2-acetylaminofluorene: A metabolite of 2-acetylaminofluorene with increased carcinogenic activity in the rat. *Cancer Res.,* 21:815–824.
82. Miller, E. C., and Miller, J. A. (1966): Mechanisms of chemical carcinogenesis: Nature of proximate carcinogens and interactions with macromolecules. *Pharmacol. Rev.,* 18:805–838.
83. Miller, J. A., and Miller, E. C. (1969): The metabolic activation of carcinogenic aromatic amines and amides. *Prog. Exp. Tumor Res.,* 11:273–301.
84. Miller, J. A., and Miller, E. C. (1967): In: *Carcinogenesis: A Broad Critique.* University of Texas, M. D. Anderson Hospital and Tumor Institute, at Houston, pp. 397–420. The Williams and Wilkins Co., Baltimore.

85. Miller, J. A. (1970): Carcinogenesis by chemicals: An overview. G. H. A. Clowes Memorial Lecture. *Cancer Res.,* 30:559–576.

86. Miller, E. C., and Miller, J. A. (1976): The metabolism of chemical carcinogenesis to reactive electrophiles and their possible mechanisms of action in carcinogenesis. In: *Chemical Carcinogens,* edited by C. E. Searle, p. 737. American Chemical Society, Washington, D.C.

87. Mirvish, S. S. (1975): Formation of N-nitroso compounds: Chemistry, kinetics and in vivo occurrence. *Toxicol. Appl. Pharmacol.,* 31:325–351.

88. Moodie, R. L. (1927): Tumors in Lower Carboniferous. *Science,* 66:540.

89. Moodie, R. L. (1918): Pathologic lesions among extinct animals. *Surg. Clin. Chicago,* 2:319–331.

90. Nagata, C., Tagashira, Y., and Kodama, M. (1974): Metabolic activation of benzo(a)pyrene: Significance of the free radical. In: *Chemical Carcinogenesis,* edited by P. O. P. T'so, and J. A. DiPaolo, p. 87. Dekker, New York.

91. Nebert, D. W., Boobis, A. R., Yagi, H., Jerina, D. M., and Kouri, R. E. (1977): Genetic differences in benzo(a)pyrene carcinogenic index *in vivo* and in mouse cytochrome P_1-450-mediated benzo(a)pyrene metabolite binding to DNA *in vitro.* In: *Biological Reactive Intermediates,* edited by D. J. Jollow, J. J. Kocsis, R. Snyder, and H. Vainio, p. 125. Plenum Press, New York.

92. Newberne, P. M. (1965): In: *Mycotoxin in Foodstuffs,* edited by G. W. Wogan, p. 187. MIT Press, Cambridge.

93. Oesch, F., Bently, P., and Glatt, H. R. (1977): Epoxide hydratase: Purification to apparent homogeneity as a specific probe for the relative importance of epoxides among other reactive metabolites. In: *Biological Reactive Intermediates,* edited by D. J. Jollow, J. J. Kocsis, R. Snyder, and H. Vainio, p. 181. Plenum Press, New York.

94. Patterson, D. S. P., and Roberts, B. A. (1971): The *in vitro* reduction of aflatoxins B_1 and B_2 by soluble avian liver enzymes. *Food Cosmet. Toxicol.,* 9:829–837.

95. Pitot, H. C., and Heidelberger, C. (1963): Metabolic regulatory circuits. *Cancer Res.,* 23:1694–1700.

96. Poirier, L. A., Miller, J. A., Miller, E. C., and Sato, K. (1967): N-benzoyloxy-N-methyl-4-aminoazobenzene: Its carcinogenic activity in the rat and its reactions with proteins and nucleic acids and their constituents *in vitro. Cancer Res.,* 27:1600–1613.

97. Pott, P. (1775): Chirurgical Observations, Reprinted in *Natl. Cancer Inst. Monog.,* 10:7 (1963).

98. Public Health Service Survey of Compounds Which Have Been Treated For Carcinogenic Activity, *Publ. No. 149.* Public Health Service, Washington, D.C.

99. Pullman, A., and Pullman, B. (1955): Electronic structure and carcinogenic activity of aromatic molecules. New Developments. *Adv. Cancer Res.,* 3:117–169.

100. Purchase, I. F. H. (1967): Acute toxicity of aflatoxins M_1 and M_2 in one-day-old ducklings. *Food Cosmet. Toxicol.,* 5:339–342.

101. Purchase, I. F. H., and Vortser, L. J. (1968): Aflatoxin in commercial milk samples. *S. Afr. Med. J.,* 42:219.

102. Rehn, L. (1895): Über Blasengeschwülste bei fuchsin-arbeiten. *Arch. Klin. Chir.,* 50:588–600.

103. Sander, J., and Schweinsberg, F. (1972): Wechselbeziehungen zwischen Nitrat, Nitrit und Kanzerogen. *Zentralbl. Bakt. Hyg. B,* 156:299–320.

104. Sargeant, K., O'Kelly, J., Carnaghan, R. B. A., and Allcroft, R. (1961): The assay of a toxic principle in certain ground nut meals. *Vet. Rec.,* 73:1219–1223.

105. Schoental, R., and Magee, P. N. (1962): Induction of squamous carcinomas of the lung and of the stomach and esophagus by diazomethane and N-methyl-N-nitroso-urethane, respectively. *Br. J. Cancer,* 16:92–100.

106. Schoental, R. (1970): Hepatotoxic activity of retrosine, senkirkine and hydroxysenkirkine in newborn rats and the role of epoxides in carcinogenesis by pyrrolizidine alkaloids and aflatoxins. *Nature,* 227:401–402.

107. Selkirk, J. K., Croy, R. G., and Gelboin, H. V. (1974): Benzo(a)pyrene metabolites: Efficient and rapid separation by high-pressure liquid chromatography. *Science,* 184:169–171.

108. Selkirk, J. K., Croy, R. G., Roller, P. P., and Gelboin, H. V. (1974): High-pressure liquid chromatographic analysis of benzo*(a)*pyrene metabolism and covalent binding and the mechanism of action of 7,8-benzoflavone and 1,2-epoxy-3,3,3-trichloropropane. *Cancer Res.,* 34:3474–3480.

109. Selkirk, J. K., Croy, R. G., Wiebel, F. J., and Gelboin, H. V. (1976): Differences in benzo(a)py-

rene metabolism between rodent liver microsomes and embryonic cells. *Cancer Res.,* 36:4476–4479.

110. Selkirk, J. K., Croy, R. G., and Gelboin, H. V. (1976): High-pressure liquid chromatographic separation of 10-benzo(a)pyrene phenols and the identification of 1-phenol and 7-phenols as new metabolites. *Cancer Res.,* 36:922–926.

111. Selkirk, J. K. (1977): Benzo(a)pyrene carcinogenesis: A Biochemical Selection Mechanism. *J. Toxicol. Environ. Health,* 2:1245–1258.

112. Sims, P., Grover, P. L., Swaisland, A., Pal, K., and Hewer, A. (1974): Metabolic activation of benzo(a)pyrene proceeds by a diol-epoxide. *Nature,* 252:326–328.

113. Sims, P., and Grover, P. L. (1974): Epoxides in polycyclic aromatic hydrocarbon metabolism and carcinogenesis. *Adv. Cancer Res.,* 20:165–274.

114. Slaga, T. J., Viaje, A., Berry, D. L., Bracken, W. M., Buty, S. G., and Scribner, J. D. (1976): Skin tumor initiating ability of benzo(a)pyrene 4,5′, 7,8-, and 7,8-diol-9,10-epoxide on 7,8-diol. *Cancer Lett.* 2:115–122.

115. Slaga, T. J., Bracken, W. M., Viaje, A., Levin, W., Yagi, H., Jerina, D. M., and Conney, A. H. (1977): Comparison of the tumor-initiating activities of benzo(a)pyrene arene oxides and diol epoxides. *Cancer Res.,* 37:4130–4133.

116. Slaga, T. J., Viaje, A., Bracken, W. M., Berry, D. L., Fischer, S. M., Miller, D. R., and LeClerc, S. M. (1977): Skin-tumor-initiating ability of benzo(a)pyrene-7,8-diol-9,10-epoxide (anti) when applied topically in tetrahydrofuran. *Cancer Lett.* 3:23–30.

117. Slaga, T. J. (1978): In: *Mechanisms of Tumor Promotion and Co-Carcinogenesis,* edited by T. J. Slaga, R. K. Boutwell, and A. Sivak, p. 1. Raven Press, New York.

118. Swann, P. F., and Magee, P. N. (1971): The alkylation of N-7 of guanine of nucleic acids of the rat by diethylnitrosamine, N-ethyl-N-nitrosourea and ethyl methanesulfonate. *Biochem. J.,* 125:841–847.

119. Swenson, D. H., Miller, J. A., and Miller, E. C. (1975): The reactivity and carcinogenicity of aflatoxin B_1-2,3-dichloride. A model for the putative 2,3-oxide metabolite of aflatoxin B_1. *Cancer Res.,* 35:3811–3823.

120. Thiede, T., and Christensen, B. C. (1969): Bladder tumors induced by chlornaphazine: A five-year follow-up study of chlornaphazine treated patients with polycythemia. *Acta Med. Scand.,* 185:133–137.

121. Trager, W. T., Stoloff, L., and Campbell, A. D. (1964): A comparison of assay procedures for aflatoxin in peanut products. *J. Assoc. Off. Agr. Chem.,* 47:993–1001.

122. T'so, P. O. P., Caspary, W. J., Cohen, B. I., Leavitt, J. C., Lesko, S. A., Lorentzen, R. J., and Schechtman, L. M. (1974): Basic mechanisms in polycyclic hydrocarbon carcinogenesis. In: *Chemical Carcinogenesis,* edited by P. O. P. T'so and J. A. DiPaolo, p. 113. Dekker, New York.

123. Vesselinovitch, S. D., Mihsilovich, N., Lombard, L. L., and Wogan, G. N. (1972): Aflatoxin B_1, a hepatocarcinogen in the infant mouse. *Cancer Res.,* 32:2289–2291.

124. Weinstein, I. B., Jeffrey, A. M., Hennette, K. W., Blobstein, S. H., Harvey, R. G., Harris, C., Autrup, H., Kasai, H., and Nakanishi, K. (1976): Benzo(a)pyrene diol epoxides as intermediates in nucleic acid binding *in vitro* and *in vivo. Science,* 193:592–595.

125. Weissburger, E. K., and Weissburger, J. H. (1958): Chemistry, carcinogenicity and metabolism of 2-fluorenamine and related compounds. *Adv. Cancer Res.,* 5:331–431.

126. Williams, M. H. (1962): Environmental and industrial bladder cancer, preventive measures. *Acta Unio Int. Contra Cancrum.,* 18:676–683.

127. Wilson, R. H., DeEds, F., and Cox, A. J. (1941): The toxicity and carcinogenic activity of 2-acetaminofluorene. *J. Cancer Res.,* 1:595–608.

128. Wislocki, P. G., Wood, A. W., Chang, R. L., Levin, W., Yagi, H., Hernandez, O., Dansette, P. M., Jerina, D. M., and Conney, A. H. (1976): Mutagenicity and cytotoxicity of benzo(a)pyrene arene oxides, phenols, quinones and dihydrodiols in bacterial and mammalian cells. *Cancer Res.,* 36:3350–3357.

129. Wislocki, P. G., Chang, R. L., Wood, A. W., Levin, W., Yagi, H., Hernandez, O., Mah, H. D., Dansette, P. M., Jerina, D. M., and Conney, A. H. (1977): High carcinogenicity of 2-hydroxybenzo(a)pyrene on mouse skin. *Cancer Res.,* 37:2608–2611.

130. Wogan, G. N. (1973): Aflatoxin carcinogenesis. *Methods Cancer Res.,* 7:309–344.

131. Wolf, H., and Jackson, E. W. (1963): Hepatomas in rainbow trout: Descriptive and experimental epidemiology. *Science,* 142:676–678.

132. Wood, A. W., Chang, R. L., Levin, W., Yagi, H., Thakker, D. R., Jerina, D. M., and Conney,

A. H. (1977): Differences in mutagenicity of the optical enantiomers of the diasteneomeric benzo(a)pyrene 7,8-diol-9,10-epoxides. *Biochem. Biophys. Res. Commun.,* 77:1389–1396.

133. Yamiagiwa, K., and Ichikawa, K. (1915): Experimentalle Studie üker die Pathogenese der Epitelialgeschwülste. *Kaiserl. Univ. Tokyo,* 15:295–344.

134. Yang, S. K., McCourt, D. M., Roller, P. R., and Gelboin, H. V. (1976): Enzymatic conversion of benzo(a)pyrene leading predominantly to the diol-epoxide r-7,t-8-dihydroxy-9,10-oxy-7, 8,9,10-tetrahydrobenzo(a)pyrene through a single enantiomer of r-7, t-8-dihydroxy-7,8-dihydro-benzo(a)pyrene. *Proc. Natl. Acad. Sci. (USA),* 73:2594–2598.

Carcinogenesis, Vol. 5: Modifiers of Chemical
Carcinogenesis, edited by T. J. Slaga.
Raven Press, New York, 1980.

2

Tumor Promotion and Preneoplastic Progression

Nancy H. Colburn

*Laboratory of Viral Carcinogenesis, National Cancer Institute,
Bethesda, Maryland 20205*

The subjects of tumor promotion and cocarcinogensis have been reviewed periodically (138,20). This review focuses primarily on recent studies of carcinogenesis as a multistage process with attention to what has been learned about the phenotypes of neoplastic and preneoplastic cells and their determinants and to how progression to malignancy can be halted or delayed.

Carcinogenesis has been known to occur by a stagewise process since Rous (110,44), Berenblum (10), Mottram (84), Boutwell (19), and co-workers demonstrated the effectiveness of hyperplasiogenic agents in eliciting tumors following a subcarcinogenic exposure of skin to polycyclic aromatic hydrocarbons. Croton oil, containing the most active of hyperplasiogenic or tumor-promoting agents, was introduced by Berenblum (10). The isolation and characterization by Hecker (52) and Van Duuren (135) of phorbol esters as the active components of croton oil has made possible the recent studies of the action of tumor-promoting agents in cell culture.

Although most studies of two-stage carcinogenesis have been carried out on skin, recent studies have made it clear that tumor promotion is a general phenomenon that extends to a number of tissues including liver (42,94,98,99,114,122, 147), lung (149), colon (106), and bladder (56). There have been a few reports of tumor promotion by phorbol esters or phorbol in organs such as liver and lung (see for example Armuth and Berenblum, 2). Other classes of agents also appear to be active as promotors. These include phenobarbital (94), bile acids (106), sodium cyclamate (56), and other compounds shown on Table 1.

TUMOR PROMOTION AS A MULTISTAGE PROCESS

In Vivo Studies

Studies of rat liver carcinogenesis have indicated that cells undergo a series of morphologic and biochemical alterations during preneoplastic stages (1,8,

TABLE 1. *Some nonphorbol agents shown to have tumor-promoting and/or carcinogenesis enhancing activity*

Agent	System	Reference
Phenobarbital	Rat liver	(94)
Polychlorinated biphenyls	Rat liver	(59)
DDT	Rat liver	(94,95)
Thioacetamide	Rat liver	(25)
α-Hexachlorocyclohexane	Rat liver	(25)
Butylated hydroxytoluene	Rat liver	(25)
Butylated hydroxytoluene	Mouse lung	(149)
Bile acids	Rat colon	(106)
Sodium cyclamate	Rat bladder	(56)
Sodium saccharin	Rat bladder	(56)
Epidermal growth factor	Mouse skin	(109)

41,61,66,114,146). Scherer and Emmelot (114), using formulations proposed by Druckrey (39) based on determination of tumor incidence as a function of time and dose, estimated the number of steps involved in carcinogenesis to be about six. They proposed that some of the seven stages distinguishable during experimental liver carcinogenesis might be candidates, namely steps leading to "islands, reversible hyperplastic nodules, irreversible hyperplastic nodules, highly differentiated carcinoma containing glycogen," and three less differentiated tumors.

Burns and co-workers (23,24) have obtained evidence for a similar number of stages in mouse skin carcinogenesis. These premalignant stages include steps leading to promoter-dependent clones, autonomous clones, promoter-dependent papillomas, autonomous papillomas, and squamous cell carcinomas. Some of these steps may occur as parts of alternative pathways. In at least one pathway papillomas appear to constitute preneoplastic lesions (23,24). There is evidence presented in earlier reports that some (20,45,117,127), but not all (51,113,137) papillomas are precursors of carcinomas. Burns et al. (23) found that about 5% of papillomas produced after 100 days of promotion by 12-*O*-tetradecanoyl-phorbol-13-acetate (TPA) persisted for an additional 24 weeks in the absence of phorbol ester. These promoter-independent or "autonomous papillomas" (24) may be immediate precursors to carcinomas. The other 95% which regressed appear to be promoter-dependent or "conditional papillomas" (24) and may be precursors to autonomous papillomas. They appear, however, not to be direct precursors of carcinomas as indicated by the observation that with long-term promotion, in which a high proportion of papillomas were conditional, the conversion rate to carcinomas was lower than with shorter promotion in which most papillomas were autonomous (24). Furthermore, another treatment scheme which preferentially yields autonomous papillomas, namely low initiator dose, gives a high conversion rate to carcinomas, thus further substantiating the role of autonomous but not of conditional papillomas as direct precarcinomatous lesions.

In spite of the demonstrated preneoplastic role of some papillomas, they appear not to be obligatory. A single application of a carcinogenic aromatic hydrocarbon at high dose yields carcinomas, some of which occur without prior evidence of a palpable papilloma (134 and Burns et al., *personal communication*). Burns and co-workers *(personal communication)* have postulated that an alternative precarcinoma pathway may include conditional and autonomous clones of cells analogous to conditional and autonomous papillomas.

Carcinogenesis In Vitro as a Multistage Process: Evidence for Promoter-Dependent Stages

Relatively little is known about the critical processes that occur in preneoplastic cells during the interval between the initial carcinogen-cell interaction and the onset of malignancy. *In vivo* investigations have been hampered by the fact that in intact tissues preneoplastic cells constitute a minority population in a heterogeneous mass and are often difficult to identify. Recent tissue culture studies, on the other hand, offer promising approaches to studying cloned populations of cells at various preneoplastic stages and their responses to tumor promoters.

Using a hybrid *in vivo–in vitro* transformation system of fetal rat brain cells treated with ethylnitrosourea, Laerum and Rajewsky (68) have identified five preneoplastic stages characterized primarily by growth and morphologic criteria. The acquisition of anchorage independence (stage IV) preceded the acquisition of tumorigenicity (stage V) by one to twelve passages. Yet another *in vivo–in vitro* system, a rat liver epithelial cell system, has been described by Borenfreund et al. (18) who found that preneoplastic cells were characterized by the presence of structures which appeared to be Mallory bodies, inclusions found in livers of chronic alcoholics.

Although the *in vivo–in vitro* systems offer certain advantages, they have not yet provided a means of studying promoter-dependent steps during carcinogenesis. Recently Steele et al. (125) and V. E. Steele *(personal communication)* have demonstrated a phorbol ester-dependent second stage of transformation following organ culture exposure of rat tracheal epithelium to a subcarcinogenic concentration of N-methyl-N′-nitro-N-nitrosoguanidine (MNNG). The treated organ cultures gave rise to primary cell cultures which, in turn, yielded cell lines that acquired tumorigenicity some 6 months after the initial MNNG exposure. This tracheal epithelial system retains some of the advantages of the *in vivo–in vitro* systems, e.g., availability of appropriate target cells for the initiator and capacity to yield differentiated carcinomas resembling those induced *in vivo*.

The heterogeneity of organ cultures, however, poses a problem for identifying and isolating target cells for the tumor promoter. For this purpose cell cultures appear promising. Evidence suggesting a phorbol ester-dependent second stage in the transformation of rat embryo cells initiated with benzo *(a)* pyrene (BP) has been reported by Lasne et al. (70). In this system, however, the promoting effect of 14 passages of phorbol ester exposure appeared to be replaceable by 22 to 25 passages without phorbol ester as indicated by growth in agar and tumorigenicity. This suggests that the TPA was enhancing or speeding up complete carcinogenesis induced by the initial exposure to BP and therefore may have been acting not as a tumor promoter but as another type of cocarcinogen. More recently Mondal et al. (81) and Heidelberger et al. (54) have demonstrated initiation and promotion stages during chemical transformation of C3H/ 10T1/2 cells. Initial exposure to low concentrations (0.1 μg/ml) of the polycyclic aromatic hydrocarbons 3-methylcholanthracene (MCA) or BP yielded less than 2% dishes with type III transformed foci after 6 weeks. Continuous exposure to TPA (0.1 μg/ml), beginning at 5 days following initiator, yielded 47% and 30% dishes with transformed foci 6 weeks after MCA and BP, respectively. These data do not, however, rule out the possibility that TPA could have speeded up a process which might have occurred without it in a period longer than 6 weeks. An alternative interpretation is that promoter-mediated acceleration of transformation, which appeared to occur in the experiments of Lasne et al. (70) and may occur in the 2-stage transformation of 10T1/2 cells (81,63), may be analogous to the demonstrated shortening of the latent period for tumor formation by tumor promoters *in vivo* (19,20).

Promotion of transformation by phorbol ester treatment of 10T1/2 cells previously initiated by ultraviolet irradiation (83) or X-radiation (63) has also been demonstrated. Although TPA promotion following a subeffective dose of X-radiation (400 rads) yielded a significant level of type III foci, the level of type II foci (about one-third of which are nontumorigenic (107)) was much higher. The authors suggested that the nonmalignant type II foci may be analogous to benign papillomas produced during skin carcinogenesis.

Recent studies in our laboratory (30,33,34a), using cell lines derived from mouse primary epidermal cell cultures exposed to carcinogen or to solvent alone, have led to the identification of cells that respond to TPA by irreversibly acquiring anchorage-independent growth. Such acquisition of neoplastic phenotype did not occur during some 60 passages in the absence of TPA. These TPA-responsive cells have the advantage of being derived from normal mouse epidermal cells (33,34) and, therefore, of offering the possibility of studying the same target cells for tumor-promoting phorbol esters which occur *in vivo* in mouse epidermis. This system is currently being used to study the mechanism of TPA-dependent irreversible changes leading to malignancy.

Yet another promising *in vitro* system for studying preneoplastic progression has been described by Barrett et al. (6,7). They found that during transformation of hamster embryo cells by BP, morphologic transformation, enhanced fibrinolytic activity, and anchorage-independent growth occurred sequentially with predictable numbers of population doublings required for each shift. Although promoter-dependent changes have not been reported for this system, it does allow precise definition of preneoplastic phenotypes and their sequential relationships.

PHENOTYPIC EFFECTS OF TUMOR PROMOTERS

Tumor Promoters Inhibit Differentiation

In 1954, Berenblum (11) proposed that tumor promotion involved a nonspecific proliferative stimulus and a specific inhibition of maturation. Following that, studies in many laboratories demonstrated that tumor promoters stimulate cell proliferation in normal or previously initiated epidermis (19). Furthermore, a number of studies using mouse epidermis provided support for the inhibited maturation hypothesis. Ultrastructure studies by Raick (102) indicated that after exposure to TPA putative committed cells regained the nuclear and cytoplasmic organization characteristic of epidermal basal cells. Raick also found that TPA induced the appearance of "dark cells," a phenotypic variant also found in wound healing, and he suggested that tumor promoters not only inhibit normal maturation but induce an abnormal pathway of differentiation.

Krieg et al. (67) demonstrated that chalone responsiveness, a marker of normal adult epidermal functionalization absent from newborn epidermis (13), showed a transient disappearance in response to TPA. Colburn et al. (31,32) found that the activity of histidase, an enzyme present in normal adult epidermis and liver but low or absent from newborn fetal epidermis and from all other tissues tested, was decreased after treatment by tumor-promoting phorbol esters. In another study of biochemical markers, Balmain (4,5) showed that TPA induced the appearance of two proteins found at high levels in normal newborn but not in normal adult epidermis.

More recently, phorbol esters have been shown to inhibit terminal differentiation in cell culture systems. The processes inhibited include myogenesis in chick myoblasts (28), erythroid differentiation in Friend erythroleukemia cells (111,151), adipocyte induction from 3T3 cells (37), chondrogenesis in chick chondroblasts (93), neurite induction in neuroblastoma cells (58), and melanogenesis in melanoma cells (85). Studies with primary mouse epidermal cell cultures (46,152) have shown that phorbol esters suppress keratinization as determined by phase microscopy. In nearly all of the studies described above, both *in vivo* and *in vitro* suppression of differentiation were transient with reversal occurring after removal of TPA. In some systems, for example, melanogenesis (85) TPA appeared to delay rather than inhibit differentiation since reversal occurred eventually even in the presence of TPA. Exceptions to this reversibility, however, were found when previously initiated epidermis (31,32,87,103) was exposed to TPA. In these cases, dark cells and ultrastructural features characteristic of a more embryonic type (103), low histidase activity (31,32), and high ornithine decarboxylase (ODC) activity (87) persisted into papillomas and carcinomas that arose later.

Tumor Promoters Induce Transient Mimicry of the Neoplastic Phenotype

Tumor promoters have been found to transiently induce in epidermal and other cells a set of phenotypic changes that resemble those found in malignant cells. Raick (103) and Raick and Burdzy (104) found that tumor-promoting agents, but not nonpromoting (or weakly promoting) mitogens, induced in basal cells certain morphologic changes resembling those found in papillomas and carcinomas. Histidase activity, likewise lowered by promoting but not by nonpromoting agents (31,32), is low or absent in epidermal tumors (3,31). Recently, G_1 chalone responsiveness, which is decreased by TPA, has been reported to be very low in a transplantable epidermal carcinoma (13a). Epidermal ornithine decarboxylase, transiently induced by TPA (90,91), is also elevated in mouse epidermal papillomas and carcinomas (87). Based on these and other data, O'Brien et al. (87,90) proposed that tumor promoters, acting as irreversible derepressors, transitorily induce the tumor phenotype in normal cells.

In 1967, Sivak and Van Duuren (120) reported that TPA produced in 3T3 cells a release from density-dependent inhibition of growth similar to that found in transformed 3T3 cells. Recent cell-culture studies have demonstrated that a number of biochemical features of the neoplastic phenotype are also transiently mimicked after exposure to TPA. Lichti et al. (75) and Yuspa et al. (154) found that tumor-promoting phorbol esters induced ornithine decarboxylase in primary epidermal cell cultures with maximal induction at 6 to 12 hr posttreatment and a return to normal levels by 24 to 48 hr.

TPA treatment of chick embryo cells was found to transiently decrease cell surface LETS protein (fibronectin) (14) and cell volume (38), to increase plasminogen activator levels (145), sugar transport, and saturation density (38), and to produce changes in cell-surface glycyoprotein profiles (142). All of these changes resemble those found in chick cells after transformation by oncogenic viruses (142). Induction of plasminogen activator (144), increased sugar transport and saturation density, and loss of LETS protein (38) have also been found to occur in response to other tumor-promoting phorbol esters but not in response to certain nonphorbol tumor promoters such as anthralin, cantharidin, and tobacco leaf extract (144) (Blumberg et al., *personal communication*).

In addition to producing mimicry of the transformed phenotype, phorbol esters also produce synergy in induction of fibrinolytic activity and membrane glycoprotein shifts which occur in chick embryo fibroblasts after transformation by Rous Sarcoma virus (142). TPA has been postulated to activate the src gene product (M. H. Wigler, *personal communication*). TPA also produces synergistic induction of ornithine decarboxylase in chemically transformed hamster embryo fibroblasts (88).

One aspect of the neoplastic phenotype which appears to show neither synergy nor mimicry in response to tumor promoters is anchorage-independent growth. Although certain cells have been found to respond to TPA by acquiring anchorage-independent growth (30,33,54,63), this appears to involve not a mimicry of neoplasia but an acquisition of it by initiated or preneoplastic cells.

THE MECHANISM OF TUMOR PROMOTION

Stimulation of Cell Proliferation

That tumor promoters stimulate cell proliferation in epidermal target tissue is well established (for review, see Boutwell, 20). That tumor-promoting phorbol esters stimulate DNA (deoxyribonucleic acid) synthesis in the cell culture analog, namely primary epidermal cell cultures, is also clear (46,55,152,154). Promoter-stimulated cell division appears to be a general phenomenon that extends to a number of tumor promoters in a variety of tissues. Thioacetamide, α-hexachloro-cyclohexane, or butylated hydroxytoluene when administered following exposure to hepatocarcinogens induced stimulated proliferation and conversion of carcinogen-resistant cells to preneoplastic liver foci (25) (see Table 2).

Although stimulated proliferation has for some time appeared to be insufficient for promotion (see, for example, 20,22,102,103), recent *in vitro* studies suggest that it may even be unnecessary. Peterson et al. (96) found that the doubling time of previously initiated 10T1/2 cells was unaffected by exposure to TPA under conditions that led to malignant transformation. Nor was the plateau density significantly increased by TPA. However, treatment of cells during log or stationary phase produced a two- to threefold mid-stationary phase increase in the rate of tritiated thymidine incorporation and in the labeling index. This finding was interpreted by the authors as indicating a delayed and partially synchronized arrival at stationary phase induced by the TPA, but alternatively might reflect a DNA synthesis stimulation.

Similarly, Colburn et al. (30,33) found that the doubling times and the plateau densities of preneoplastic epidermal cell lines showed little or no increase after exposure to TPA under conditions that led to malignant transformation. TPA did, however, increase the plateau density of preneoplastic epidermal cells when the serum concentration was decreased (Colburn et al., *unpublished observations*) and of 10T1/2 cells when the medium was changed from Eagles basal to Dulbeccos (142). Unlike Peterson et al. (96) we found significant stimulation of tritiated thymidine incorporation during log phase of some but not all TPA-responsive cell lines (30,33).

Although the data on initiated TPA-responsive mouse 10T1/2 cells and epidermal cells may suggest the lack of a requirement for stimulated cell proliferation during promotion, a more likely interpretation may be the lack of such a requirement during a substage of promotion, presumably a late phase. During tumor promotion *in vivo* there may be early substage(s) during which a proliferative stimulus is critical and for which an *in vitro* analog has not yet been demonstrated. Perhaps *in vitro* the critical proliferation stimulus is provided by growth in

TABLE 2. Cellular and molecular responses to tumor promoters that occur during tumor promotion in vivo or in vitro

System	DNA ↑ synthesis	ODC ↑	SCEs ↑	Protease[a] ↑	PGs ↑	PL ↑	Histidase ↓
Mouse epidermis	+(20)	+(90)	ND	+(132)	+(140)[g] (121)[g]	+(108)	+(32)
Rat liver							
10T1/2 Cells	+(25) −(96) + (142)	ND ND	ND	ND	ND ND	ND ND	+(97)[h] NR
Preneoplastic epidermal cells	+(30) (33)	−(d)	+(86)	+(62)[e] I.P.[f]	ND	ND	NR[i]
Balb/c 3T3 cells	+(119)[b],(c)	+(c)	ND	ND	+(92)	+(126)	NR

[a] PA and other proteases.
[b] By implication since plateau density is increased.
[c] O'Brien and Diamond (unpublished data).
[d] T. Ben, N. Colburn, and U. Lichti (unpublished data).
[e] By implication since protease inhibitors block promotion of transformation.
[f] W. Laug and N. Colburn (in progress).
[g] By implication since indomethacin blocks promotion and ODC induction by TPA.
[h] By implication since histidase decreases progressively during carcinogenesis.
[i] The histidase level is decreased to 1% of the level in intact epidermis on cultivation of the cells Colburn et al. (unpublished data).
↑ Indicates an increase produced by tumor promoters; ↓ indicates a decrease.
Numbers in parentheses indicate references.
SCEs: sister chromatid exchanges, PGs: prostaglandin levels, ND, not determined, NR, not relevant, absent from untreated cells.

culture in the absence of tumor promoters, in which case the *in vitro* analog may not be forthcoming.

Ornithine Decarboxylase Induction

Studies by Boutwell et al. (21,90,91) and Lichti et al. (75) have demonstrated that for mouse epidermis both *in vivo* and *in vitro* there is a strong correlation between tumor-promoting activity and ODC-inducing activity for a series of phorbol esters. The observation has been extended to wounding which promotes carcinogenesis and induces ODC and skin massage which does neither (27). Such a specific correlation suggests that ODC induction plays a causal role in tumor promotion, or is a parallel result of a determinant of promotion. Evidence suggesting a noncausal or even nonessential role of induced ODC comes from the observation that glucocorticoids, which inhibit tumor promotion (121), fail to inhibit induction of ODC by promoters (155).

Alternatively, there may be necessary events unrelated to ODC induction which are glucocorticoid sensitive. Such an interpretation says nothing of the role or lack of it for ODC. In fact, there have been several reports which demonstrated that tumor-promotion inhibiting steroids also inhibited promoter-stimulated DNA, RNA, and protein synthesis (116,155). This dissociation of macromolecular stimulation from ODC induction (155; and T. G. O'Brien et al., *personal communication*) rules out any obligatory links between the ODC induction and the stimulated cell proliferation which occur in response to tumor promoters. As for the role of ODC induction in tumor promotion, it may play a role or it may simply serve as a useful marker of tumor-promoting activity which is tightly coupled but not causally related.

Proteases and Inflammation

Various other molecular events have been proposed as mediators of tumor promotion (see Table 2). These include induction of certain proteases including plasminogen activator (PA) (132) and induction of inflammatory mediators, notably prostaglandins (140).

Protease action was implicated in promotion by Troll et al. in 1970 (130) who found that the protease inhibitor N-α-tosyl-L-lysylchloromethane when applied to mouse skin during promotion with TPA also inhibited the tumor yield and increased the average time for tumor appearance. Promotion inhibition was also observed for the competitive protease inhibitors tosyl arginine methyl ester and leupeptin (131). Studies with both phorbol ester and ingenol tumor promoters have demonstrated a consistent correlation between tumor-promoting activity and activity in inducing PA in cell cultures (142,144,145). Whether tumor-promotion inhibitory doses of leupeptin also inhibit plasminogen activator *in vivo* is unknown. In fact, PA induction during tumor promotion *in vivo* has not been demonstrated although induction of partially characterized proteinase(s) has been shown to occur *in vivo* after TPA treatment (132). Transient PA induction has been shown to occur during transformation of hamster embryo cells by BP (6). This change occurs subsequent to morphologic alteration and prior to acquisition of anchorage independence. Although transformed 10T1/2 mouse embryo cells show elevated PA levels (60), PA elevation during tumor promotion *in vitro* by phorbol esters has not been reported. An independent indication that PA may play a role in tumor promotion comes from the finding that promotion-inhibiting glucocorticoids also inhibit the induction of PA in hepatoma HTC cells by TPA (141).

The inflammatory activity of tumor promoters has been known since long before the "ear redness" test was utilized to monitor the purification of croton-oil factors (Hecker and co-workers, 53). Cutaneous inflammation appears to be mediated by a variety of substances including prostaglandins (49). Ohuchi and Levine (92) have shown that tumor-promoting phorbol esters stimulate phospholipid deacylation and prostaglandin synthesis in canine kidney cells. Prostaglandin synthesis stimulation was inhibited by retinol (K. Ohuchi and L. Levine, *personal communication*) that also inhibits skin tumor promotion by phorbol esters (36,139). The prostaglandin biosynthesis inhibitor indomethacin inhibits tumor promotion (121), ODC induction (140), and histidase decrease (72 and Colburn et al., *unpublished*). However, the inhibitor levels used were very high for only moderate promotion inhibition and could have blocked promotion by mechanisms unrelated to prostaglandin biosynthesis.

Cell Surface Alterations

The first indication that tumor-promoting activity may be mediated by cell-surface interactions came from the work of Sivak et al. (118) who demonstrated changes in the activities of several plasma membrane enzymes. Phorbol esters were also shown to stimulate the synthesis and phosphorylation of membrane phospholipids (108,126). Subsequently, Van Duuren et al. (136) reported evidence for conformational changes in plasma membrane proteins after exposure to tumor promoting but not nonpromoting phorbol esters. Recently, P. B. Fisher and I. B. Weinstein *(personal communication)* have reported that tumor promoters rapidly alter the fluorescence polarization of membranes, a parameter which may reflect membrane lipid fluidity. Tumor-promoting phorbol diesters and mezerein induced a decrease in fluorescence polarization whereas the nonpromoters phorbol and 4-phorbol-12,13-didecanoate did not. Whether these membrane shifts are involved in the mechanism of tumor promotion remains to be demonstrated.

There have been several reports of promoter-induced shifts in cell-surface receptors, shifts which might be involved in mediating the altered growth regulation associated with preneoplastic and neoplastic phenotypes. Marks and co-workers (67,77,76) showed that tumor-promoting phorbol esters produced a transient loss of chalone response and a transient decrease in β-adrenergic response. Both chalones and β-adrenergic agonists appear to be active in restricting the growth rate of epidermal cells via binding to cell-surface receptors (67,76). Recently Lee and Weinstein (73) have reported that TPA and other phorbol and nonphorbol promoters inhibit the binding of epidermal growth factor (EGF) to EGF receptors by a mechanism that appears to involve neither competition nor decreased affinity. Apparently promoters inactivate EGF receptors and consequently decrease the number available for binding to EGF.

Todaro and co-workers (128) have reported that cells transformed by RNA (ribonucleic acid) tumor viruses lose the ability to bind EGF to cell-surface receptors. A similar loss of EGF binding has been reported for chemically transformed Syrian hamster embryo fibroblasts (57). This loss appears not to be the general case for chemical transformation (Todaro, *personal communication*) or for DNA virus transformation (128). These workers have proposed that transformed cells which lose EGF or other growth-factor receptors acquire the capacity to synthesize growth factors to which they themselves inappropriately respond, thus giving rise to a locked-in stimulated growth and an escape from normal growth-factor regulation. Recently De Larco and Todaro (35) have reported that a human fibrosarcoma line, which has lost multiplication stimulating activity (MSA), synthesizes MSA-related peptides of 7,000 and 11,000 molecular weight that show mitogenic activity. To the extent that tumor promoters induce a mimicry of the transformed state, they may function to abolish regulation by EGF and substitute an inappropriate growth stimulation similar to that mediated by sarcoma growth factors, a change which may be reversible early in promotion but may become constitutive late in promotion.

A number of reports have dealt with the possibility that the interaction of phorbol esters with cells may resemble the interaction of polypeptide hormones with receptors. (See, for example, Estensen et al., 40.) It has been suggested (142) that TPA may be able to utilize polypeptide hormone receptors in much the same way the opiates utilize receptors for endogenous enkephalins or endorphins. Although TPA appears not to compete for EGF receptors (73), one can postulate that TPA competes with other, as yet untested, growth factors for binding to their receptors. A direct demonstration of a receptor for TPA has not as yet been reported. The finding of clonal heterogeneity of cells for TPA responsiveness (43 and N. H. Colburn, *unpublished*) appears promising for discerning critical interactions of TPA with cellular receptors.

Induction versus Selection

The first demonstration that the process of carcinogenesis may be inductive rather than selective came from the work of Mondal and Heidelberger (82) who reported malignant transformation of mouse prostate cells after exposure of single cells to polycylic aromatic hydrocarbons. That observation does not, however, rule out the possibility that promotion may involve selection. Premalignant colonies produced after single-cell exposure to carcinogen could be heterogeneous with respect to responses leading to malignancy.

Mondal et al. (81) reported that neither 10T1/2 cells nor a transformed clone derived from 10T1/2 cells showed decreased plating efficiency in the presence of 0.1 μg/ml TPA, the concentration used for promotion. This lack of differential cytotoxicity led the authors to rule out selection as accounting for promotion *in vitro* by TPA.

Research in our laboratory (34a) also suggests that TPA is inducing preneoplastic changes leading to malignancy rather than selecting for preexisting but unexpressed malignant cells. Recently we have found that concentrations of TPA which induce anchorage-independent growth in preneoplastic cells are without effect on the plating efficiency in monolayer of either the preneoplastic cells or their transformed derivatives. Furthermore, TPA was found to induce anchorage independence in single cells (34a) thus indicating an inductive rather than a selective mechanism whereby tumor promoters mediate late premalignant conversion. The possibility that promotion involves selection in addition to induction cannot be ruled out.

The Irreversible Steps in Tumor Promotion: Possible Mechanisms

The irreversibility of some stages of tumor promotion has been well established by the work of Burns and co-workers (23,24) who demonstrated irreversible formation of carcinomas from autonomous papillomas and irreversible formation of autonomous papillomas from one or more precursors in response to TPA exposure. How promoters can impact genes without being mutagenic and constitutively alter gene expression without undergoing covalent interactions is a major unsolved problem of tumor promotion. In 1963, Pitot and Heidelberger (100) proposed a nonmutational mechanism of carcinogenesis whereby interlocking operons could respond to the carcinogen with a locked-in derepression of an oncogene. Perhaps tumor promoters might act in a similar way on the repressor of a gene previously mutated by an initiator. Alternatively, if initiators act to induce a mutagenic change, then promoters may act in part to increase the mutation frequency without themselves being mutagenic. Evidence for phorbol ester enhancement of ultraviolet light-induced mutation frequency has been presented by Trosko et al. (133) and for enhancement of chemically induced mutation frequency by Lankas et al. (69).

Radman and co-workers (101) have proposed that the transformed state is a state of permanent derepression triggered by an inducer protease. Phorbol esters, they postulate, could interact with the inducer protease repressor and inactivate it giving rise to expression of previously repressed genes which if appropriately mutated by the initiator can specify the malignant phenotype. Evidence for protease inactivation of a repressor has been presented by Meyn et al. (80). As discussed earlier, TPA is known to induce proteases. More recently Kinsella and Radman (65) have proposed that tumor promoters permit the expression of an initiator-induced recessive mutation by inducing aberrant mitotic segregation which leads to haploid gene copies or to double recessives. Such genetic recombination might be effected by sister chromatid exchange or a similar process. Radman and co-workers (65 and *personal communication*) have shown that TPA, but not nonpromoting phorbol esters, induced elevated levels of sister chromatid exchanges in the absence of DNA damage or mutagenesis. A suggestion that this might lead to genetic recombination came from the finding that TPA stimulated the segregation of two recessive traits from a heterozygous cell hybrid. Evidence for induction of sister chromatid exchanges in 10T1/2 cells by TPA has been obtained by Nagasawa and Little (86). Both this group and Radman and co-workers found that protease inhibitors inhibited the induction of sister chromatid exchanges by TPA. Protease inhibitors also inhibited promotion by TPA in 10T1/2 cells initiated by low doses of X-ray (62). Of interest is the recent report that saccharin, which shows tumor promoting activity in bladder (29,56), also induces sister chromatid exchanges (150).

Other Aspects of Tumor-Promotion Mechanism

Certain responses to tumor promoters, namely changes in cyclic nucleotide levels and induction of viruses, have not been discussed so far in this review of tumor-promotion mechanism. Suffice it to say that as indicated by Garte et al. (47) the data on the effects of phorbol esters on cyclic nucleotide levels have been conflicting but suggest no change in cyclic AMP levels. Regarding the role of viruses, although chemical transformation of mouse embryo cells by polycyclic aromatic hydrocarbons appeared to occur independently of virus production (105), the possibility exists that tumor promoters may function by inducing virus or viral oncogenes. Zur Hausen et al. (157) have reported that TPA induces Epstein-Barr virus.

A final note on promotion mechanism deals with the metabolism of tumor promoters. Recent studies of TPA metabolism in mouse epidermis (12) indicate that metabolic activation of TPA does not occur and that the half-life of TPA *in vivo* appears to be 18 hr or less, depending on whether metabolites are determined after single or multiple applications of TPA. This half-life is consistent with the observation that for maximal tumor yield the frequency of tumor promotion must be about once per 3 days (19,20), and suggests a time frame during which the critical responses to tumor promoters must occur. TPA metabolism studies have also been carried out in hamster fibroblasts which metabolize it rapidly and human fibroblasts which do not (89).

INHIBITION OF TUMOR PROMOTION: POSSIBILITIES FOR CANCER PREVENTION

Anti-inflammatory Steroids

For more than 20 years, it has been known that cortisone inhibits tumor promotion by croton oil in mouse skin (19,48,129). Since then the observation

TABLE 3. *Biochemical effects of tumor-promotion inhibitors*

Tumor-promotion inhibitor	DNA ↑	ODC ↑	Proteases[a] ↑	Histidase ↓	PGs ↑	SCEs ↑
Glucocorticoids	↓ (121)	NE or ↑ (155)	↓ (141,142)	NE[d]	NE (156,92)	↓ (65)
Protease inhibitors	ND	ND		NE[d]	↓[e]	↓ (65)(86)
Retinoids	NE[b](36)	↓ (140,36)	NE (143) ↑ (148)	ND	↓[e]	ND
PG synthesis inhibitors	↓ (141)[c]	↓ (140)	↓ (141)[c]	↑ (72)		ND

[a] Including PA.
[b] No effect.
[c] Magnitude of the effect is relatively small.
[d] N. Colburn *et al.* (unpublished data).
[e] K. Ohuchi and L. Levine (personal communication).

An arrow in the opposite direction from that showing the promoter effect indicates that the promotion inhibitor blocks or antagonizes the promoter effect; an arrow in the same direction indicates enhancement.
For abbreviations and symbols, see Table 2.

has been extended to other glucocorticoids. Belman and Troll (9), Scribner and Slaga (116), and Slaga and co-workers (115,121) have demonstrated that dexamethasone and fluocinolone acetonide (FA) applied simultaneously with TPA were potent inhibitors of tumor promotion. FA doses as low as 0.1µg per mouse given together with 2µg TPA per mouse produced almost complete inhibition of tumor promotion. The latter investigators (121) found that the FA-sensitive events were taking place subsequent to the first 4 weeks of promotion, and suggested that the steroid has no effect on the conversion of initiated cells into latent tumor cells postulated to occur (19) during the first phase of promotion. The mechanism of promotion inhibition by glucocorticoids is not known. Like most hormones their effects are pleotropic. As summarized in Table 3, phorbol ester stimulated DNA, RNA, and protein synthesis and PA induction (116,121,141) are all inhibited by these steroids but ODC induction is not (155). The inhibitory effect on promotion may be mediated primarily through counteracting hyperplasia (121), a hyperplasia that may be needed for the conversion of latent tumor cells into gross tumors (19). However, other modes of action, such as inhibition of sister chromatid exchange induction or plasminogen activator induction, cannot be ruled out.

Retinoids

A number of synthetic vitamin A derivatives or retinoids have been shown to prevent the development of cancer when administered after initiation during preneoplastic progression of skin (16,17), respiratory tract (112), mammary gland (50), and urinary bladder (124). Bollag (15) demonstrated that epidermal papillomas and carcinomas initiated by dimethylbenz*(a)*anthracene and promoted by croton oil could be prevented by oral administration of retinoic acid during the promotion phase. Not only can retinoids prevent the induction of premalignant lesions in epidermis (15–17) and bladder epithelium (124), but they can reverse premalignant lesions of epidermis (16) and prostate (26,71) after they are already formed. Although low doses prevent cancer in a variety of tissues, high doses of retinoids appear to enhance tumor promotion or even function as tumor promoters in hamster cheek pouch (74,78). These effects may be associated with toxicity which can unspecifically produce enhancement of carcinogenesis.

Recently retinoids have been shown to inhibit *in vitro* transformation of 10T1/2 cells by MCA (79). The retinoids were active at concentrations that affected neither plating efficiency nor growth rate of MCA-treated cells. When the start of retinoid exposure was delayed as long as 3 weeks after MCA treatment, the extent of inhibition of transformation was 80%. Since 6 to 8 weeks are required for transformation (107), this implies that the retinoid acts primarily or entirely on progression or promotion rather than initiation. The effect was reversible; given sufficient time, the transformation frequency approached that attained without retinoids (J. S. Bertram, *personal communication*).

Recent results in our laboratory (34a) indicate that retinoids inhibit the TPA-dependent acquisition of anchorage independence by preoplastic epidermal cells. The inhibitory activity of several retinoids parallels their activity for inhibiting tumor promotion *in vivo* (139). Thus, retinoids can inhibit one or more phases of tumor promotion by phorbol esters both *in vivo* and *in vitro*. Whether the inhibition of epidermal carcinogenesis *in vivo* represents a delay rather than an irreversible or long-term prevention remains to be determined.

The mechanism whereby retinoids prevent or reverse preoplastic progression is not known. Retinoids are known to influence the balance between cell proliferation and differentiation in epithelial tissues (123) and cells in culture (153). Verma and Boutwell (139) have shown that retinoic acid inhibits ODC induction by TPA under conditions in which tumor promotion is inhibited. Ninety percent inhibition of promotion occurs with greater than 90% inhibition of ODC induction but little inhibition of DNA synthesis rate (36). In contrast, retinoic acid was found to inhibit the comitogenic action of phorbol esters in bovine lymphocytes (64).

CONCLUSION

Although the multistage nature of carcinogenesis in a variety of tissues is much better understood than it was 10 years ago, a number of basic questions about preoplastic progression and tumor promotion remain to be answered:

1. What properties of initiated cells render them responsive to tumor promoters?

2. Does tumor promotion involve induction of new cell types or selection of preexisting ones or both?

3. If the mechanism is selective, what is the basis for selection?

4. Can tumor promotion be subdivided into a sequential series of qualitatively different substages? If so, what characterizes the preoplastic target cells that respond to promoters at each of these stages and what critical changes do they undergo?

5. Is there one set of sequential changes that must occur during preoplastic progression or are there alternative pathways for converting initiated cells to malignant tumors?

6. Although the central dogma of chemical carcinogenesis holds that initiation is irreversible and promotion reversible, recent reports have made it clear that promotion includes some irreversible steps. How can promoters, themselves nonmutagenic, impact genes postulated to have been mutated by initiators to give rise to irreversible expression of malignancy?

Recent advances in tumor promotion research have made it clear that tumor promotion is a general phenomenon which occurs in a variety of tissues in response to a number of different chemicals. Extensive work with *in vivo* and *in vitro* systems has yielded considerable information on molecular responses to tumor-promoting phorbol esters. What remains is the difficult pursuit of discerning which molecular events determine the progression to malignancy. To this end stable preneoplastic cells which respond to phorbol esters by acquiring a later-stage premalignant or malignant (30,54) phenotype may be useful. Finally, attempts to arrest or delay tumor promotion by exposure to retinoids or steriods appear promising, both for elucidation of promotion mechanism and for cancer prevention.

REFERENCES

1. Anthony, P. P. (1976): Precursor lesions for liver cancer in humans. *Cancer Res.,* 36:2579–2583.
2. Armuth, V., and Berenblum, I. (1972): Systemic promoting action of phorbol in liver and lung carcinogenesis in AKR mice. *Cancer Res.,* 32:2259–2262.
3. Baden, H. P., Sviokla, S., Mittler, B., and Pathak, M. A. (1968): Histidase activity in hyperplastic and neoplastic rat epidermis and liver. *Cancer Res.,* 28:1463–1467.
4. Balmain, A. (1976): The synthesis of specific proteins in adult mouse epidermis during phases of proliferation and differentiation induced by the tumor promoter TPA, and in basal and differentiating layers of neonatal mouse epidermis. *J. Invest. Dermatol.,* 67:246–253.
5. Balmain, A. (1978): Synthesis of specific proteins in mouse epidermis after treatment with the tumor promoter TPA. In: *Carcinogenesis, Vol. 2, Mechanisms of Tumor Promotion and Cocarcinogenesis,* edited by T. J. Slaga, A. Sivak, and R. K. Boutwell, pp. 153–172. Raven Press, New York.
6. Barrett, J. C., Crawford, B. D., Grady, D. L., Hester, L. D., Jones, P. A., Benedict, W. F., and Ts'o, P. O. (1977): Temporal acquisition of enhanced fibrinolytic activity by Syrian hamster embryo cells following treatment with benzo(a)pyrene. *Cancer Res.,* 37:3815–3823.
7. Barrett, J. C., and Ts'o, P. O. P. (1978): Evidence for the progressive nature of neoplastic transformation *in vitro. Proc. Natl. Acad. Sci. USA,* 75:3761–3765.
8. Becker, F. F. (1976): Sequential phenotypic and biochemical alterations during chemical hepatocarcinogenesis. *Cancer Res.,* 36:2563–2566.
9. Belman, S., and Troll, W. (1972): The inhibition of croton oil-promoted mouse skin tumorigenesis by steroid hormones. *Cancer Res.,* 32:450–454.
10. Berenblum, I. (1941): The cocarcinogenic action of croton resin, *Cancer Res.,* 1:44–48.
11. Berenblum, I. (1954): Carcinogenesis and tumor pathogenesis. *Adv. Cancer Res.,* 2:129–175.
12. Berry, D. L., Bracken, W. M., Fischer, S. M., Viaje, A., and Slaga, T. J. (1978): Metabolic conversion of 12-*O*-tetradecanoylphorbol-13-acetate in adult and newborn mouse skin and mouse liver microsomes. *Cancer Res.,* 38:2301–2306.
13. Bertsch, S., and Marks, F. (1974): Lack of an effect of tumor-promoting phorbol esters and of epidermal G_1 chalone on DNA synthesis in the epidermis of newborn mice. *Cancer Res.,* 34:3283–3288.
13a. Bertsch, S., and Marks, F. (1979): Effects of epidermal chalone and epidermal growth factor on a transplantable epidermal carcinoma (Hewitt) of the mouse in vivo. *Cancer Res.,* 39:239–243.
14. Blumberg. P. M., Driedger, P. E., and Rossow, P. W. (1976): Effect of phorbol ester on a transformation-sensitive surface protein of chick fibroblasts. *Nature,* 264:446–447.
15. Bollag, W. (1972): Prophylaxis of chemically induced benign and malignant epithelial tumors by vitamin A acid (retinoic acid). *Eur. J. Cancer,* 8:689–693.
16. Bollag, W. (1974): Therapeutic effects of an aromatic retinoic acid analog on chemically induced skin papillomas and carcinomas of mice. *Eur. J. Cancer,* 10:731–737.
17. Bollag, W. (1975): Therapy of epithelial tumors with an aromatic retinoic acid analog. *Chemotherapy,* 21:236–247.
18. Borenfreund, E., Higgins, P. J., and Bendich, A. (1977): *In vivo* initiated rat liver carcinogenesis studied *in vitro;* formation of alcoholic hyaline-type bodies. *Cancer Lett.,* 3:145–150.
19. Boutwell, R. K. (1964): Some biological aspects of skin carcinogenesis. *Prog. Exp. Tumor Res.,* 4:207–250.

20. Boutwell, R. K. (1974): The function and mechanism of promoters of carcinogenesis. *CRC Crit. Rev. Toxicol.,* 2:419–443.

21. Boutwell, R. K. (1977): The role of the induction of ornithine decarboxylase in tumor promotion. In: *Origins of Human Cancer, Book B,* edited by H. H. Hiatt, J. D. Watson, and J. A. Winsten, pp. 49–58. Cold Spring Harbor Laboratory, New York.

22. Boutwell, R. K. (1978): Biochemical Mechanism of Tumor Promotion. In: *Carcinogenesis Vol. 2. Mechanisms of Tumor Promotion and Cocarcinogenesis,* edited by T. J. Slaga, A. Sivak, and R. K. Boutwell, pp. 49–58. Raven Press, New York.

23. Burns, F. J., Vanderlaan, M., Sivak, A., and Albert, R. E. (1976): Regression kinetics of mouse skin papillomas. *Cancer Res.,* 36:1422–1427.

24. Burns, F. J., Vanderlaan, M., Snyder, E., and Albert, R. E. (1978): Induction and progression kinetics of mouse skin papillomas. In: *Carcinogenesis, Vol. 2. Mechanisms of Tumor Promotion and Cocarcinogenesis,* edited by T. J. Slaga, A. Sivak, and R. K. Boutwell, pp. 91–96. Raven Press, New York.

25. Cameron, R., Lee, G., and Farber, E. (1978): Chemical mitogens as effective alternatives to partial hepatectomy in the new model for the sequential analysis of hepatocarcinogenesis. *Proc. Am. Assoc. Cancer Res.,* 19:56.

26. Chopra, D. P., and Wilkoff, L. J. (1976): Inhibition and reversal by B-retinoic acid of hyperplasia induced in cultured mouse prostate tissue by 3-methylcholanthrene or N-methyl-N'-nitro-N-nitrosoguanidine. *J. Natl. Cancer Inst.,* 56:583–589.

27. Clark-Lewis, I., and Murray, A. W. (1978): Tumor promotion and the induction of epidermal ornithine decarboxylase activity in mechanically stimulated mouse skin. *Cancer Res.,* 38:494–497.

28. Cohen, R., Pacifici, M., Rubinstein, N., Beihl, J., and Holtzer, H. (1977): Effect of tumour promoter on myogenesis, *Nature,* 266:538–540.

29. Cohen, S. M., Arai, M., and Friedell, G. H. (1978): Promoting effect of DL-Tryptophan and saccharin in urinary bladder carcinogenesis in the rat. *Proc. Am. Assoc. Cancer Res.,* 19:4.

30. Colburn, N. H., Former, B., and Warren, L. (1978): Tumor promoting phorbol esters induce anchorage independent growth in some epidermal cell strains. *Proc. Am. Assoc. Cancer Res.,* 19:65.

31. Colburn, N. H., Head, R. A., and Lau, S. (1975): The relationship of epidermal histidase levels to tumor promotion, hyperplasia and neoplasia. *Proc. Am. Assoc. Cancer Res.,* 16:46.

32. Colburn, N. H., Lau, S., and Head, R. (1975): Decrease of epidermal histidase activity by tumor-promoting phorbol esters. *Cancer Res.,* 35:3154–3159.

33. Colburn, N. H., Vorder Bruegge, W. F., Bates, J., and Yuspa, S. H. (1978): Epidermal cell transformation in vitro. In: *Carcinogenesis, Vol. 2. Mechanisms of Tumor Promotion and Cocarcinogenesis,* edited by T. J. Slaga, A. Sivak, and R. K. Boutwell, pp. 257–271. Raven Press, New York.

34. Colburn, N. H., Vorder Bruegge, W. F., Bates, J. R., Gray, R. H., Rossen, J. D., Kelsey, W. H., and Shimada, T. (1978): Correlation of anchorage-independent growth with tumorigenicity of chemically transformed mouse epidermal cells. *Cancer Res.,* 38:624–634.

34a. Colburn, N. H. (1979): The use of tumor promoter responsive epidermal cell lines to study preneoplastic progression. In: *Neoplastic Transformation in Differentiated Epithelial Cell Systems In Vitro,* edited by L. M. Franks and C. B. Wigley. Academic Press, New York *(in press).*

35. De Larco, J. E., and Todaro, G. J. (1978): A human fibrosarcoma cell line producing multiplication stimulating activity (MSA)-related peptides. *Nature,* 272:356–358.

36. De Young, L., Weeks, R. G., Verma, A., and Boutwell, R. K. (1978): A dissociation of TPA induced epidermal ornithine decarboxylase activity and cellular proliferation and its relevance to the mechanism of skin tumor formation. *Cancer Res. (in press).*

37. Diamond, L., O'Brien, T. G., and Rovera, G. (1978): Tumor promoters inhibit terminal cell differentiation in culture. In: *Carcinogenesis Vol. 2. Mechanisms of Tumor Promotion and Cocarcinogenesis,* edited by T. J. Slaga, A. Sivak, and R. K. Boutwell, pp. 173–195. Raven Press, New York.

38. Driedger, P. E., and Blumberg, P. M. (1977): The effect of phorbol diesters on chicken embryo fibroblasts. *Cancer Res.,* 37:3257–3265.

39. Druckrey, H. (1967): Quantitative Aspects in Chemical Carcinogenesis. In: *Potential Carcino-*

genic Hazards from Drugs, UICC Monograph Series, Vol. 7, edited by R. Truhaut. Springer Verlag, Berlin.

40. Estensen, R. D., Drazich, B. F., and Hadden, J. W. (1978): Phorbol myristate acetate as a lymphocyte mitogen: Quantitation of effects in culture and relationship to binding and inhibition by analogs. In: *Carcinogenesis, Vol. 2. Mechanisms of Tumor Promotion and Cocarcinogenesis,* edited by T. J. Slaga, A. Sivak, and R. K. Boutwell, pp. 379–388. Raven Press, New York.

41. Farber, E. (1976): Hyperplastic areas, hyperplastic nodules, and hyperbasophilic areas as putative precursor lesions. *Cancer Res.,* 36:2532–2533.

42. Farber, E., and Solt, D. (1978): A new liver model for the study of promotion. In: *Carcinogenesis. Vol. 2. Mechanisms of Tumor Promotion and Cocarcinogenesis,* edited by T. J. Slaga, A. Sivak, and R. K. Boutwell, pp. 443–448. Raven Press, New York.

43. Fibach, E., Yamasaki, H., Weinstein, I. B., Bank, A., Rifkind, R. A., and Marks, P. A. (1978): Clonal heterogeneity of murine erythroleukemia cells (MELC) to tumor promoter mediated inhibition of cell differentiation. *Proc. Am. Assoc. Cancer Res.,* 19:238.

44. Friedewald, W. F., and Rous, P. (1944): The initiating and promoting elements in tumor production. An analysis of the effects of tar benzpyrene and methylcholanthrene on rabbit skin. *J. Exp. Med.,* 80:101–126.

45. Friedewald, W. F., and Rous, P. (1950): Pathogenesis of deferred cancer, study of after-effects of methylcholanthrene upon rabbit skin. *J. Exp. Med.,* 91:459–483.

46. Fusenig, N. E., and Samsel, W. (1978): Growth promoting activity of phorbolester TPA on cultured mouse skin keratinocytes, fibroblasts and carcinoma cells. In: *Carcinogenesis Vol. 2. Mechanisms of Tumor Promotion and Cocarcinogenesis,* edited by T. J. Slaga, A. Sivak, and R. K. Boutwell, pp. 173–195. Raven Press, New York.

47. Garte, S. J., Troll, W., and Belman, S. (1978): Effect of phorbol myristate acetate on cyclic nucleotide levels in normal and stimulated mouse epidermis in vivo (meeting abstract). *Proc. Am. Assoc. Cancer Res.,* 19:7.

48. Ghadially, R. N., and Green, H. N. (1954): The effect of cortisone on chemical carcinogenesis in the mouse skin. *Br. J. Cancer,* 8:291–295.

49. Greaves, M. W., and McDonald-Gibson, W. (1973): Effect of non-steroid anti-inflammatory drugs on prostaglandin biosynthesis by skin. *Br. J. Dermatol.,* 88:47–50.

50. Grubbs, C. J., Moon, R. C., Sporn, M. B., and Newton, D. L. (1977): Inhibition of mammary cancer by retinyl methyl ether. *Cancer Res.,* 37:599–602.

51. Haran-Ghera, N., and Lurie, M. (1971): Effect of heterologous antithymocyte serum on mouse skin tumorigenesis. *J. Natl. Cancer Inst.,* 46:103–112.

52. Hecker, E. (1968): Cocarcinogenic principles from the seed oil of croton tigluim and from other euphorbraceae. *Cancer Res.,* 28:2338–2349.

53. Hecker, E., and Schmidt, R. (1974): Phorbol esters—the irritants and cocarcinogens of croton tigluim L. *Prog. Chem. Org. Natur. Prod.,* 31:377–467.

54. Heidelberger, C., Mondal, S., and Peterson, A. R. (1978): Initiation and promotion in cell cultures. In: *Carcinogenesis Vol. 2. Mechanisms of Tumor Promotion and Cocarcinogenesis,* edited by T. J. Slaga, A. Sivak, and R. K. Boutwell, pp. 197–202. Raven Press, New York.

55. Hennings, H., Yuspa, S. H., Michael, D., and Lichti, U. (1978): Modification of epidermal cell response to 12-*O*-tetradecanoylphorbol-13-acetate by serum level, culture temperature and pH. In: *Carcinogenesis, Vol. 2. Mechanisms of Tumor Promotion and Cocarcinogenesis,* edited by T. J. Slaga, A. Sivak, and R. K. Boutwell, pp. 233–243. Raven Press, New York.

56. Hicks, R. M., Chowaniec, J., and Wakefield, J. St. J. (1978): Experimental Induction of Bladder Tumors by a Two-Stage System. In: *Carcinogenesis, Vol. 2. Mechanisms of Tumor Promotion and Cocarcinogenesis,* edited by T. J. Slaga, A. Sivak, and R. K. Boutwell. pp. 475–489. Raven Press, New York.

57. Hollenberg, M. D., and Barrett, J. C. (1978): Selective reduction in the binding of epidermal growth factor-urgastrone by chemically transformed Syrian hamster embryonic fibroblasts. *Proc. Am. Assoc. Cancer Res.,* 19:70.

58. Ishii, D. N., Fibach, E., Yamasaki, H., and Weinstein, I. B. (1978): Tumor promoters inhibit morphological differentiation in cultured mouse neuroblastoma cells. *Science,* 200:556–559.

59. Ito, N., Nagasaki, H., Arai, M., Makiura, S., Sugihara, S., and Hirao, K. (1973): Histopathologic studies on liver tumorigenesis in mice by technical polychlorinated biphenyls and its promoting effect on liver tumors induced by benzene hexachloride. *J. Natl. Cancer Inst.,* 51:1637–1646.

60. Jones, P. A., Laug, W. A., Gardner, A., Nye, C. A., Fink, L. M., and Benedict, W. F.

(1976): In vitro correlates of transformation in C3H/10T1/2 clone 8 mouse cells. *Cancer Res.,* 36:2863–2867.

61. Karasaki, S. (1976): Ultrastructural and cytochemical studies on hyperbasophilic foci with special reference to the demonstration of cell alterations in hepatocarcinogenesis. *Cancer Res.,* 36:2567–2572.

62. Kennedy, A. R., and Little, J. (1978): Protease inhibitors suppress radiation induced malignant transformation in vitro. *Nature,* 276:825–826.

63. Kennedy, A. R., Mondal, S., Heidelberger, C., and Little, J. B. (1978): Enhancement of x-ray transformation by 12-*O*-tetradecanoylphorbol-13-acetate in a cloned line of C3H mouse embryo cells. *Cancer Res.,* 38:439–443.

64. Kensler, T. W., and Mueller, G. C. (1978): Retinoic acid inhibition of the comitogenic action of mezerein and phorbol esters in bovine lymphocytes. *Cancer Res.,* 38:771–775.

65. Kinsella, A., and Radman, M. (1978): Tumor promoter induces sister chromatid exchanges: Relevance to mechanism of carcinogenesis. *Proc. Natl. Acad. Sci. USA,* 75:6149–6153.

66. Kitagawa, T. (1976): Sequential phenotypic changes in hyperplastic area during hepatocarcinogenesis in the rat. *Cancer Res.,* 36:2534–2539.

67. Krieg, L., Kuhlmann, J., and Marks, F. (1974): Effect of tumor-promoting phorbol esters and of acetic acid on mechanisms controlling DNA synthesis and mitosis (chalones) and on the biosynthesis of histidine-rich protein in mouse epidermis. *Cancer Res.,* 34:3135–3146.

68. Laerum, O. D., and Rajewsky, M. F. (1975): Neoplastic transformation of fetal rat brain cells in culture after exposure to ethylnitrosourea in vivo. *J. Natl. Cancer Inst.,* 55:1177–1187.

69. Lankas, G. R., Christian, R. T., and Baxter, C. S. (1977): Effect of tumor promoting agents on mutation frequencies in cultured V79 Chinese hamster cells. *Mutat. Res.,* 45:153–156.

70. Lasne, C., Gentil, A., and Chouroulinkov, I. (1974): Two-stage malignant transformation of rat fibroblasts in tissue culture. *Nature,* 247:490–491.

71. Lasnitzki, I. (1955): The influence of A hypervitaminosis on the effect of 20-methylcholanthrene on mouse prostate glands grown in vitro. *Br. J. Cancer,* 9:434–441.

72. Lau, S., and Colburn, N. (1975): Prostaglandins as possible mediators of the action of tumor-promoting phorbol esters. *Clin. Res.,* 23:558A.

73. Lee, L. S., and Weinstein, I. B. (1978): Tumor-promoting phorbol esters inhibit binding of epidermal growth factor to cellular receptors. *Science,* 202:313–315.

74. Levij, I. S., and Polliack, A. (1968): Potentiating effect of vitamin A on 9-10 dimethyl-1-2-benzanthracene carcinogenesis in the hamster cheek pouch. *Cancer,* 22:300–306.

75. Lichti, U., Yuspa, S. H., and Hennings, H. (1978): Ornithine and *S*-adenosylmethionine decarboxylases in mouse epidermal cell cultures treated with tumor promoters. In: *Carcinogenesis, Vol. 2. Mechanisms of Tumor Promotion and Cocarcinogenesis,* edited by T. J. Slaga, A. Sivak, and R. K. Boutwell, pp. 221–232. Raven Press, New York.

76. Marks, F. (1976): Epidermal growth control mechanisms, hyperplasia, and tumor promotion in the skin. *Cancer Res.,* 36:2636–2643.

77. Marks, F., Bertsch, S., Grimm, W., and Schweizer, J. (1978): Hyperplastic transformation and tumor promotion in mouse epidermis: Possible consequences of disturbances of endogenous mechanisms controlling proliferation and differentiation. In: *Carcinogenesis,* Vol. 2. *Mechanisms of Tumor Promotion and Cocarcinogenesis,* edited by T. J. Slaga, A. Sivak, and R. K. Boutwell, pp. 97–116. Raven Press, New York.

78. McGaughey, C., Jensen, J. L., and Stowell, E. C. (1977): Effects of adenosine and guanosine cyclic phosphates and their corresponding nucleotides and nucleosides on vitamin A-induced epidermal tumor promotion and growth in hamster cheek pouch. *J. Med.,* 8:443–456.

79. Merriman, R. L., and Bertram, J. S. (1978): Inhibition *in vitro* of 3-methylcholanthrene (MCA) induced malignant transformation of C3H/10 T 1/2 Cl 8 (10T1/2) mouse fibroblasts by retinoids. *Proc. Am. Assoc. Cancer Res.,* 19:236.

80. Meyn, M. S., Rossman, T., and Troll, W. (1977): A protease inhibitor blocks SOS functions in escherichia coli: Antipain prevents repressor inactivation, ultraviolet mutagenesis, and filamentous growth. *Proc. Natl. Acad. Sci. USA,* 74:1152–1156.

81. Mondal, S., Brankow, D. W., and Heidelberger, C. (1976): Two-stage chemical oncogenesis in cultures of C3H/10T1/2 cells. *Cancer Res.,* 36:2254–2260.

82. Mondal, S., and Heidelberger, C. (1970): *In vitro* malignant transformation by methylcholanthrene of the progeny of single cells derived from C3H mouse prostate. *Proc. Natl. Acad. Sci. USA,* 65:219–225.

83. Mondal, S., and Heidelberger, C. (1976): Transformation of C3H/10T1/2C18 mouse embryo fibroblasts by ultraviolet irradiation and a phorbol ester. *Nature*, 260:710–711.

84. Mottram, J. C. (1944): A developing factor in experimental blastogenesis. *J. Pathol. Bacteriol.*, 56:181–187.

85. Mufson, R. A., Fisher, P. B., and Weinstein, I. B. (1978): Phorbol Esters produce a delay in the expression of melanogenesis by B-16 melanoma cells. *Proc. Am. Assoc. Cancer Res.*, 19:183.

86. Nagasawa, H., and Little, J. B. (1979): Effect of tumor promoters, protease inhibitors and repair processes on x-ray induced sister chromatid exchanges in mouse cells. *Proc. Natl. Acad. Sci. USA*, 76:1943–1947.

87. O'Brien, T. G. (1976): The induction of ornithine decarboxylase as an early possibly obligatory, event in mouse skin carcinogenesis. *Cancer Res.*, 36:2644–2653.

88. O'Brien, T. G., and Diamond, L. (1978): Ornithine decarboxylase polyamines and tumor promoters. In: *Carcinogenesis, Vol. 2, Mechanisms of Tumor Promotion and Cocarcinogenesis*, edited by T. J. Slaga, A. Sivak, and R. K. Boutwell, pp. 273–287. Raven Press, New York.

89. O'Brien, T. G., and Diamond, L. (1978): Metabolism of tritium-labeled 12-O-tetradecanoyl-phorbol-13-acetate by cells in culture. *Cancer Res.*, 38:2562–2566.

90. O'Brien, T. G., Simsiman, R. C., and Boutwell, R. K. (1975): Induction of the polyamine-biosynthetic enzymes in mouse epidermis and their specificity for tumor promotion. *Cancer Res.*, 35:2426–2433.

91. O'Brien, T. G., Simsiman, R. C., and Boutwell, R. K. (1975): Induction of the polyamine-biosynthetic enzymes in mouse epidermis by tumor-promotion agents. *Cancer Res.*, 35:1662–1670.

92. Ohuchi, K., and Levine, L. (1978): Stimulation of prostaglandin synthesis by tumor-promoting phorbol 12,13 diesters in canine kidney (MDCK) cells. *J. Biol Chem.*, 253:4783–4790.

93. Pacifici, M., and Holtzer, H. (1977): Effects of a tumor-promoting agent on chondrogenesis. *Am. J. Anat.*, 150:207–212.

94. Peraino, C., Fry, M. R. J., and Grube, D. D. (1978): Drug-induced enhancement of hepatic tumorigenesis. In: *Carcinogenesis, Vol. 2. Mechanisms of Tumor Promotion and Cocarcinogenesis* edited by T. J. Slaga, A. Sivak, and R. K. Boutwell, pp. 421–432. Raven Press, New York.

95. Peraino, C., Fry, R. J. M., Staffeldt, E., and Christopher, J. P. (1975): Comparative enhancing effect of phenobarbital, amobarbital, diphenylhydantoin, and dichlorodiphenyltrichloroethane on 2-acetylaminofluorene-induced hepatic tumorigenesis in the rat. *Cancer Res.*, 35:2884–2890.

96. Peterson, A. R., Mondal, S., Brankow, D. W., Thon, W., and Heidelberger, C. (1977): Effects of promoters on DNA synthesis in C3H/10T1/2 mouse fibroblasts. *Cancer Res.*, 37:3223–3227.

97. Poirier, M. C., Poirier, L. A., and Lepage, R. (1972): The hepatic activities of 1-carbon enzymes during chronic administration of diethylnitrosamine, 2-acetylaminofluorene and N,N-dimethyl-4-aminoazobenzene to rats. *Cancer Res.*, 32:1104–1107.

98. Pitot, H. C. (1977): The natural history of neoplasia. *Am. J. Pathol.*, 89:192–201.

99. Pitot, H. C., Barsness, L., and Kitagawa, T. (1978): Stages in the process of hepatocarcinogenesis in rat liver. In: *Carcinogenesis, Vol. 2. Mechanisms of Tumor Promotion and Cocarcinogenesis*, edited by T. J. Slaga, A. Sivak, and R. K. Boutwell, pp. 433–442, Raven Press, New York.

100. Pitot, H. C., and Heidelberger, C. (1963): Metabolic regulatory circuits and carcinogenesis. *Cancer Res.*, 23:1694–1700.

101. Radman, M., Villani, G., Boiteux, S., Defais, M., Caillet-Fauquet, P., and Spadari, S. (1977): On the mechanism and genetic control of mutagenesis induced by carcinogenic mutagens. In: *Origins of Human Cancer*, edited by H. H. Hiatt, J. D. Watson, and J. A. Winsten, pp. 903–922. Cold Spring Harbor Laboratory, New York.

102. Raick, A. N. (1973): Ultrastructural, histological, and biochemical alterations produced by 12-O-tetradecanoyl-phorbol-13-acetate on mouse epidermis and their relevance to skin tumor promotion. *Cancer Res.*, 33:269–286.

103. Raick, A. N. (1974): Cell differentiation and tumor promoting activity in skin carcinogenesis. *Cancer Res.*, 34:2915–2925.

104. Raick, A. N., and Burdzy, K. (1973): Ultrastructural and biochemical changes induced in mouse epidermis by a hyperplastic agent, ethylphenylpropiolate. *Cancer Res.*, 33:2221–2230.

105. Rapp, U. R., Nowinski, R. C., Reznikoff, C. A., and Heidelberger, C. (1975): The role of endogenous oncornaviruses in chemically-induced transformation: I. Transformation independent of virus production. *Virology*, 65:392–409.

106. Reddy, B. S., Weisburger, J. H., and Wynder, E. L. (1978): Colon cancer: bile salts as tumor promoters. In: *Carcinogenesis, Vol. 2. Mechanisms of Tumor Promotion and Cocarcinogenesis,* edited by T. J. Slaga, A. Sivak, and R. K. Boutwell. pp. 453–464. Raven Press, New York.

107. Reznikoff, C. A., Bertram, J. S., Brankow, D. W., and Heidelberger, C. (1973): Quantitative and qualitative studies of chemical transformation of cloned C3H mouse embryo cells sensitive to postconfluence inhibition of cell division. *Cancer Res.,* 33:3239–3249.

108. Rohrschneider, L. R., O'Brien, D. H., and Boutwell, R. K. (1972): The stimulation of phospholipid metabolism in mouse skin following phorbol ester treatment. *Bichem. Biophys. Acta,* 280:57–70.

109. Rose, S. P., Stahn, R., Passovoy, D. S., and Herschman, H. (1976): Epidermal growth factor enhancement of skin tumor induction in mice. *Experientia,* 32:913–915.

110. Rous, P., and Kidd, J. G. (1941): Conditional neoplasms and subthreshold neoplastic states. A study of the tar tumors of rabbits. *J. Exp. Med.,* 73:365–390.

111. Rovera, G., O'Brien, Thomas G., and Diamond, L. (1977): Tumor promoters inhibit spontaneous differentiation of friend erythroleukemia cells in culture. *Proc. Natl. Acad. Sci., USA* 74:2894–2898.

112. Saffiotti, U., Montesano, R., Sellakumar, A. R., and Borg, S. A. (1967): Experimental cancer of the lung. Inhibition by vitamin A of the induction of tracheobronchial squamous metaplasia and squamous cell tumors. *Cancer,* 20:857–864.

113. Salaman, M. H., and Roe, R. J. C. (1964): Carcinogenesis. *Br. Med. Bull.,* 20:139–144.

114. Scherer, E., and Emmelot, P. (1976): Kinetics of induction and growth of enzyme-deficient islands involved in hepatocarcinogenesis. *Cancer Res.,* 36:2544–2554.

115. Schwarz, J. A., Viaje, A., and Slaga, T. J. (1977): Fluocinolone acetonide: A potent inhibitor of mouse skin tumor promotion and epidermal DNA synthesis. *Chem. Biol. Interact.,* 17:331–347.

116. Scribner, J. D., and Slaga, T. J. (1973): Multiple effects of dexamethasone on protein synthesis and hyperplasia caused by a tumor promoter. *Cancer Res.,* 33:542–546.

117. Shubik, P., Baserga, R., and Ritchie, A. C. (1953): The life and progression of induced skin tumors in mice. *Br. J. Cancer,* 7:342–351.

118. Sivak, A., Mossman, B. T., and Van Duuren, B. L. (1972): Activation of cell membrane enzymes in the stimulation of cell division. *Biochem. Biophys. Res. Commun.,* 46:605–609.

119. Sivak, A., Rudenko, L., and Simons, I. (1978): Carcinogen-induced neoplastic transformation in Balb/C 3T3 cells. *Proc. Am. Assoc. Cancer Res.,* 19:36.

120. Sivak, A., and Van Duuren, B. L. (1967): Phenotypic expression of transformation: Induction in cell culture by a phorbol ester. *Science,* 157:1443–1444.

121. Slaga, T. J., Fischer, S. M., Viaje, A., Berry, D. L., Bracken, W. M., Le Clerc, S., and Miller, D. R. (1978): Inhibition of tumor promotion by antiinflammatory agents: An approach to the biochemical mechanism of promotion. In: *Carcinogenesis, Vol. 2. Mechanisms of Tumor Promotion and Cocarcinogenesis,* edited by T. J. Slaga, A. Sivak, and R. K. Boutwell, pp. 173–195, Raven Press, New York.

122. Solt, D. B., Medline, A., and Farber, E. (1977): Rapid emergence of carcinogen-induced hyperplastic lesions in a new model for the sequential analysis of liver carcinogenesis. *Am. J. Pathol.,* 88:595–618.

123. Sporn, M. B., Dunlop, N. M., Newton, D. L., and Smith, J. M. (1976): Prevention of chemical carcinogenesis by vitamin A and its synthetic analogs (retinoids). *Fed. Proc.,* 35:1332–1338.

124. Sporn, M. B., Squire, R. A., Brown, C. C., and Smith J. M. (1977): Retinoic acid: Inhibition of bladder carcinogenesis in the rat. *Science,* 195:487–489.

125. Steele, V. E., Marchok, A. C., and Nettesheim, P. (1978): An organ culture system for studying multistage carcinogenesis in respiratory epithelium. In: *Carcinogenesis. Vol. 2. Mechanisms of Tumor Promotion and Cocarcinogenesis,* edited by T. J. Slaga, A. Sivak, and R. K. Boutwell, pp. 289–300, Raven Press, New York.

126. Suss, R., Kinzel, V., and Kreibich, G. (1971): Cocarcinogenic croton oil factor A stimulates lipid synthesis in cell cultures. *Experientia,* 27:46–47.

127. Tarin, D. (1967): Sequential electron microscopical study of experimental mouse skin carcinogenesis. *Int. J. Cancer,* 2:195–211.

128. Todaro, G. J., De Larco, J. E., Nissley, S. P., and Rechler, M. M. (1977): MSA and EGF receptors on sarcoma virus transformed cells and human fibrosarcoma cells in culture. *Nature,* 267:526–528.

129. Trainin, N. (1963): Adrenal imbalance in mouse skin carcinogenesis. *Cancer Res.,* 23:415–419.

130. Troll, W., Klassen, A., and Janoff, A. (1970): Tumorigenesis in mouse skin: Inhibition by synthetic inhibitors of proteases. *Science,* 169:1211–1213.

131. Troll, W., Meyn, M. S., and Rossman, T. G. (1978): Mechanisms of protease action in carcinogenesis. In: *Carcinogenesis. Vol. 2. Mechanisms of Tumor Promotion and Cocarcinogenesis,* edited by T. J. Slaga, A. Sivak, and R. K. Boutwell, pp. 301–312. Raven Press, New York.

132. Troll, W., Rossman, T., Katz, J., Levitz, M., and Sugimura, M. (1975): Proteinases in tumor promotion and hormone action. In: *Proteases and Biological Control,* edited by E. Reich, D. B. Rifkin, and E. Shaw, pp. 977–987. Cold Spring Harbor Laboratory, New York.

133. Trosko, J. E., Chang, C., Yotti, L. P., and Chu, E. Y. H. (1977): Effect of phorbol myristate acetate on the recovery of spontaneous and ultraviolet-light induced 6-thioguanine and ouabain-resistant Chinese Hamster cells. *Cancer Res.,* 37:188–193.

134. Turusov, V., Day, N., Andrianov, L., and Jain, D. (1971): Influence of dose on skin tumors induced in mice by single application of 7,12-dimethylbenz*(a)*anthracene. *J. Natl. Cancer Inst.,* 47:105–111.

135. Van Duuren, B. L. (1969): Tumor-promoting agents in two-stage carcinogenesis. *Prog. Exp. Tumor Res.,* 11:31–68.

136. Van Duuren, B. L., Banerjee, S., and Witz, G. (1976): Fluorescence studies on the interaction of the tumor promoter phorbol myristate acetate and related compounds with rat liver plasma membranes. *Chem. Biol. Interact.,* 15:233–246.

137. Van Duuren, B. L., Sivak, A., Segal, A., Seidman, I., and Katz, C. (1973): Dose-response studies with a pure tumor-promoting agent, phorbol myristate acetate. *Cancer Res.,* 33:2166–2172.

138. Various authors (1978): In: *Carcinogenesis Vol. 2: Mechanisms of Tumor Promotion and Cocarcinogenesis,* edited by T. J. Slaga, A. Sivak, and R. K. Boutwell. Raven Press, New York.

139. Verma, A. K., and Boutwell, R. K. (1977): Vitamin A acid (retinoic acid), a potent inhibitor of 12-*O*-Tetradecanoyl-phorbol-13-acetate-induced ornithine decarboxylase activity in mouse edpidermis. *Cancer Res.,* 37:2196–2201.

140. Verma, A. K., Rice, H. M., and Boutwell, R. K. (1977): Prostaglandins and skin tumor promotion: Inhibition of tumor promoter-induced ornithine decarboxylase activity in epidermis by inhibitors of prostaglandin synthesis. *Biochem. Biophys. Res. Commun.,* 79:1160–1166.

141. Viaje, A., Slaga, T. J., Wigler, M., and Weinstein, B. (1977): Effects of antiinflammatory agents on mouse skin tumor promotion, epidermal DNA synthesis, phorbol ester-induced cellular proliferation, and production of plasminogen activator. *Cancer Res.,* 37:1530–1536.

142. Weinstein, I. B., Wigler, M., and Pietropaolo, C. (1977): The action of tumor-promoting agents in cell culture. In: *Origins of Human Cancer,* edited by H. H. Hiatt, J. D. Watson, and J. A. Winsten, pp. 751–772. Cold Spring Harbor Laboratory, New York.

143. Weinstein, I. B., Wigler, M., Fisher, P. B., Sisskin, E., and Pietropaolo, C. (1978): Cell culture studies on the biologic effects of tumor promotors. In: *Carcinogenesis, Vol. 2 Mechanisms of Tumor Promotion and Cocarcinogenesis,* edited by T. J. Slaga, A. Sivak, and R. K. Boutwell, pp. 313–333. Raven Press, New York.

144. Wigler, M., De Feo, D., and Weinstein, I. B. (1978): Induction of plasminogen activator in cultured cells by macrocyclic plant diterpene esters and other agents related to tumor promotion. *Cancer Res.,* 38(5):1434–1437.

145. Wigler, M., and Weinstein, I. B. (1976): Tumour promotor induces plasminogen activator. *Nature,* 259:232–233.

146. Williams, G. M. (1976): Functional markers and growth behavior of preneoplastic hepatocytes. *Cancer Res.,* 36:2540–2543.

147. Williams, G. M. (1978): Enhancement of hyperplastic lesions in the rat liver by the tumor promoter phenobarbital. In: *Carcinogenesis, Vol. 2. Mechanisms of Tumor Promotion and Cocarcinogenesis,* edited by T. J. Slaga, A. Sivak, and R. K. Boutwell, pp. 449–451. Raven Press, New York.

148. Wilson, E. L. and Reich, E. (1979): Plasminogen activator in chick fibroblasts: Induction of synthesis by retinoic acid; synergism with viral transformation and phorbol ester. *Cell,* 15:385–392.

149. Witschi, H., and Lock, S. (1978): Butylated hydroxytoluene: A possible promoter of adenoma formation in mouse lung. In: *Carcinogenesis, Vol. 2. Mechanisms of Tumor Promotion and*

Cocarcinogenesis, edited by T. J. Slaga, A. Sivak, and R. K. Boutwell, pp. 465–474. Raven Press, New York.

150. Wolff, S., and Rodin, B. (1978): Saccharin-induced sister chromatid exchanges in chinese hamster and human cells. *Science,* 200:543–545.

151. Yamasaki, H., Fibach, E., Nudel, U., Weinstein, I. B., Rifkind, R. A., and Marks, P. A. (1977): Tumor promoters inhibit spontaneous and induced differentiation of murine erythroleukemia cells in culture. *Proc. Natl. Acad. Sci. USA,* 74:3451–3455.

152. Yuspa, S. H., Ben, T., Patterson, E., Michael, D., Elgjo, K., and Hennings, J. (1976): Stimulated DNA synthesis in mouse epidermal cell cultures treated with 12-*O*-tetradecanoyl-phorbol-13-acetate. *Cancer Res.,* 36:4062–4068.

153. Yuspa, S. H., Elgjo, K., Morse, J. A., and Wiebel, F. J. (1977): Retinyl acetate modulation of cell growth kinetics and carcinogen-cellular interaction in mouse epidermal cell cultures *Chem. Biol. Interact,* 16:251–264.

154. Yuspa, S. H., Lichti, U., Ben, T., Patterson, E., Hennings, H., Slaga, T. J., Colburn, N., and Kelsey, W. (1976): Phorbol esters stimulate DNA synthesis and ornithine decarboxylase activity in mouse epidermal cell cultures. *Nature,* 262:402–404.

155. Yuspa, S. H., Lichti, U., Hennings, H., Ben, T., Patterson, E., and Slaga, T. J. (1978): Tumor promoter stimulated proliferation in mouse epidermis *in vivo* and *in vitro:* Mediation by polyamines and inhibition by the anti-promoter steroid fluocinolone acetonide. In: *Carcinogenesis Vol. 2: Mechanisms of Tumor Promotion and Cocarcinogenesis,* edited by T. J. Slaga, A. Sivak, and R. K. Boutwell, pp. 245–255. Raven Press, New York.

156. Ziboh, V. A. (1973): Biosynthesis of prostaglandin E_2 in human skin: Subcellular localization and inhibition by unsaturated fatty acids and anti-inflammatory drugs. *J. Lipid Res.,* 14:377–384.

157. Zur Hausen, H. Z., O'Neill, F. J., and Freese, U. K. (1978): Persisting oncogenic herpesvirus induced by the tumour promoter TPA. *Nature,* 272:373–375.

Carcinogenesis, Vol. 5: Modifiers of Chemical
Carcinogenesis, edited by T. J. Slaga.
Raven Press, New York © 1980.

3

Activation and Inactivation of Carcinogens by Microsomal Monooxygenases: Modification by Benzoflavones and Polycyclic Aromatic Hydrocarbons

Friedrich J. Wiebel

Gesellschaft für Strahlen- und Umweltforschung, Institute of Toxicology and Biochemistry, München-Neuherberg, West Germany

METABOLISM OF CARCINOGENS BY MULTIPLE FORMS OF MONOOXYGENASES

Over the last few decades, it has become increasingly apparent that the metabolism of chemicals leads to the formation of both biologically inert and highly reactive products. In fact, numerous studies have established that most chemicals have to be metabolically activated to become cytotoxic, mutagenic, or carcinogenic. The primary group of enzymes involved in the activation and detoxification of chemicals are the microsomal monooxygenases.[1] These enzymes oxidize a wide variety of exogenous and endogenous compounds to more polar derivatives which usually undergo secondary enzymic reactions such as hydration or conjugation. Although these secondary reactions have also been shown to be involved in the activation process of some chemical carcinogens, they generally yield products that are less harmful than the parent compound (for reviews on the metabolic activation of carcinogens, see refs. 38,40,41,89,116,140).

A key determinant in the biological activity of a chemical is the steady-state level of its reactive intermediates which, in the framework of these considerations, depends on the rate of formation by the monooxygenases and on the rate of disappearance by any of a number of mechanisms, secondary enzymic reactions, nonenzymatic breakdown, or some form of binding or sequestration. It is apparent that a change in the rate of any of these reactions may alter the steady-state level of the reactive intermediate and that they deserve equal attention.

---

[1] The enzyme system is also known as mixed-function oxidase, microsomal hydroxylase, or microsomal drug-metabolizing enzyme.

However, because the initial oxidation step seems to be rate limiting in the metabolism of many compounds its modification has to be a prime aspect in the activation and detoxification of chemical carcinogens and will be the focus of the following discussion.

The microsomal monooxygenases are membrane-bound, multicomponent systems consisting of two enzymes, a hemoprotein, cytochrome P-450, and a flavoprotein, NADPH-cytochrome C reductase (for review, see refs. 18,20,82,86,118). An essential feature in drug metabolism and its alteration by chemicals is the existence of multiple forms of monooxygenases. In recent studies several forms of cytochrome P-450 have been separated and partially characterized by catalytic, spectral, electrophoretic, and immunological properties (7,51,57,82,84,86,115, 141). The different species of the cytochrome seem to have a broad but overlapping substrate specificity (57,82–84,86). A second important fact recently established by a number of investigations is that the different cytochrome species preferentially oxygenate substrates in specific positions of the molecule. This has been shown for such diverse compounds as biphenyl (28), 2-acetylaminofluorene (79,80), bromobenzene (146), benzo(a)pyrene (BP) (55,104,141), or n-hexane (39).

Distribution and activity of different forms of cytochrome P-450 are currently subject to intensive investigation. From observations to date it appears that the amounts of the different monooxygenase forms may vary between species and strains of animals, their age and sex, tissue, cellular and possibly subcellular localization, and external factors such as diet (see reviews in refs. 13,24,25,43, 47,86,118,134).

MODIFICATION OF MONOOXYGENASE ACTIVITY BY CHEMICALS

Chemicals alter monooxygenase activity by at least three mechanisms. They may:

1. trigger a series of intracellular regulatory and biosynthetic steps that lead to an increase or decrease of enzymic activity,
2. directly interfere with the catalytic process, or
3. cause the inactivation or destruction of the cytochrome.

All three modes of interference with monooxygenase activity may be important in the activation of chemical carcinogens.

INDUCTION

Application of numerous compounds (25,105) to animals or to cells in culture results in an increase in monooxygenase activity usually referred to as *induction*; but it has to be kept in mind that treatment with an "inducer" may also cause a depression of monooxygenase activity. For a detailed discussion of the mechanism and the biological significance of monooxygenase induction the reader is referred to a number of comprehensive reviews (18,25,26,40).

The inducing chemicals fall into two major groups that are typified by phenobarbital and 3-methylcholanthrene (MC). The first group includes a large number of bulky and nonpolar compounds such as barbiturates, dichlorodiphenyltrichloroethane (DDT), certain polychlorinated biphenyls, etc. The second group comprises chemicals that are planar and larger than naphthalene. To this group belong the polycyclic aromatic hydrocarbons (25), phenothiazines (132), indoles (81), and 2,3,7,8-tetrachlorodibenzo-*p*-dioxin (TCDD) (99). The group also includes a number of flavonoids (22,131) of which the noncarcinogenic 5,6-benzoflavone (5,6-BF) (6,17,67,68,120,129) is increasingly replacing the carcinogenic MC as a "routine" inducer of monooxygenase activity (15,22,51,88). Although the inducing potency of these heterogeneous compounds differs by several orders of magnitude their qualitative effects on the monooxygenase(s) appear to be identical (15,51). Polychlorinated biphenyls, which were thought to possibly combine the properties of phenobarbital- and MC-type inducers (2), were later shown to consist of a mixture of chlorobiphenyl congeners each of which produces either an MC-like response or a phenobarbital-like response or is devoid of both activities (44,98). A number of observations however indicate that a third group of inducers may exist represented by pregnenolone-16 α-carbonitrile (PCN) which induces monooxygenase activities different from those induced by phenobarbital or MC (85).

Four aspects in the different modes of phenobarbital- and MC-type induction deserve attention in regard to the metabolism of carcinogens and their manipulation in experimental models: the degree of induction, their time course, response of specific monooxygenase forms, and tissue specificity.

Phenobarbital induces a plethora of changes in structural and functional components of the cell including most enzymes and cofactors involved in the metabolism of xenobiotics. The monooxygenases induced by phenobarbital are generally of the cytochrome P-450 type[2] although the level of cytochrome P-448 (see below) might also be slightly elevated (51). Induction of cytochrome P-450-containing enzymes by phenobarbital appears to occur in tissues which contain an appreciable constitutive level of the enzyme, i.e., predominantly in liver and to a minor degree in extrahepatic tissues of some species, e.g., lung of rabbit (47) or small intestine of mouse (75). Maximum levels of monooxygenase activity are attained several days after repeated application of the inducer and usually do not exceed the constitutive level by more than two- to fourfold.

3-Methylcholanthrene induces only a small number of enzymes. The monooxygenases induced by MC belong to the group of "cytochrome P-448," i.e., cytochromes that are characterized by a hypochromic shift of the Soret peak of the reduced hemoprotein carbon monoxide complex. Their induction takes place

---

[2] The nomenclature is inadequate for the many forms of monooxygenases of which at least six have been isolated (115). In this review "cytochrome P-450" refers to the monooxygenase species which predominate in liver of untreated animals, have their Soret peak at 450 nm or above, and are not inducible by MC. "Cytochrome P-448" (also called P$_1$-450) denotes the monooxygenase species which are inducible by MC and have a Soret peak at about 448 nm in liver microsomes. This nomenclature is also applied to monooxygenases of extrahepatic tissues which might exhibit different Soret peaks (7).

in liver and in virtually all extrahepatic tissues. Following application of the inducer, monooxygenase activity increases within a few hours and reaches a maximum after about 24 hr. The degree of induction of cytochrome P-448-dependent reactions by MC differs greatly in various tissues and cells but is usually greater than the induction by phenobarbital; maximum induced levels may be 50 to 100 times higher than the constitutive activities. As noted above, inducer treatment may also lower the level of some monooxygenase activities. For example, treatment with MC type inducers caused a decrease in the *O*-deethylation of 7-ethoxycoumarin in rabbit liver (9), the *N*-demethylation of dimethylnitrosamine in rat liver (4,5) and the epoxidation of aldrine in newly isolated hepatocytes (102).

INHIBITION

Chemicals that directly modify monooxygenase activity share with the substrates an overlapping specificity for the different forms of the enzyme. This, of course, applies to chemicals that function as competitive inhibitors but may also apply to compounds which affect monooxygenase activity by other mechanisms, e.g., compounds that may alter the environment of the catalytic center of the enzyme such as chaotropic agents, organic solvents, or detergents. Many of the monooxygenase inhibitors can be divided into two groups which preferentially inhibit either phenobarbital-inducible, cytochrome P-450-dependent reactions or MC-inducible, cytochrome P-448-dependent reactions. Compounds typical of the former group are 2-diethylaminoethyl-2,2-diphenyl valerate (SKF 525-A) and metyrapone (46,117). There is an array of compounds that have similarly been shown to interfere more strongly with the activity of cytochrome P-450 than cytochrome P-448: DDT, pyridine, *n*-octylamine, various imidazoles, steroids, tetrahydrocannabinol (46), aliphatic alcohols, dimethylsulfoxide (140), butylated hydroxytoluene and hydroxyanisole (142), or ethoxyquin (64).

A representative of the inhibitors of cytochrome P-448-dependent reactions is the synthetic flavone 7,8-benzoflavone (7,8-BF) (α-naphthoflavone). The effects of 7,8-BF on monooxygenase activity and on carcinogenesis of aromatic polycyclic hydrocarbons have been extensively studied and will be presented in more detail in the following to provide a basis for the discussion of the possibilities and limitations that are likely to be encountered in the modification of carcinogen metabolism by monooxygenases and of tumor initiation in experimental animals and man.

DEGRADATION

Evidence is rapidly growing which indicates that many chemicals are capable of degrading cytochrome P-450 (29,30,48,59,60,61,76,93,100). A variety of compounds, e.g., secobarbital and other barbiturates containing allyl groups (76), allylisopropylacetamide (29), 2,2,2-trifluoroethylvinyl ether (61) and vinyl chlo-

TABLE 1. *Effect of 7,8-benzoflavone on BP hydroxylase activity in hepatic microsomes from untreated, phenobarbital- or methylcholanthrene-treated rats*

	pmol of product formed/mg protein/min		
Addition	Untreated	Phenobarbital	MC
None	150	410	1880
7,8-BF (10^{-5})	210 ($+$ 42)[a]	450 ($+$ 11)	990 ($-$ 53)
7,8-BF (10^{-4})	220 ($+$ 45)	460 ($+$ 12)	440 ($-$ 78)

[a]Values in parentheses give the percentage of inhibition ($-$) or stimulation ($+$). Substrate concentration was 10^{-4} M BP. Adapted from Wiebel et al. (140).

ride (48,60,100) have been shown to destroy cytochromes P-450 *in vivo* (61,100) and *in vitro* (48,60,76). Another group of chemicals which have been shown to reduce the level of cytochrome(s) P-450 is comprised of thionosulfur-containing compounds (59), including disulfiram and diethyldithiocarbamate, both inhibitors of tumor initiation induced by polycyclic aromatic hydrocarbons (PAH) or azoxymethane (16,127). Since the process of destruction involves the oxidative metabolism of many or all of these chemicals they are also likely to exhibit some degree of specificity for the different forms of cytochrome P-450.

It is evident that all chemicals which interfere with the activity of monooxygenases potentially alter tumor initiation by carcinogens that have to be activated; indeed, such structurally diverse compounds as antioxidants, steroids, organic thiocyanates, disulfiram, SKF 525-A, polychlorinated biphenyls, or barbiturates, all of which affect the monooxygenases, have been found to modify chemical tumorigenesis (16,124–127). The discussion following will focus on the effects of two groups of modifiers of monooxygenases, the benzoflavones and polycyclic hydrocarbons. For the action of other types of compounds inhibiting chemical carcinogenesis, the reader is referred to the comprehensive reviews by Wattenberg (121,126).

INHIBITION OF MONOOXYGENASE ACTIVITY BY 7,8-BENZOFLAVONE

A number of studies have established that 7,8-BF is a potent inhibitor of the MC-inducible form of monooxygenases in liver and has little inhibitory effect on the hepatic "constitutive" cytochrome P-450-dependent enzyme predominating in untreated or phenobarbital-treated animals (31,140). For example, 7,8-BF at equimolar concentrations with the substrate BP increases or does not significantly affect BP-hydroxylation[3] in microsomes from phenobarbital-treated or untreated (male) rats (Table 1). In contrast, BP-hydroxylation in

---

[3] The conversion of BP to phenolic products has been widely employed as general measure for the metabolism of PAH by monooxygenases and is frequently called "aryl hydrocarbon hydroxylase."

microsomes from MC-treated rats is about 50% inhibited by 7,8-BF at a concentration one-tenth that of the substrate (140).

The differential effect of 7,8-BF has been used to probe for the presence of the two forms of monooxygenases in liver (Table 2), extrahepatic tissues, and cells in culture (Table 3) of many species and strains of animals and to study their dependency on age, sex, diet, and the state of induction. 7,8-BF invariably inhibited monooxygenase activity induced by MC-type inducers irrespective of the source of the enzyme or the mode of enzyme preparation, i.e., in isolated cells, homogenates, nuclei, microsomes, and purified cytochrome P-448 fractions. This is also pertinent for the different substrates and seemingly different reactions of the MC-induced monooxygenase. Thus, 7,8-BF inhibits MC-induced oxygenation of naphthalene, 4-hydroxylation of acetanilide, 4- and 2-hydroxylation of biphenyl (8), and *O*-deethylation of 7-ethoxycoumarine (145). Whenever MC treatment failed to induce monooxygenase activity, 7,8-BF also was ineffective as an inhibitor. For example, MC-treatment does not induce hepatic BP-hydroxylase activity and cytochrome P-448 in DBA/2N mice which are poorly responsive to PAH-inducers (46,99). Under these conditions 7,8-BF increases rather than inhibits the monooxygenase activity (46,99). BP-hydroxylase activity in DBA/2N mice elicited by the more powerful MC-type inducer TCDD is again highly sensitive to the inhibitory action of the flavone (99).

The rule that 7,8-BF inhibits MC-induced monooxygenase seems also to apply

TABLE 2. *Effect of 7,8-benzoflavone on hepatic monooxygenase activity in vitro*[a]

Tissue preparation	Species	Age	Un-treated	PAH-treated	Ref.
Microsomes	Rat	Adult	↑↓[b]	↓↓	31,140
Microsomes	Mouse C57B1	Adult	↑	↓↓	46
Microsomes	Mouse DBA	Adult	↑	↑	46,99
			↑	↓↓[d]	99
Microsomes	Rabbit	Adult	↑	↑↓	7
Microsomes	Rabbit	Newborn	↑↑	↓↓	7
8,000 × *g* supernatant	Rat	Adult	↑↓	↓↓	62
8,000 × *g* supernatant	Rat	Newborn	↑↑	↓↓	95,137
Partially purified mono-oxygenase	Rat	Adult	↑↓	↓↓	83
Nuclei	Rat	Adult	↓	↓	19
Homogenates	Human	Adult	↑	ND[c]	65,97[e]
Homogenates	Human	Fetal	↑↑	ND	95
Perfused organ	Rat	Adult	↑↓	↓↓	63

[a] Monooxygenase activity was determined by the metabolism of benzo(*a*)pyrene if not noted otherwise.

[b] Arrows denote the stimulation (↑), inhibition (↓), or the lack of a significant effect (↑↓) in the presence of 7,8-BF. The number of arrows gives a relative measure of the extent of the 7,8-BF effect in a given tissue but not in different tissues or in different species.

[c] Not determined.

[d] *In vivo* induction with TCDD.

[e] F. J. Wiebel, J. K. Selkirk, and H. V. Gelboin (*unpublished results*).

TABLE 3. *In vitro effect of 7,8-benzoflavone on monooxygenase activity of extrahepatic tissues and cells in culture*[a]

Tissue	Species	Un-treated	PAH-treated	Ref.
Lung	Rat	↓[b]	↓↓	140
Lung	Mouse, C57B1	↓	↓↓	70
Lung	Syrian hamster	↓↓	↓↓	23
Kidney	Rat	↓↓	↓↓	140
Small intestine	Rat	↑↑	↓↓	113
Small intestine	Mouse	↑↓	ND[c]	145[d]
Colon, mucosa	Rat	ND	↓↓	36
Skin	Mouse, Swiss-NIH	↓	↓↓	140
Skin	Mouse, CD-1	↓	↓↓	109
Skin	Mouse, C3H/He	↓	↓↓	120
Skin	Mouse, DBA/2N	↓	↓	120
Harderian gland	Mouse, C57B1	↑↓	↓	71
Harderian gland	Syrian hamster	↓	ND	71
Bone marrow	Rabbit	ND	↓	3
Adrenal gland	Human	↑↓	ND	95
Placenta	Human	↓	ND	95[e]
Cells in culture				
Freshly isolated from				
Liver	Rat	↑	↓	119
Small intestine	Rat	↑	↓	114
Colon (explant)	Rat	ND	↓	10
Short-term cultures				
Primary hepatocytes	Rat,fetal	↓	↓	94
Primary hepatocytes	Human,fetal	↑	↓↓	96
Primary placenta	Human	↓	↓	45
Secondary embryo	Syrian hamster	↓	↓↓	140
Lymphocytes	Human	↓	↓	135[f]
Established cell line				
H-4-II-E hepatoma	Rat	↓	↓	g

[a-c] See footnote in Table 2.

[d] Microsomes from phenobarbital-treated animals; the mouse strain used is not responsive to PAH-type inducers; 7-ethoxycoumarin *O*-dealkylation.

[e] Placenta from smokers.

[f] A. Pawlack et al. *(unpublished results).*

[g] F. J. Wiebel *(unpublished results).*

where more than one form of the cytochrome is inducible by MC treatment. As shown by Atlas and co-workers (7), MC induces two different forms of hepatic cytochrome in rabbits which can be distinguished by their specificity for the substrates *N*-acetylaminofluorene and BP, their electrophoretic banding, and their varying activity during different developmental stages. 7,8-BF independently inhibits the activities of both MC-induced *N*-acetylaminofluorene-*N*-hydroxylase and MC-induced BP-hydroxylase.

In preparations of extrahepatic tissues 7,8-BF generally inhibited not only the MC-induced but also the "constitutive" BP-hydroxylase (Table 3) although frequently to a lesser extent (140). This indicates that extrahepatic tissues contain predominantly a cytochrome P-448-dependent monooxygenase similar to that induced by MC and only a minor fraction of the cytochrome P-450-dependent form, if any. Similar conclusions have been drawn from spectral and kinetic analysis of extrahepatic monooxygenases (147). Wattenberg and Leong (122,123) have shown that the presence of the 7,8-BF-"sensitive" monooxygenase in untreated animals may largely be due to fortuitous MC-type inducers in the diet.[4]

Only a few data are available on the inhibitory activity of 7,8-BF *in vivo.* Indirect evidence that the flavone may reduce the metabolism of PAH in mouse skin *in vivo* will be presented below. The effect of 7,8-BF on the systemic metabolism of drugs, i.e., largely hepatic activity, was examined using the duration of zoxazolamine paralysis and hexobarbital hypnosis as an indicator (143). Hexobarbital and zoxazolamine served as model substrates for the phenobarbital- and MC-inducible monooxygenase(s), respectively. The selective inhibition of zoxazolamine paralysis after MC-pretreatment (143) was in good agreement with the results obtained *in vitro.*

The reason for the stimulatory effect of 7,8-BF on hepatic BP-hydroxylation *in vitro,* which is particularly strong in newborn animals (7,95,137) and somewhat variable in adult animals (137,140), is not known. It is interesting that hydroxylase activity in the small intestine from untreated animals was increased in the presence of 7,8-BF (145) in view of observations by Ullrich and co-workers (75) who showed that the small intestine may contain cytochrome P-450 which is inducible by phenobarbital.

The mechanism of monooxygenase inhibition by 7,8-BF is still a matter of controversy. Kinetic data suggest that 7,8-BF at low concentrations, i.e., below 3.3 μM, might act as a competitive inhibitor of BP hydroxylation but at higher concentrations (3.3 and 10 μM) inhibits the oxygenation reaction by a more complex mechanism (137). Kinetic analysis of the effect of 7,8-BF (1, 20, and 100 μM) on MC-induced 4- and 2-biphenyl hydroxylation led Atlas and Nebert (8) to conclude that 7,8-BF inhibits the reactions by a noncompetitive mechanism. The seemingly discrepant results and interpretations might largely be due to the different range of inhibitor concentrations used. Recent results by Waechter suggest that 7,8-BF is rapidly metabolized to phenolic products by rat liver microsomes (119a).

A large series of naturally occurring and synthetic flavonoids has been tested for their potency as modifiers of monooxygenase activity (139). Some of these compounds showed a stronger stimulatory activity on the constitutive hepatic monooxygenase than 7,8-BF; others were equally potent inhibitors of the MC-

---

[4] It has to be kept in mind that 7,8-BF might affect other cellular functions. Thus, 7,8-BF was found to (a) inhibit prostaglandin synthesis (77) possibly by inhibiting fatty acid cyclooxygenase (50), (b) prevent BP-induced increase in prostaglandin F_2 synthesis (50), and (c) reduce the activity of DT-diaphorase(s) (72,78). The flavone also inhibited prostaglandin A_1 hydroxylation in liver microsomes from untreated guinea pigs (73). The relationship of this monooxygenase to the 7,8-BF-inhibitable monooxygenase in rat is not clear.

induced enzyme or had effects opposite to those of 7,8-BF. However, none of these derivatives equaled 7,8-BF in its distinct differential effect on the two forms or groups of monooxygenases.

It has to be emphasized that the two flavones most frequently used to modify chemical carcinogenesis, 5,6-BF and 7,8-BF, are both inhibitors and inducers of the monooxygenases and differ only in their relative potencies. Generally, 5,6-BF is the better inducer of the enzyme (32,109,129), whereas 7,8-BF is the more potent inhibitor (32,140).

EFFECT OF BENZOFLAVONES ON TUMORIGENESIS

The discovery of the inhibitory and inducing properties of benzoflavones on monooxygenase activity (31,131,140) was soon followed by the examination of their effect on tumorigenesis using a variety of carcinogenic polycyclic hydrocarbons, experimental regimens or animals (Table 4). Gelboin and co-workers (42) applied the "inhibitor" 7,8-BF simultaneously with the tumor initiator 7,12-dimethylbenz[*a*]anthracene (DMBA) to the skin of mice and observed that the flavone strongly inhibited tumor formation caused either by a single application of DMBA followed by croton oil treatment or by repeated application (42,68). These observations were later confirmed by others under similar experimental conditions (17,109). Inhibition occurred only when the inhibitor was applied within a few hours of the initial action of the carcinogen (67), supporting the notion that the flavone interferes with an initiation step of tumorigenesis. To differentiate between the inhibitory and inducing effect of the flavone on the activating enzymes, Gelboin and co-workers (42) examined the action of benz*(a)*anthracene which is a strong inducer of monooxygenase activity in skin (42,138) but a weak inhibitor of the enzyme *in vitro* (42). Application of benz*(a)*anthracene also exerted some inhibitory effect on tumor formation by DMBA; however, inhibition by benz*(a)*anthracene was much weaker than that by 7,8-BF and was largely limited to the first weeks of tumor development (67). 5,6-BF has similar but weaker inhibitory effects on PAH tumorigenesis than its isomer 7,8-BF (17,67,109). Two naturally occurring flavonoids, nobiletin which is a very weak inhibitor of MC-inducible monooxygenase and apigenin which strongly inhibits the constitutive and MC-inducible monooxygenase (139), were both found to be ineffective as inhibitors of DMBA-induced tumor formation (67).

It soon became apparent that 7,8-BF was not equally effective in inhibiting the initiation of carcinogenesis by all polycyclic hydrocarbons. Kinoshita and Gelboin (68) showed that 7,8-BF had no inhibitory effect or occasionally even enhanced BP-induced tumor formation in mouse skin under conditions where DMBA tumorigenesis was strongly inhibited. Similarly, Slaga and co-workers (17,109) observed that 7,8-BF effectively reduced tumorigenesis induced by DMBA and MC but increased or at least failed to inhibit tumorigenesis

TABLE 4. *Effect of benzoflavones and related flavones on tumor initiation by polycyclic aromatic hydrocarbons*

Modifying flavone	Carcinogen[a]	Ref.	Effect[b]	Target tissue
Simultaneous application				
7,8-BF	DMBA	(17,42,107)	↓↓	Skin
7,8-BF	MC	(107)	↓↓	Skin
7,8-BF	DBA	(17)	↑↓ or ↑	Skin
7,8-BF	BP	(68,120)	(↓) or ↑	Skin
7,8-BF	6-Methyl-BP	(108)	(↓)	Skin
7,8-BF	6-OH-methyl-BP	(108)	↑↓	Skin
7,8-BF	7-OH-methyl-BA	(68,107)	(↓) or ↑	Skin
7,8-BF	15,16-H-11-methyl-CPP	(77)	↓↓	Skin
5,6-BF	MC	(107)	↓	Skin
5,6-BF	DBA	(17)	↑↓	Skin
4′,5,7-trihydroxyflavone (apigenin)	DMBA	(68)	↑↓	Skin
3′,4′,5,6,7,8-hexa-methoxyflavone (nobiletin)				
3,3′,4′,5,7-pentahy-droxyflavone (quercetin)	DMBA	(68)	↑↓	Skin
	BP	(108)	(↓)	Skin
Pretreatment				
7,8-BF	DMBA	(32)	↓↓	Lung
5,6-BF	DMBA	(32,128)	↓↓	Lung
5,6-BF	BP	(129)	↓↓	Lung, skin
5,6-BF	DMBA	(128)	↓↓	Mammary gland[c]
3,3′,4′,5,7-penta-methoxyflavone (quercetin-pentamethyl ether)	BP	(129)	↓	Lung

[a] Abbreviations: 7-OH-methyl-BA = 7-hydroxymethylbenz(a)anthracene, 6-OH-methyl-BP = 6-hydroxymethylbenzo(a)pyrene; 6-methyl-BP = 6-methylbenzo(a)pyrene; 15,16-H-11-methyl-CPP = 15,16-dihydro-11-methylcyclopenta(a)phenanthrene-17-one.
[b] Arrows denote the *in vitro* inhibition -↓-, or stimulation -↑-, or the lack of a significant effect -↑↓-. The numbers of arrows give a relative measure of the strength of the 7,8-BF effects. (↓) = weak inhibition.
[c] All studies listed in this table were performed with mice except this experiment in which rats were used (128).

by 7-hydroxymethyl-12-methylbenz*(a)*anthracene and dibenz*(a,h)*anthracene (DBA), respectively. In all studies described so far the modifier and tumor initiator were applied simultaneously or within a short time period.

A different approach was chosen by Wattenberg and co-workers (128–131) who pretreated animals with 5,6-BF for various days prior to the application of the carcinogen with the rationale of preinducing "detoxifying" enzyme activity. This treatment was also found to be effective in reducing tumor formation. Topical application of 18 mg 5,6-BF to the skin of mice over a 3-day period inhibited tumorigenesis initiated by subsequent "painting" of 0.01 mg BP by more than 50% (129). Likewise, feeding of 5,6-BF or 7,8-BF to mice for about 2 weeks prior to oral application of DMBA or BP markedly inhibited the formation of pulmonary adenoma in mice (32,128,129). Similar results were obtained for DMBA-induced mammary tumors in Sprague–Dawley rats (128).

In parallel experiments, treatment with benzoflavones was found to increase BP-hydroxylase activity in lung and skin (129), the target tissues of the carcinogens. It was observed in separate studies that BP-hydroxylase is also inducible by MC-type compounds in mammary gland of rats (F. J. Wiebel, *unpublished results*). Although the reduction in tumor formation can be reasonably attributed to induction of carcinogen metabolizing enzymes, it is not clear whether enzyme induction in the liver or in the extrahepatic target tissues is the critical event. The study (129) in which the systemic metabolism of the carcinogen is circumvented by application of the "inducing" benzoflavone directly to the target tissue, i.e., the skin, is difficult to interpret because of the large excess of the benzoflavone over the tumor-initiating polycyclic hydrocarbon (see above).

In earlier experiments Hoch-Ligeti and co-workers (54) observed that pretreatment of rats with MC inhibited the hepatocarcinogenicity of dimethylnitrosamine. In this case, the inhibitory effect may be attributable to a depression of the primary activation reaction, the *N*-demethylation of the nitrosamine that occurs after MC treatment (4). Surprisingly, later experiments (6) showed that pretreatment with 5,6-BF an equally potent suppressor of dimethylnitrosamine demethylase (5) did not inhibit but increased dimethylnitrosamine-induced hepatocarcinogenesis. The reasons for these seemingly contradictory results are obscure.

INHIBITION AND STIMULATION OF CELLULAR TRANSFORMATION AND BACTERIAL MUTAGENESIS BY 7,8-BENZOFLAVONE

Only a few studies are concerned with the effect of 7,8-BF on malignant transformation of cells *in vitro* by polycyclic hydrocarbons. Although these reports agree in that the benzoflavone strongly inhibits the cytotoxicity of the transforming agents, they disagree on the effect of the flavone on their cell-transforming activity (33,87). Marquardt and co-workers (87) observed a complete suppression by 7,8-BF of colony formation by MC in an established line of mouse fibroblasts but did not find a significant effect on cellular transformation by DMBA or 7-hydroxymethylbenz(a)anthracene. Inhibition of 7-hydroxymethylbenz(a)anthracene- and DMBA-induced transformation by 7,8-BF may be obscured by the increased number of surviving cells in the presence of the benzoflavone.

In contrast, DiPaolo and co-workers (33) reported that 7,8-BF as well as benz(a)anthracene enhances MC- and BP-induced transformation of secondary hamster embryo cells up to two- and fivefold, respectively, even taking into account the reduction in cytotoxicity by the flavone. The reasons for these discrepancies are not clear. They might be due to a number of variables in experimental regimen, materials, or cell lines used.

In a bacterial mutagenesis system in which "promutagens" are activated by inclusion of hepatic microsomes ("Ames system") 7,8-BF alters mutagenicity in a fashion predictable from its effects on the different monooxygenase forms (37). 7,8-BF effectively inhibited mutagenicity of MC mediated by microsomes from MC-treated C57BL/6N mice that respond to the inducer but increased or did not affect mutagenicity mediated by microsomes from phenobarbital-treated C57BL/6N mice or from MC-treated DBA/2N mice that do not respond to pretreatment with the PAH. Likewise, in the Ames system using homogenates of human liver, 7,8-BF markedly increased the mutagenicity of aflatoxin B_1 (21) which is in keeping with its stimulatory effect on the oxidative metabolism of BP, zoxazolamine, or antipyrene observed earlier (65). In a system containing nuclei from liver of MC-treated C57BL/6N mice, 7,8-BF inhibited the NADPH-stimulated mutagenicity of N-hydroxy-2-acetylamino-fluorene suggesting the involvement of a cytochrome P-448 form in this process (101).

EFFECT OF 7,8-BENZOFLAVONE ON THE METABOLISM OF POLYCYCLIC HYDROCARBONS

The complex metabolism of PAH by microsomal monooxygenases and hydrases and its biological implications have been extensively studied during the last decade and are comprehensively described elsewhere (38,41,92). Significant progress has been made with the finding that the probable ultimate carcinogen derived from BP is the BP-7,8-dihydrodiol-9,10-oxide which arises through a sequence of highly stereoselective monooxygenation and hydration steps (38). Recent studies indicate that other carcinogenic PAH such as DMBA (91) or MC (66) undergo the same process of metabolic activation to vicinal dihydrodiol oxides as BP.

Selkirk and co-workers (103) analyzed the effect of 7,8-BF on the metabolism of BP to dihydrodiols, phenols, and quinones in hepatic microsomes from MC-treated rats. The overall metabolism of BP was strongly inhibited by the flavone in agreement with the inhibition of BP-hydroxylase activity. The metabolism of BP to dihydrodiols was inhibited to a greater extent (75–80%) than the formation of phenols (61–69%) or of quinones (55%). Similar results were obtained by Alexandrov and co-workers (1) using nuclei of liver from MC-treated rats as the source of monooxygenase activity. The formation of dihydro-diols was also inhibited by about 25% in nuclei from untreated and phenobarbi-tal-treated animals under conditions where the overall metabolism of BP was not significantly reduced. Pelkonen and co-workers (97) observed that 7,8-BF stimulated the formation of BP-phenols but did not affect the formation of BP-dihydrodiols in homogenates of human liver. Berry *et al.* (14) noted that 7,8-BF caused a general reduction of the formation of phenols, quinones, and dihydrodiols in mouse epidermal homogenates from MC-treated mice. BP-me-tabolism in epidermal homogenates from untreated mice was too low to be measurable. Apparently the flavone interferes with the monooxygenase complex *in vitro* to inhibit the oxygenation in all sites of the BP-molecule. Differences in the degree of inhibition of various metabolic pathways might be due to the presence of more than one monooxygenase form which preferentially attack specific sites of the BP-molecule and exhibit a different sensitivity to the benzofla-vone. Generally, it appears that the formation of BP-phenols, i.e., largely of the 3-OH-BP (55,69,103), is less sensitive to the inhibitory effect of 7,8-BF than the formation of the other metabolite fractions. Sloane (112) reported that microsome-mediated 6-hydroxymethylation was increased several fold in the presence of 7,8-BF. These observations and the occasional stimulatory effect of 7,8-BF on BP tumorigenesis in skin (68) suggested that 6-hydroxymethylation may be involved in 7,8-BF stimulated BP-tumorigenesis (109). However, recent studies by Slaga and co-workers (108) showed a weak inhibitory effect of 7,8-BF on BP and 6-methyl-BP tumorigenesis, lending little support to the notion that direct hydroxymethylation is an essential step in the metabolic activation of BP to the ultimate carcinogenic form(s).

The effect of 7,8-BF on the metabolism of DMBA has not been studied in detail. In hepatic microsomes from MC-treated rats, 7,8-BF (10 μM) reduced the overall metabolism of ^{3}H-DMBA (10 μM) by about 50% (F. J. Wiebel, J. K. Selkirk, and H. V. Gelboin, *unpublished observations*). The conversion to products that were extractable into water and alkali or remained in organic solvents was affected to a similar degree. In microsomes from untreated rats, 7,8-BF increased somewhat the alkali-soluble fraction but had no significant effect on other metabolite fractions.

Coombs and co-workers (27) observed that 7,8-BF slightly increased but did not qualitatively change the metabolism of 15,16-dihydro-11-methylcyclopenta-*(a)*phenanthrene-17-one in microsomes from untreated rats. Topical application of this compound to skin has been shown to lead to tumor formation which is strongly suppressed by simultaneous application of 7,8-BF (27).

At present, our knowledge on the effects of 7,8-BF on carcinogen metabolism is very limited. No clear evidence is available which shows that the benzoflavone specifically increases or suppresses a cutaneous "detoxifying" or "activating" pathway for any of the carcinogenic PAH. Further studies in this area are needed to gain more insight into the mechanism by which the flavone inhibits tumorigenesis and to resolve the question of why it suppresses tumor initiation by some carcinogens but not by others.

MODIFICATION OF CARCINOGEN BINDING
IN MOUSE SKIN BY 7,8-BENZOFLAVONE

The analysis of covalent binding of activated chemicals to cellular macromolecules is of major interest in view of two aspects. In the general context of xenobiotic metabolism, covalent binding may serve as an indirect measure of the steady state of reactive intermediates and may be a useful criterion for the interference by modifiers of monooxygenases with drug activation. In the context of chemical carcinogenesis, covalent binding might give specific indications for the nature of the "ultimate" carcinogenic form.

Kinoshita and Gelboin (67) observed a significant reduction of [³H]DMBA binding to mouse skin macromolecules 24 hr after simultaneous application of 7,8-BF and the radioactively labeled carcinogen. The binding of [³H]BP to protein and RNA was similarly inhibited by 7,8-BF; however, there was only a small reduction in the binding of [³H]BP to DNA. Likewise, Bowden and co-workers (17) showed that 7,8-BF at high doses strongly decreased the level of [³H]DMBA binding to protein, RNA, and DNA of mouse skin but had no significant effect on the binding of [³H]DBA to any of the cutaneous macromolecules. Thus there appears to be a rough correlation between the effect of 7,8-BF on tumorigenesis of DMBA, BP, and DBA and those on their binding *in vivo* at least to DNA, supporting the notion that the inhibitor acts on the level of metabolic activation to binding species.

In vivo binding of the carcinogen might be inhibited in various ways. The flavone may interfere with the induction of the cutaneous monooxygenase by the carcinogen and reduce the relative amounts of "activating enzymes." Observations by Kinoshita and Gelboin (67) argue against this possibility, since simultaneous application of 100 nmoles of 7,8-BF with equimolor amounts of the "inducer" DMBA does not alter the time course and extent of BP-hydroxylase induction found after DMBA alone. 7,8-BF itself has no apparent inducing activity in skin when applied topically, although it induces the hydroxylase activity in all tissues examined (32,120), including skin (42), when applied intraperitoneally or with the diet. Induction by 7,8-BF in skin might be obscured by *in vitro* inhibition of enzyme activity due to the carry-over of residual 7,8-BF in the tissue preparation (17,67). Another mechanism postulated for the inhibition of binding by the flavone is direct interference with the activation of the carcinogen. Evidence for this notion comes from binding studies *in vitro*. In agreement with the strong suppression of cutaneous monooxygenase activity *in vitro* (42,140), binding of BP, DMBA, MC, and DBA to DNA by epidermal homogenates was inhibited by 50% in the presence of equimolar concentrations of 7,8-BF (14,109). It has to be noted that the epidermal homogenates used were derived from mice that had been pretreated with 100 nmol of the unlabeled carcinogen for 18 hr, i.e., after induction of the 7,8-BF-sensitive monooxygenase form. Although those results clearly demonstrate the potentially strong inhibitory action of 7,8-BF on the activation of polycyclic hydrocarbons in skin, at least of inducer-pretreated animals, they do not help to clarify the apparent discrepancy in the effects of 7,8-BF on MC and DMBA versus DBA- and BP-induced tumorigenesis. A better correlation of tumorigenesis and *in vitro* binding was obtained again in experiments that more closely resemble the *in vivo* conditions of metabolic activation (109). Mice were treated topically with unlabeled DMBA, MC, or DBA alone or together with 7,8-BF, and then the *in vitro* binding capacity of epidermal homogenates for tritiated DMBA, MC, and DBA, respectively, was examined at various times after application. *In vivo* treatment with the carcinogens alone increased their subsequent *in vitro* binding two- to fourfold after a few hours. However, simultaneous *in vivo* treatment with 7,8-BF inhibited the *in vitro* binding only of [^{3}H]DMBA and [^{3}H]MC but not of [^{3}H]DBA in accordance with the effects of 7,8-BF on tumor initiation by these agents. The inhibitory effect on DMBA and MC binding was limited to the first 6 hr of *in vivo* treatment. At later times, 7,8-BF was without effect or even increased [^{3}H]DMBA binding.

These observations support the notion that the inhibition of carcinogen binding in skin by 7,8-BF is caused by a reduction in the potential for carcinogen activation rather than a direct inhibition of carcinogen metabolism. The mechanism by which 7,8-BF alters the capacity of skin to activate carcinogens to binding species remains a matter of speculation. It may be possible, for example, that the benzoflavone inactivates cytochrome P-450, as has been shown for a variety of chemicals (see above and refs. 30,48,59,60,76,100); however, this has not been explored yet.

EFFECTS OF 7,8-BENZOFLAVONE ON CARCINOGEN BINDING IN CELLS IN CULTURE AND IN NUCLEAR PREPARATIONS

The effect of 7,8-BF on the binding of BP or DMBA in cell systems *in vitro* generally follows the pattern of the flavone effect on BP-hydroxylase activity. Inhibition of monooxygenase activity in human and rat cultured colon by 7,8-BF was accompanied by a reduction in the overall binding of tritiated BP to cellular protein during a 24 hr period of exposure (10,11). Similarly, inhibition of BP-metabolism in freshly isolated hepatocytes from MC-treated rats roughly matched the inhibition of binding to endogeneous DNA (23). A good correlation of [^{3}H]BP metabolism and [^{3}H]BP binding was also observed in hepatic microsomes from MC-treated rats (103). It should be noted that in all these experiments the activating enzymes were induced by MC treatment *in vivo* or by exposure to the binding PAH in culture, i.e., the 7,8-BF-sensitive cytochrome P-448 was most likely the predominant monooxygenase form. In autoradiographic studies,

Harris and co-workers (49) found that 7,8-BF also inhibits the binding of [³H]BP in epithelial cells of trachea maintained in short-term organ culture (3 hr) from hamsters that had not been pretreated with any inducer.

Hill and Shih (52,106) noted that 7,8-BF strongly inhibits the binding of BP in microsomes from lungs of PAH-treated mice and hamsters but only weakly from untreated animals. These results together with the observations of others on the lack of inhibition of BP-tumorigenesis by 7,8-BF (68) suggested to them that a reaction catalyzed by the "constitutive," cytochrome P-450-dependent monooxygenase might be the critical event in BP-induced lung carcinogenesis.

Baird and Diamond (12) examined in more detail the effect of 7,8-BF on BP binding to DNA in secondary cultures of embryo cells from Syrian hamster. They observed that the benzoflavone significantly reduces the level of binding. Separation of hydrocarbon-DNA adducts into two fractions did not show any qualitative differences between untreated and 7,8-BF treated cells. This is in keeping with the observation that secondary hamster cells in culture, like established cell lines, contain predominantly, if not solely, one form of the monooxygenase, i.e., the form that is associated with cytochrome P-448 and is inducible by MC (136). Increasing concentrations of the inhibitor reduced the degree of BP-binding much more than that of BP metabolism yielding a semilogarithmic relationship between the inhibition of BP metabolism and BP binding. From these results Baird and Diamond (12) concluded that the flavone inhibits two metabolic steps involved in the activation of BP to binding species which is compatible with the notion that the binding metabolite of BP and of other polycyclic hydrocarbons may arise through two successive oxygenation steps (38).

In contrast to the findings in cell cultures, the binding pattern of BP in nuclei of rat liver was found to be considerably more complex presumably because of the multiplicity of monooxygenase(s) present in the nuclear preparations (1,19). It is interesting that 7,8-BF preferentially inhibited the binding products derived from 9-hydroxy-BP and 7,8-dihydro-7,8-dihydroxy-BP-9,10-oxide, which are formed in nuclei from both phenobarbital- and MC-treated animals (1). Under conditions where the overall binding of BP and DNA was not inhibited by the flavone, the formation of DNA-adducts derived from 7,8-dihydroxy-BP-9,10-oxide, which comprises only a small fraction, was largely suppressed. In view of the apparent lack of major effects of 7,8-BF on BP metabolism *in vitro* described above, these findings at least give some indication that 7,8-BF may selectively inhibit a particular pathway of BP. The data also point out that great caution has to be taken in attempting to directly correlate the effects of a modifier on the overall DNA-binding of carcinogens with its effect on tumorigenicity. The question why 7,8-BF inhibits BP tumorigenesis so poorly but seems to selectively suppress the formation or binding of just those reactive BP metabolites which are believed to be the ultimate carcinogenic forms (cf. ref. 38) remains to be resolved.

INTERFERENCE OF POLYCYCLIC HYDROCARBONS WITH CARCINOGEN METABOLISM AND TUMOR INITIATION

Polycyclic hydrocarbons, either carcinogenic or noncarcinogenic, have frequently been found to inhibit the tumor-initiating activity of other carcinogenic chemicals (35,53,90,111; for discussions see refs. 34,40,56,121). Tumor initiation by various types of carcinogens, e.g., substituted and unsubstituted aromatic hydrocarbons, aromatic amines, or azo dyes in liver, skin, ear, mammary gland, and small intestine, could be reduced by simultaneous application of usually smaller amounts of PAH (Table 5). It is apparent that PAH interfere with each other on the level of oxidative metabolism either by their nature as inducers or as substrate "inhibitors" of monooxygenases and will therefore alter the carcinogenic activity. In most of these studies the mechanism of inhibition has not been clarified and is obscured by the multiple role of PAH in monooxygenase activity. Studies by Miller and co-workers (90) have thrown some light on the complex mechanism of the protective action of PAH in azo dye and acetylaminofluorene tumorigenesis in liver. They observed that feeding of 3′-methyl-4-dimethylaminoazobenzene decreased the hepatic capacity for azo dye N-demethylation and reduction, and that MC counteracts this loss of enzyme activities resulting in lower levels of free azo dye in the liver and blood and of protein-bound dye in the liver. In the case of MC-inhibited acetylaminofluorene tumorigenesis in rats (90), the protective PAH may preferentially induce the ring hydroxylation of acetylaminofluorene (79,80) thought to be an inactivation pathway (89,133). Recent observations indicated that MC-pretreatment may also promote the biliary excretion of the N-hydroxy derivative to decrease the concentration of the reactive intermediate in the liver cells (80).

Thus, the mode of PAH "protection" might differ, depending on the type of carcinogen used. Generally, induction of *hepatic* carcinogen metabolism by the modifying PAH will reduce the effective dose of the carcinogen in *extrahepatic* target tissues. This, for example, might be the case for the reduced tumor initiation induced by DMBA in the mammary gland after pretreatment of rats with small amounts of PAH (58). However, a protective role of monooxygenase induction in the mammary gland itself cannot be excluded in these experiments. The significance of induction by the protecting PAH is even more difficult to evaluate in experimental models of carcinogenesis in which the carcinogenic and the inhibitory agents are simultaneously applied to the target tissue, e.g., topically to the skin. Although the protecting PAH are capable of inducing cutaneous monooxygenase activity at small doses (138), it is not evident how this could appreciably alter the increase in enzyme activity resulting from the simultaneous application of the carcinogen which is itself usually an efficient inducer. Under these conditions, the protective effect of PAH might rather be sought in a modification of metabolic pathways of the carcinogen or by a competition for the activating enzyme. In an approach to resolve this issue, Slaga and co-workers (110) studied the effect of dibenz*(a,c)*anthracene, a potent inhibitor

TABLE 5. *Mutual interference of polycyclic aromatic hydrocarbons and related compounds in tumor formation*

"Modifier"	Carcinogen[a]	Ratio modifier to carcinogen	Inhibition	Target	Ref.
Naphthalene	DMBA	4/1 [b]	−	Skin	(53)
Anthracene[c]					
Phenanthrene[c]	BP	10/1	+	Skin	(35)
Pyrene[c]					
Pyrene	3′-CH₃-DAB	1/20	−	Liver	(90)
Chrysene	MC	1/1	+	Skin	(74)
Chrysene	BP	1/6	+	Skin	(35)
Benz[a]anthracene	3′-CH₃-DAB	1/20	+	Liver	(90)
Benz[a]anthracene	DMBA	2/1 [b]	+	Skin	(53)
BP	3′-CH₃-DAB	1/20	+	Liver	(90)
Perylene	BP	1/10	+	Skin	(35)
Dibenz[a,h]anthracene	3′-CH₃-DAB	1/20	+	Liver	(90)
Dibenz[a,c]anthracene	DMBA	2/1	+	Skin	(110)
DMBA	3′-CH₃-DAB	1/20	+	Liver	(90)
MC	3′-CH₃-DAB	1/20	+	Liver	(90)
MC	AAF	1/8	+	Liver	(90)
MC	7-Fluoro-AAF	1/3	+	Liver	(90)
Fluorene	DMBA	2/1 [b]	−	Skin	(53)
Benzo(a)fluorene	BP	1/10	+	Skin	(35)
Dibenzo(a,g)fluorene	DMBA	2/1 [b]	+	Skin	(53)
Dibenzo(a,g)fluorene	MC	1/1	+	Skin	(74)
Benzo(k)fluoranthene	BP	1/1	+	Skin	(35)
Naphthol	BP	5/1	+	Skin	(35)
Benzo(a)carbazole	BP	1/6	+	Skin	(35)

[a] Abbreviations: AAF = 2-acetylaminofluorene; 3′-CH₃-DAB = 3′-methyl-4-dimethylaminoazobenzene.
[b] Approximate ratios.
[c] Anthracene, phenanthrene, and pyrene were applied together at a modifier to carcinogen ratio of 10:1 each.

of DMBA-induced tumorigenesis (107,110), on the activation of DMBA to binding species in mouse skin. Topical application of 200 nmoles of dibenz-*(a,c)*anthracene increased *in vitro* binding of [³H]DMBA to DNA by skin preparations. However, when dibenz*(a,c)*anthracene was applied together with equimolar amounts of unlabeled DMBA, the *in vitro* binding of [³H]DMBA was lower than that after pretreatment with DMBA alone. Dibenz*(a,c)*anthracene apparently alters the effect of DMBA on the cutaneous capacity for its own activation. In view of these data, the modifying PAH is unlikely to exert its effect by a general induction of cutaneous monooxygenases. It remains to be established whether the inhibitory action of dibenz*(a,c)*anthracene occurs by protection of inactivating pathways or suppression of activating pathways, if at all by modification of monooxygenase activity.

In contrast to the qualitatively uniform induction of monooxygenase by PAH, these compounds appear to interfere with each other's oxidative metabolism in a more complex manner (139,144). As shown in Table 6, PAH exert widely varying effects on BP hydroxylation in hepatic microsomes from untreated and MC-treated rats. At equimolar concentrations some of the compounds inhibit the two forms of "BP-hydroxylases" to the same degree; others have no inhibitory effect; and a third group more strongly affects one type of enzyme(s) than the other.

Among a large number of chemicals tested for their potency as modulators of PAH-metabolism two compounds, 9-chloro-7*H*-dibenzo*(a,g)*carbazole and 6-aminochrysene, were found to be particularly powerful inhibitors and were studied in more detail (139). 9-Chloro-7*H*-dibenzo*(a,g)*carbazole inhibits MC-induced enzyme activity by 50% at 5×10^{-7} M concentration, i.e., one-hundredth

TABLE 6. *Inhibition of BP hydroxylase by various homo- and heterocyclic aromatic hydrocarbons in hepatic microsomes of rat*[a]

Addition	BP-hydroxylase activity, % of solvent control	
	Untreated	MC-treated
Naphthalene	96	100
Anthracene	86	96
Phenanthrene	69	89
Perylene	100	93
DMBA	62	68
Dibenz[*a,h*]anthracene	103	90
Dibenz[*a,h*]anthracene	90	60
MC	100	49
6-Aminochrysene	20	20
9-Chloro-7H-dibenzo[*a,g*]-carbazole	62	5

[a]Concentration of the substrate BP and of the polycyclic hydrocarbons added was 80 μM. MC-treatment induced BP-hydroxylase about sixfold. For other conditions, see ref. 144. Adapted from Williams et al. (144) and Wiebel et al. (139).

of the substrate concentration. In contrast, enzyme activity in microsomes from untreated animals is two orders of magnitude less sensitive to the inhibitor. Such a differential effect is not found with 6-aminochrysene that inhibits the enzyme(s) from untreated and MC-treated animals with equal efficiency, e.g., 50% at 5×10^{-6} M concentration. The observations suggest that some polycyclic hydrocarbons might strongly inhibit the metabolism of carcinogens *in vivo* and modify the carcinogenic response. The data further indicate that the interference with the activity of different monooxygenases differs considerably between different hydrocarbons and will be difficult to predict.

CONCLUSIONS AND PROSPECTS

Although the present treatise has largely been focused on a single group of carcinogens, the polycyclic hydrocarbons, and on a very few modifiers of monooxygenase activity, principal problems and considerations associated with the inhibition of tumor initiation by chemicals become apparent. Evidently, monooxygenases play a crucial role in the activation of carcinogens; however, their exact function in the activation process is extremely difficult to evaluate because of the multiplicity of enzyme forms each of which may oxygenate molecules in various positions to a number of biologically active or inactive products. It is clear that the biological effectiveness of modifiers is largely governed by their specificity for the many different forms of the monooxygenases. In view of the multiplicity of enzyme forms and their dual role in carcinogen metabolism, the search for a "universal" inhibitor of chemical carcinogenesis on the level of oxidative activation is likely to be futile. Chemicals, whether they are inducers or inhibitors of the enzymes, will have to fit the metabolism of each individual carcinogen, its dose, mode of application, and target tissue in order to exert a protective effect. At present there are very few carcinogens of which we know the "activating" and "inactivating" oxidative pathways to make such a selection. Accordingly, the prospects to inhibit chemical carcinogenesis by modifying monooxygenase activity in man are not bright. The large number and variety of both known and suspected carcinogens in the human environment and the lack of information on their oxidative metabolism are obstacles that appear insurmountable at present and will be difficult to overcome in the near future.

However, modifiers of monooxygenase activity may prove to be very useful to elucidate the activation of compounds in experimental models of chemical carcinogenesis. A number of potent inhibitors and inducers of the enzyme system are available which have been shown to markedly alter the course of tumor initiation by chemicals. A major drawback of these modifiers, which greatly hampers the analysis of their effects *in vivo,* is their ability to function as both inducers and inhibitors of the monooxygenases. Development of compounds that possess only one of these functions would mean a significant advance in this field. Another important factor, as pointed out above, is the specificity of the modifier for different forms of monooxygenases. A promising beginning has been made in exploring the differential effects of modifiers, such as 7,8-BF, which shows some degree of specificity for one group of monooxygenases. Further studies are required to characterize the various forms of monooxygenases, their regulation, substrate specificity, tissue distribution, and cellular localization. Based on this information, selective inducers or inhibitors of the monooxygenases may be identified providing valuable tools to untangle the complex oxidative metabolism of procarcinogens to their "ultimate" carcinogenic form and to probe for the role of monooxygenase activity in the organ specificity of chemical carcinogens.

REFERENCES

1. Alexandrov, K., and Thompson, M. H. (1977): Influence of inducers and inhibitors of mixed-function oxidases on benzo(a)pyrene binding to the DNA of rat liver nuclei. *Cancer Res.*, 37:1443–1449.
2. Alvares, A. P., Bickers, D. R., and Kappas, A. (1973): Polychlorinated biphenyls: A new type of inducer of cytochrome P-448 in the liver. *Proc. Natl. Acad. Sci. USA*, 70:1321–1325.
3. Andrews, L. S., Sonawane, B. R., and Yaffe, S. J. (1976): Characterization and induction of aryl hydrocarbon (benzo(a)pyrene) hydroxylase in rabbit bone marrow. *Res. Commun. Chem. Pathol. Pharmacol.*, 15:319–330.
4. Arcos, J. C., Bryant, G. M., Venkatesan, N., and Argus, M. F. (1975): Repression of dimethylnitrosamine-demethylase by typical inducers of microsomal mixed-function oxidases. *Pharmacology*, 24:1544–1547.
5. Arcos, J. C., Valle, R. T., Bryant, G. M., Buu-Hoi, N. P., and Argus, M. F. (1976): Dimethylnitrosamine-demethylase: Molecular size-dependence of repression by polynuclear hydrocarbons. Nonhydrocarbon repressors. *J. Toxicol. Environ. Health*, 1:395–408.
6. Argus, M. F., Hoch-Ligeti, C., Arcos, J. C., and Conney, A. H. (1978): Differential effects of β-naphthoflavone and pregnenolone-16α-carbonitrile on dimethylnitrosamine-induced hepatocarcinogenesis. *J. Natl. Cancer Inst.*, 61:441–449.
7. Atlas, S. A., Boobis, A. R., Felton, J. S., Thorgeirsson, S. S., and Nebert, D. W. (1977): Ontogenetic expression of polycyclic aromatic compound-inducible monooxygenase activities and forms of cytochrome P-450 in rabbit. *J. Biol. Chem.*, 252:4712–4721.
8. Atlas, S. A., and Nebert, D. W. (1976): Genetic association of increases in naphthalene, acetanilide, and biphenyl hydroxylations with inducible aryl hydrocarbon hydroxylase in mice. *Arch. Biochem. Biophys.*, 175:495–506.
9. Atlas, S. A., Thorgeirsson, S. S., Boobis, A. R., Kumaki, K., and Nebert, D. W. (1975): Differential induction of murine Ah locus-associated monooxygenase activities in rabbit liver and kidney. *Biochem. Pharmacol.*, 24:2111–2116.
10. Autrup, H., Harris, C. C., Fugaro, S., and Selkirk, J. K. (1977): Effect of various chemicals on the metabolism of benzo(a)pyrene by cultured rat colon. *Chem. Biol. Interact.*, 18:337–347.
11. Autrup, H., Harris, C. C., Stoner, G. D., Jesudason, M. L., and Trump, B. F. (1977): Binding of chemical carcinogens to macromolecules in cultured human colon: Brief communication. *J. Natl. Cancer Inst.*, 59:351–354.
12. Baird, W. M., and Diamond, L. (1976): Effect of 7,8-benzoflavone on the formation of benzo-(a)pyrene-DNA-bound products in hamster embryo cells. *Chem. Biol. Interact.*, 13:67–75.
13. Bend, J. R., and Hook, G. E. R. (1977): Hepatic and extrahepatic mixed-function oxidases. In: *Handbook of Physiology. Reactions to Environmental Agents*, edited by D. H. K. Lee, pp. 419–440. Williams and Wilkins Co., Baltimore.
14. Berry, D. L., Bracken, W. R., Slaga, T. J., Wilson, N. M., Buty, S. G., and Juchau, M. R. (1977): Benzo(a)pyrene metabolism in mouse epidermis. Analysis by high pressure liquid chromatography and DNA binding. *Chem.-Biol. Interact.*, 18:129–142.
15. Boobis, A. R., Nebert, D. W., and Felton, J. S. (1977): Comparison of β-naphthoflavone

and 3-methylcholanthrene as inducers of hepatic cytochrome(s) P-448 and aryl hydrocarbon (benzo(a)pyrene) hydroxylase activity. *Mol. Pharmacol.*, 13:259–268.

16. Borchert, P., and Wattenberg, L. W. (1976): Inhibition of macromolecular binding of benzo-(a)pyrene and inhibition of neoplasia by disulfiram in the mouse forestomach. *J. Natl. Cancer Inst.*, 57:173–179.

17. Bowden, G. T., Slaga, T. J., Shapas, B. G., and Boutwell, R. K. (1974): The role of aryl hydrocarbon hydroxylase in skin tumor initiation by 7,12-dimethylbenz(a)anthracene and 1,2,5,6-dibenzanthracene using DNA binding and thymidine-^{3}H incorporation into DNA as criteria. *Cancer Res.*, 34:2634–2642.

18. Boyd, J. S., and Smellie, R. M. S., editors (1972): *Biological Hydroxylation Mechanisms.* Academic Press, New York.

19. Bresnick, E., Vaught, J. B., Chuang, A. H. L., Stoming, T. A., Bockman, D., and Mukhtar, H. (1977): Nuclear aryl hydrocarbon hydroxylase and interaction of polycyclic hydrocarbons with nuclear components. *Arch. Biochem. Biophys.*, 181:257–269.

20. Brodie, B. B., Gillette, J. R., editors (1971): *Concepts in Chemical Pharmacology,* Part II. Springer, New York.

21. Buening, M. K., Fortner, J. G., Kappas, A., and Conney, A. H. (1978): 7,8-benzoflavone stimulates the metabolic activation of aflatoxin B_1 to mutagens by human liver. *Biochem. Biophys. Res. Commun.*, 82:348–355.

22. Bürki, K., Liebelt, A. G., and Bresnick, E. (1973): Expression of aryl hydrocarbon hydroxylase induction in mouse tissues in vivo and in organ culture. *Arch. Biochem. Biophys.*, 158:641–649.

23. Burke, M. D., Vadi, H., Jernström, B., and Orrenius, S. (1977): Metabolism of benzo(a)pyrene with isolated hepatocytes and the formation and degradation of DNA-binding derivatives. *J. Biol. Chem.*, 252:6424–6431.

24. Campbell, T. C., and Hayes, J. R. (1974): Role of nutrition in the drug-metabolizing enzyme system. *Pharmacol. Rev.*, 26:171–197.

25. Conney, A. H. (1967): Pharmacological implications of microsomal enzyme induction. *Pharmacol. Rev.*, 19:317–366.

26. Conney, A. H., and Burns, J. J. (1972): Metabolic interactions among environmental chemicals and drugs. *Science,* 178:576–586.

27. Coombs, M. M., Bhatt, T. S., and Vose, D. W. (1975): The relationship between metabolism, DNA-binding, and carcinogenity of 15,16-dihydro-11-methylcyclopenta(a)phenanthrene-17-one in the presence of a microsomal enzyme inhibitor. *Cancer Res.*, 35:305–309.

28. Creaven, P. J., and Parke, D. V. (1966): The stimulation of hydroxylation by carcinogenic and non-carcinogenic compounds. *Biochem. Pharmacol.*, 15:7–16.

29. De Matteis, F. (1971): Loss of haem in rat liver caused by the porphyrogenic agent 2-allyl-2-isopropylacetamide. *Biochem. J.*, 124:767–777.

30. De Matteis, F. (1974): Covalent binding of sulfur to microsomes and loss of cytochrome P-450 during the oxidative desulfuration of several chemicals. *Mol. Pharmacol.*, 10:849–854.

31. Diamond, L., and Gelboin, H. V. (1969): Alpha-naphthoflavone: An inhibitor of hydrocarbon cytotoxicity and microsomal hydroxylase. *Science,* 166:1023–1025.

32. Diamond, L., McFall, R., Miller, J., and Gelboin, H. V. (1972): The effects of two isomeric benzoflavones on aryl hydrocarbon hydroxylase and the toxicity and carcinogenicity of poly-cyclic hydrocarbons. *Cancer Res.*, 32:731–736.

33. DiPaolo, J. A., Donovan, P. J., and Nelson, R. L. (1971): Transformation of hamster cells *in vitro* by polycyclic hydrocarbons without cytotoxicity. *Proc. Natl. Acad. Sci. USA,* 68:2958–2961.

34. Falk, H. L. (1971): Anticarcinogenesis—an alternative. *Prog. Exp. Tumor Res.*, 14:105–137.

35. Falk, H. L., Kotin, P., and Thompson, S. (1964): Inhibition of carcinogenesis. The effect of polycyclic hydrocarbons and related compounds. *Arch. Environ. Health,* 9:169–179.

36. Fang, W., and Strobel, H. W. (1978): The drug and carcinogen metabolism system of rat colon microsomes. *Arch. Biochem. Biophys.*, 186:128–138.

37. Felton, J. S., and Nebert, D. W. (1975): Mutagenesis of certain activated carcinogens *in vitro* associated with genetically mediated increases in monooxygenase activity and cytochrome P_1-450. *J. Biol. Chem.*, 250:6769–6778.

38. Freudenthal, R., and Jones, P. W., editors (1976): *Polynuclear aromatic hydrocarbons: Chemistry, metabolism and carcinogenesis.* Raven Press, New York.

39. Frommer, U., Ullrich, V., and Orrenius, S. (1974): Influence of inducers and inhibitors on the hydroxylation pattern of N-hexane in rat liver microsomes. *FEBS Lett.,* 41:14–16.

40. Gelboin, H. V. (1967): Carcinogens, enzyme induction, and gene action. *Adv. Cancer Res.,* 10:1–81.

41. Gelboin, H. V., Kinoshita, N., and Wiebel, F. J. (1972): Microsomal hydroxylases: induction and role in polycyclic hydrocarbon carcinogenesis and toxicity. *Fed. Proc.,* 31:1298–1309.

42. Gelboin, H. V., Wiebel, F., and Diamond, L. (1970): Dimethylbenzanthracene tumorigenesis and aryl hydrocarbon hydroxylase in mouse skin: Inhibition by 7,8-benzoflavone. *Science,* 170:169–171.

43. Gillette, J. R., Davis, D. C., and Sasame, H. A. (1972): Cytochrome P-450 and its role in drug metabolism. *Annu. Rev. Pharmacol.,* 12:57–84.

44. Goldstein, J. A., Hickman, P., Bergman, H., McKinney, J. D., and Walker, M. P. (1977): Separation of pure polychlorinated biphenyl isomers into two types of inducers on the basis of induction of cytochrome P-450 or P-448. *Chem. Biol. Interact.,* 17:69–87.

45. Goto, T., and Wiebel, F. J. (1979): Aryl hydrocarbon (benzo(a)pyrene) monooxygenase activity in human primary amnion cell cultures. *Eur. J. Cancer, (in press).*

46. Goujon, F. M., Nebert, D. W., and Gielen, J. E. (1972): Genetic expression of aryl hydrocarbon hydroxylase induction. IV. Interaction of various compounds with different forms of cytochrome P-450 and the effect on benzo(a)pyrene metabolism *in vitro. Mol. Pharmacol.,* 8:667–680.

47. Gram, T. E., (1973): Comparative aspects of mixed function oxidation by lung and liver of rabbits. *Drug Metab. Rev.,* 2:1–32.

48. Guengerich, F. P., and Strickland, T. W. (1977): Metabolism of vinyl chloride: Destruction of the heme of highly purified liver microsomal cytochrome P-450 by a metabolite. *Mol. Pharmacol.,* 13:993–1004.

49. Harris, C. C., Kaufman, D. G., Sporn, M. B., Boren, H., Jackson, F., Smith, J. M., Pauley, J., Dedick, P., and Saffiotti, U. (1973): Localization of benzo(a)pyrene-^{3}H and alterations in nuclear chromatin caused by benzo(a)pyrene-ferric oxide in the hamster respiratory epithelium. *Cancer Res.,* 33:2842–2848.

50. Hassid, A., and Levine, L. (1977): Induction of fatty acid cyclooxygenase activity in canine kidney cells (MDCK) by benzo(a)pyrene. *J. Biol. Chem.,* 252:6591–6593.

51. Haugen, D. A., Coon, M. J. and Nebert, D. W. (1976): Induction of multiple forms of mouse liver cytochrome P-450. Evidence for genetically controlled *de novo* protein synthesis in response to treatment with β-naphthoflavone or phenobarbital. *J. Biol. Chem.,* 251:1817–1827.

52. Hill, D. L., and Shih, T.-W. (1975): Inhibition of benzo(a)pyrene metabolism catalyzed by mouse and hamster lung microsomes. *Cancer Res.,* 35:2717–2723.

53. Hill, W. T., Stanger, D. W., Pizzo, A., Riegel, B., Shubik, P., and Wartman, W. B. (1951): Inhibition of 9,10-dimethyl-1,2-benzanthracene skin carcinogenesis in mice by polycyclic hydrocarbons. *Cancer Res.,* 11:892–897.

54. Hoch-Ligeti, C., Argus, M. F., and Arcos, J. C. (1968): Combined carcinogenic effects of dimethylnitrosamine and 3-methylcholanthrene in the rat. *J. Natl. Cancer Inst.,* 40:535–549.

55. Holder, G., Yagi, H., Dansette, P., Jerina, D. M., Levin, W., Lu, A. Y. H., and Conney, A. H. (1974): Effects of inducers and epoxide hydrase on the metabolism of benzo(a)pyrene by liver microsomes and a reconstituted system: Analysis by high pressure liquid chromatography. *Proc. Natl. Acad. Sci. USA,* 71:4356–4360.

56. Homburger, F., and Treiger, A. (1969): Modifiers of carcinogenesis. *Prog. Exp. Tumor Res.,* 11:86–99.

57. Huang, M.-T., West, S. B., and Lu, A. Y. H. (1976): Separation, purification, and properties of multiple forms of cytochrome P-450 from the liver microsomes of phenobarbital-treated mice. *J. Biol. Chem.,* 251:4659–4665.

58. Huggins, C., Grand, L., and Fukunishi, R. (1964): Aromatic influences on the yields of mammary cancers following administration of 7,12-dimethylbenz(a)anthracene. *Proc. Natl. Acad. Sci. USA,* 51:737–742.

59. Hunter, A. L., and Neal, R. A. (1975): Inhibition of hepatic mixed-function oxidase activity *in vitro* and *in vivo* by various thiono-sulfur-containing compounds. *Biochem. Pharmacol.,* 24:2199–2205.

60. Ivanetich, K. M., Atonson, I., and Katz, I. D. (1977): The interaction of vinyl chloride with rat hepatic microsomal cytochrome P-450 *in vitro. Biochem. Biophys. Res. Commun.,* 74:1411–1418.

61. Ivanetich, K. M., Marsh, J. A., Bradshaw, J. J., and Kaminsky, L. S. (1975): Fluroxene (2,2,2-trifluoroethyl vinyl ether) mediated destruction of cytochrome P-450 *in vitro*. *Biochem. Pharmacol.*, 24:1933–1936.

62. Jellinck, P. H., Smith, G., and Newcombe, A.-M. (1975): Inhibition of hepatic aryl hydrocarbon hydroxylase by 3-methylcholanthrene, 7,8-benzoflavone and other inducers added *in vitro*. *Chem. Biol. Interact.*, 11:459–468.

63. Kahl, G. R., Müller, W., Kahl, R., Jonen, H. G., and Netter, K. J. (1978): Differential inhibition of biphenyl hydroxylation in perfused rat liver. *Naunyn-Schmiedeberg's Arch. Pharmacol.*, 304:297–301.

64. Kahl, R., and Netter, K. J. (1977): Ethoxyquin as an inducer and inhibitor of phenobarbital-type cytochrome P-450 in rat liver microsomes. *Toxicol. Appl. Pharmacol.*, 40:473–483.

65. Kapitulnik, J., Poppers, P. J., Buening, M. K., Fortner, J. G., and Conney, A. H. (1977): Activation of monooxygenases in human liver by 7,8-benzoflavone. *Clin. Pharmacol. Ther.*, 22:475–484.

66. King, H. W. S., Osborne, M. R., and Brookes, P. (1978): The identification of 3-methylcholanthrene-9,10-dihydrodiol as an intermediate in the binding of 3-methylcholanthrene to DNA in cells in culture. *Chem. Biol. Interact.*, 20:367–371.

67. Kinoshita, N., and Gelboin, H. V. (1972): The role of aryl hydrocarbon hydroxylase in 7,12-dimethylbenz(a)anthracene skin tumorigenesis: On the mechanism of 7,8-benzoflavone inhibition of tumorigenesis. *Cancer Res.*, 32:1329–1339.

68. Kinoshita, N., and Gelboin, H. V. (1972): Aryl hydrocarbon hydroxylase and polycyclic hydrocarbon tumorigenesis: effect of the enzyme inhibitor 7,8-benzoflavone on tumorigenesis and macromolecule binding. *Proc. Natl. Acad. Sci. USA*, 69:824–828.

69. Kinoshita, N., Shears, B., and Gelboin, H. V. (1973): K-region and non-K-region metabolism of benzo(a)pyrene by rat liver microsomes. *Cancer Res.*, 33:1937–1944.

70. Kouri, R. E., Rude, T., Thomas, P. E., and Whitmire, C. E. (1976): Studies on pulmonary aryl hydrocarbon hydroxylase activity in inbred strains of mice. *Chem. Biol. Interact.*, 13:317–331.

71. Krieg, T., Goerz, G., Lissner, R., Bolsen, K., and Ullrich, V. (1978): Drug monooxygenase activity in the Harderian gland. *Biochem. Pharmacol.*, 27:575–577.

72. Kumaki, K., Jensen, N. M., Shire, J. G. M., and Nebert, D. W. (1977): Genetic differences in induction of cytosol reduced-NAD(P): Menadione oxidoreductase and microsomal aryl hydrocarbon hydroxylase in the mouse. *J. Biol. Chem.*, 252:157–165.

73. Kupfer, D., Navarro, J., and Piccolo, D. E. (1978): Hydroxylation of prostaglandins A$_1$ and E$_1$ by liver microsomal monooxygenase. Characteristics of the enzyme system in the guinea pig. *J. Biol. Chem.*, 253:2804–2811.

74. Lacassagne, A., Buu-Hoi, N. P., and Rudali, G. (1945): Inhibition of the carcinogenic action produced by a weakly carcinogenic hydrocarbon on a highly active carcinogenic hydrocarbon. *Br. J. Exp. Pathol.*, 26:5–12.

75. Lehrmann, C., Ullrich, V. and Rummel, W. (1973): Phenobarbital inducible drug monooxygenase activity in the small intestine of mice. *Naunyn-Schmiedeberg's Arch. Pharmacol.*, 89:89–98.

76. Levin, W., Sernatinger, E., Jacobson, M., and Kuntzman, R. (1972): Destruction of cytochrome P-450 by secobarbital and other barbiturates containing allyl groups. *Science*, 176:1341–1343.

77. Levine, L., and Hong, S. L. (1977): Analogues of anthracene, phenanthrene, and benzoflavone inhibit prostaglandin biosynthesis by cells in culture. *Prostaglandins*, 14:1–9.

79. Lotlikar, P. D., Enomoto, M., Miller, J. A., and Miller, E. C. (1967): Species variation in the N- and ring-hydroxylation of 2-acetylaminofluorene and effects of 3-methylcholanthrene pretreatment. *Proc. Soc. Exp. Biol. Med.*, 125:341–346.

80. Lotlikar, P. D., Hong, S. Y., and Baldy, W. J., Jr. (1978): Effect of 3-methylcholanthrene pretreatment on 2-acetylaminofluorene N- and ring-hydroxylation by rat and hamster liver microsomes. *Toxicol. Lett.*, 2:135–139.

81. Loub, W. D., Wattenberg, L. W. and Davis, D. W. (1975): Aryl hydrocarbon hydroxylase induction in rat tissues by naturally occurring indoles of cruciferous plants. *J. Natl. Cancer Inst.*, 54:985–988.

82. Lu, A. Y. H. (1976): Livermicrosomal drug-metabolizing enzyme system: functional components and their properties. *Fed. Proc.*, 35:2460–2463.

83. Lu, A. Y. H., Kuntzman, R., West, S., Jacobson, M., and Conney, A. H. (1972): Reconstituted

liver microsomal enzyme system that hydroxylates drugs, other foreign compounds, and endogenous substrates. II. Role of the cytochrome P-450 and P-448 fractions in drug and steriod hydroxylations. *J. Biol. Chem.,* 247:1727–1734.

84. Lu, A. Y. H., Levin, W., West, S. B., Jacobson, M., Ryan, D., Kuntzman, R., and Conney, A. H. (1973): Reconstituted liver microsomal enzyme system that hydroxylates drugs, other foreign compounds, and endogenous substrates. *J. Biol. Chem.,* 248:456–460.

85. Lu, A. Y. H., Somogyi, A., West, S., Kuntzman, R., and Conney, A. H. (1972): Pregnenolone-16α-carbonitrile: A new type of inducer of drug-metabolizing enzymes. *Arch. Biochem. Biophys.,* 152:457–462.

86. Lu, A. Y. H., and West, S. B. (1978): Reconstituted mammalian mixed-function oxidases: requirements, specificities and other properties. *Pharmacol. Ther. A.,* 2:337–358.

87. Marquardt, H., Sodergren, J. E., Sims, P., and Grover, P. L. (1974): Malignant transformation *in vitro* of mouse fibroblasts by 7,12-dimethylbenz(a)anthracene and 7-hydroxymethylbenz(a)anthracene and by their K-region derivatives. *Int. J. Cancer,* 13:304–310.

88. Matsushima, T., Sawamura, M., Hara, K., and Sugimura, T. (1976): A safe substitute for polychlorinated biphenyls as an inducer of metabolic activation system. In: *In Vitro Metabolic Activation in Mutagenesis Testing,* edited by F. J. deSerres, J. R. Fouts, J. R. Bend, and R. M. Philpot, pp. 85–88. North-Holland, Amsterdam.

89. Miller, J. A. (1970): Carcinogenesis by chemicals: An overview. *Cancer Res.,* 30:559–576.

90. Miller, E. C., Miller, J. A., Brown, R. R., and McDonald, J. M. (1958): On the protective action of certain polycyclic aromatic hydrocarbons against carcinogenesis by amino azodyes and 2-acetylaminofluorene. *Cancer Res.,* 18:469–477.

91. Moschel, R. C., Baird, W. M., and Dipple, A. (1977): Metabolic activation of the carcinogen 7,12-dimethylbenz(a)anthracene for DNA binding. *Biochem. Biophys. Res. Commun.,* 76:1092–1098.

92. Oesch, F. (1973): Mammalian epoxide hydrases: Inducible enzymes catalysing the inactivation of carcinogenic and cytotoxic metabolites derived from aromatic and olefinic compounds. *Xenobiotica,* 3:305–340.

93. Ortiz de Montellano, P. R., Mico, B. A., and Yost, G. S. (1978): Suicidal inactivation of cytochrome P-450. Formation of a heme-substrate covalent adduct. *Biochem. Biophys. Res. Commun.,* 83:132–137.

94. Owens, I. S., and Nebert, D. W. (1975): Aryl hydrocarbon hydroxylase induction in mammalian liver-derived cell cultures. Stimulation of "cytochrome $P_1$450-associated" enzyme activity by many inducing compounds. *Mol. Pharmacol.,* 11:94–104.

95. Pelkonen, O. (1977): Differential inhibition of aryl hydrocarbon hydroxylase in human foetal liver, adrenal gland and placenta. *Acta Pharmacol. Toxicol. (Kbh.),* 41:306–316.

96. Pelkonen, O., Korhonen, P., Jouppila, P., and Kärki, N. (1975): Induction of aryl hydrocarbon hydroxylase in human fetal liver cell and fibroblast cultures by polycyclic hydrocarbons. *Life Sci.,* 16:1403–1410.

97. Pelkonen, O., Sotaniemi, E., and Mokka, R. (1977): The *in vitro* oxidative metabolism of benzo(a)pyrene in human liver measured by different assays. *Chem. Biol. Interact.,* 16:13–21.

98. Poland, A., and Glover, E. (1977): Chlorinated biphenyl induction of aryl hydrocarbon hydroxylase activity: A study of the structure-activity relationship. *Mol. Pharmacol.,* 13:924–938.

99. Poland, A. P., Glover, E., Robinson, J. R., and Nebert, D. W. (1974): Genetic expression of aryl hydrocarbon hydroxylase activity. Induction of monooxygenase activities and cytochrome P_1-450 formation by 2,3,7,8-tetrachlorodibenzo-*p*-dioxin in mice genetically "nonresponsive" to other aromatic hydrocarbons. *J. Biol. Chem.,* 249:5599–5606.

100. Reynolds, E. S., Moslen, M. T., Szabo, S., and Jaeger, R. J. (1975): Vinyl chloride-induced deactivation of cytochrome P-450 and other components of the liver mixed function oxidase system: An *in vivo* study. *Res. Commun. Chem. Pathol. Pharmacol.,* 12:685.

101. Sakai, S., Reinhold, C. E., Wirth, P. J., and Thorgeirsson, S. S. (1978): Mechanism of *in vitro* mutagenic activation and covalent binding of N-hydroxy-2-acetylaminofluorene in isolated liver cell nuclei from rat and mouse. *Cancer Res.,* 38:2058–2067.

102. Schwarz, L. R., Götz, R., Wolff, T., and Wiebel, F. J. (1978): Monooxygenase and glucuronyltransferase activities in short term culture of isolated rat hepatocytes. *FEBS Lett.,* 98:203–206.

103. Selkirk, J. K., Croy, R. G., Roller, P. P., and Gelboin, H. V. (1974): High-pressure liquid

chromatographic analysis of benzo(a)pyrene metabolism and covalent binding and the mechanism of action of 7,8-benzoflavone and 1,2-epoxy-3,3,3-trichloropropane. *Cancer Res.,* 34:3474–3480.

104. Selkirk, J. K., Croy, R. G., Wiebel, F. J., and Gelboin, H. V. (1976): Differences in benzo(a)-pyrene metabolism between rodent liver microsomes and embryonic cells. *Cancer Res.,* 36:4476–4479.

105. Sher, S. P. (1971): Drug enzyme induction and drug interactions: Literature tabulation. *Toxicol. Appl. Pharmacol.,* 18:780–834.

106. Shih, T.-W., and Hill, D. L. (1977): Selective inhibition and kinetics of enzymatic reactions leading to irreversible binding of benzo(a)pyrene to microsomal macromolecules of mouse lung. *Cancer Biochem. Biophys.,* 2:55–58.

107. Slaga, T. J., and Boutwell, R. K. (1977): Inhibition of the tumor-initiating ability of the potent carcinogen 7,12-dimethylbenz(a)anthracene by the weak tumor initiator 1,2,3,4-dibenzanthracene. *Cancer Res.,* 37:128–133.

108. Slaga, T. J., Bracken, W. M., Viaje, A., Berry, D. L., Fischer, S. M., and Miller, D. R. (1978): Lack of involvement of 6-hydroxymethylation in benzo(a)pyrene skin tumor initiation in mice. *J. Natl. Cancer Inst.,* 61:451–455.

109. Slaga, T. J., Thompson, S., Berry, D. L., DiGiovanni, J., Juchau, M. R., and Viaje, A. (1977): The effects of benzoflavones on polycyclic hydrocarbon metabolism and skin tumor initiation. *Chem. Biol. Interact.,* 17:297–312.

110. Slaga, T. J., Viaje, A., Buty, S. G., and Bracken, W. M. (1978): Dibenz(a,c)anthracene: A potent inhibitor of skin-tumor initiation by 7,12-dimethylbenz(a)anthracene. *Res. Commun. Chem. Pathol. Pharmacol.,* 19:477–483.

111. Steiner, P. E., and Falk, H. L. (1951): Summation and inhibition effects of weak and strong carcinogenic hydrocarbons: 1:2-benzanthracene, chrysene, 1:2:5:6-dibenzanthracene, and 20-methylcholanthrene. *Cancer Res.,* 11:58–63.

112. Sloane, N. H. (1975): α-Naphthoflavone activation of 6-hydroxymethylbenzo(a)pyrene synthetase. *Cancer Res.,* 35:3731–3734.

113. Stohs, S. J., Grafström, R. C., Burke, M. D., Moldéus, P. W., and Orrenius, S. G. (1976): The isolation of rat intestinal microsomes with stable cytochrome P-450 and their metabolism of benzo(a)pyrene. *Arch. Biochem. Biophys.,* 177:105–116.

114. Stohs, S. J., Grafström, R. C., Burke, M. D., and Orrenius, S. (1977): Benzo(a)pyrene metabolism by isolated rat intestinal epithelial cells. *Arch. Biochem. Biophys.,* 179:71–80.

115. Thomas, P. E., Lu, A. Y. H., Ryan, D., West, S. B., Kawalek, J., and Levin, W. (1976): Immunochemical evidence for six forms of rat liver cytochrome P450 obtained using antibodies against purified rat liver cytochromes P450 and P448. *Mol. Pharmacol.,* 12:746–758.

116. Ts'o, P. O. P., and DiPaolo, J. A., editors (1974): *Chemical Carcinogenesis.* Marcel Dekker, Inc., New York.

117. Ullrich, V., Frommer, W., and Weber, P. (1973): Differences in the 0-dealkylation of 7-ethoxycoumarin after pretreatment with phenobarbital and 3-methylcholanthrene. *Hoppe Seyler's Z. Physiol. Chem.,* 354:514.

118. Ullrich, V., Roots, I., Hildebrandt, A., Estabrook, R. W., and Conney, A. H. (1977): *Microsomes and Drug Oxidations.* Pergamon Press, New York.

119. Vadi, H., Moldéus, P., Capdevila, J., and Orrenius, S. (1975): The metabolism of benzo(a)pyrene in isolated rat liver cells. *Cancer Res.,* 35:2083–2091.

119a. Waechter, F. (1978): 7,8-Benzoflavone: A substrate for microsomal mixed-function oxygenase. Abstract 26. *6th European Workshop on Drug Metabolism.* Leiden. Netherlands.

120. Watanabe, M., Watanabe, K., Konno, K., and Sato, H. (1975): Genetic differences in the induction of aryl hydrocarbon hydroxylase and benzo(a)pyrene carcinogenesis in C3H/He and DBA/2 strains of mice. *Gann,* 66:217–226.

121. Wattenberg, L. W. (1966): Chemoprophylaxis of carcinogenesis: A review. *Cancer Res.,* 26:1520–1526.

122. Wattenberg, L. W. (1971): Studies of polycyclic hydrocarbon hydroxylases of the intestine possibly related to cancer. Effect of diet on benzpyrene hydroxylase activity. *Cancer,* 28:99–102.

123. Wattenberg, L. W. (1972): Dietary modification of intestinal and pulmonary aryl hydrocarbon hydroxylase activity. *Toxicol. Appl. Pharmacol.,* 23:741–748.

124. Wattenberg, L. W. (1977): Inhibition of carcinogenic effects of polycyclic hydrocarbons by benzyl isothiocyanate and related compounds. *J. Natl. Cancer Inst.*, 58:395–398.
125. Wattenberg, L. W. (1972): Inhibition of carcinogenic and toxic effects of polycyclic hydrocarbons by phenolic antioxidants and ethoxyquin. *J. Natl. Cancer Inst.*, 48:1425–1430.
126. Wattenberg, L. W. (1978): Inhibition of chemical carcinogenesis. *J. Natl. Cancer Inst.*, 60:11–18.
127. Wattenberg, L. W., Lam, L. K., Fladmoe, A. et al (1978): Inhibitors of colon carcinogenesis. *Cancer (in press)*.
128. Wattenberg, L. W., and Leong, J. L. (1968): Inhibition of the carcinogenic action of 7,12-dimethylbenz(a)anthracene by beta-naphthoflavone. *Proc. Soc. Exp. Biol. Med.*, 128:940–943.
129. Wattenberg, L. W., and Leong, J. L. (1970): Inhibition of the carcinogenic action of benzo(a)pyrene by flavones. *Cancer Res.*, 30:1922–1925.
130. Wattenberg, L. W., Leong, J. L., and Galbraith, A. R. (1968): Induction of increased benzpyrene hydroxylase activity in pulmonary tissue *in vitro. Proc. Soc. Exp. Biol. Med.*, 127:467–469.
131. Wattenberg, L. W., Page, M. A., and Leong, J. L. (1968): Induction of increased benzpyrene hydroxylase activity by flavones and related compounds. *Cancer Res.*, 28:934–937.
132. Wattenberg, L. W., Page, M. A., and Leong, J. L. (1968): Induction of increased benzpyrene hydroxylase activity by 2-phenylbenzothiazoles and related compounds. *Cancer Res.*, 12:2539–2544.
133. Weisburger, J. H., and Weisburger, E. K. (1973): Biochemical formation and pharmacological, toxicological and pathological properties of hydroxylamines and hydroxamic acids. *Pharmacol. Rev.*, 25:1–66.
134. Weisburger, J. H., and Williams, G. M. (1975): Metabolism of chemical carcinogens. In: *Cancer A Comprehensive Treatise. 1. Etiology: Chemical and Physical Carcinogenesis.* edited by F. F. Becker, pp. 185–234. Plenum Press, New York.
135. Whitlock, J. P., Jr., Cooper, H. L., and Gelboin, H. V. (1972): Aryl hydrocarbon (benzopyrene) hydroxylase is stimulated in human lymphocytes by mitogens and benz(a)anthracene. *Science*, 177:618–619.
136. Wiebel, F. J., Brown, S., Waters, H. L., and Selkirk, J. K. (1977): Activation of xenobiotics by monooxygenases: Cultures of mammalian cells as analytical tool. *Arch. Toxicol.*, 39:133–148.
137. Wiebel, F. J., and Gelboin, H. V. (1975): Aryl hydrocarbon (benzo(a)pyrene) hydroxylases in liver from rats of different age, sex and nutritional status. *Biochem. Pharmacol.*, 24:1511–1515.
138. Wiebel, F. J., and Gelboin, H. V. (1977): Cutaneous carcinogenesis: Metabolic interaction of chemical carcinogens with skin. In: *Handbook of Physiology,* edited by A. K. Lee, pp. 337–348. Williams and Wilkins, Co., Baltimore.
139. Wiebel, F. J., Gelboin, H. V., Buu-Hoi, N. P., Stout, M. G., and Burnham, W. S. (1974): Flavones and polycyclic hydrocarbons as modulators of aryl hydrocarbon (benzo(a)pyrene) hydroxylase. In: *Chemical Carcinogenesis,* edited by P. O. P. T'so and J. A. DiPaolo, pp. 249–270. Marcel Dekker, New York.
140. Wiebel, F. J., Leutz, J. C., Diamond, L., and Gelboin, H. V. (1971): Aryl hydrocarbon (benzo-(a)pyrene) hydroxylase in microsomes from rat tissues: Differential inhibition and stimulation by benzoflavones and organic solvents. *Arch. Biochem. Biophys.*, 144:78–86.
141. Wiebel, F. J., Selkirk, J. K., Gelboin, H. V., Haugen, D. A., Van der Hoeven, T. A., and Coon, M. J. (1975): Position-specific oxygenation of benzo(a)pyrene by different forms of purified cytochrome P-450 from rabbit liver. *Proc. Natl. Acad. Sci. USA*, 72:3917–3920.
142. Wiebel, F. J., and Waters, H. L. (1978): Effect of butylated hydroxytoluene and hydroxyanisole on benzo(a)pyrene metabolism and binding. *Excerpta Medica Inter. Cong. Ser. No. 440,* Industrial and Environmental Xenobiotics, Elsevier.
143. Wiebel, F. J., Waters, H. L., Elliot, S., and Gelboin, H. V. (1976): Effect of 7,8-benzoflavone on the duration of zoxazolamine paralysis and hexobarbital hypnosis in rats. *Biochem. Pharmacol.*, 25:1431–1432.
144. Williams, D., Wiebel, F. J., Leutz, J. C., and Gelboin, H. V. (1971): Effect of polycyclic hydrocarbons *in vitro* on aryl hydrocarbon (benzo(a)pyrene) hydroxylase. *Biochem. Pharmacol.*, 20:2130–2133.
145. Wollenberg, P., and Ullrich, V. (1977): Charactcrization of thc drug monooxygenase system

in mouse small intestine. In: *Microsomes and Drug Oxidations,* edited by V. Ullrich et al., pp. 675–679. Pergamon Press, Oxford.

146. Zampaglione, N., Jollow, D. J., Mitchell, J. R., Stripp, B., Hamrick, M., and Gillette, J. R. (1973): Role of detoxifying enzymes in bromobenzene-induced liver necrosis. *J. Pharmacol. Exp. Ther.,* 187:218–227.

147. Zampaglione, N. G., and Mannering, G. J. (1973): Properties of benzpyrene hydroxylase in the liver, intestinal mucosa and adrenal of untreated and 3-methylcholanthrene-treated rats. *J. Pharmacol. Exp. Ther.,* 185:676–685.

Carcinogenesis, Vol. 5: Modifiers of Chemical Carcinogenesis, edited by T. J. Slaga. Raven Press, New York © 1980.

4

Inhibition of Chemical Carcinogenesis by Antioxidants

Lee W. Wattenberg

Department of Laboratory Medicine and Pathology, University of Minnesota, Minneapolis, Minnesota 55455

Increasing numbers of chemical carcinogens are being identified. In some instances, this identification originates from considerations of chemical structure and in others the initial information is derived from empirical observations. The basic work of James and Elizabeth Miller, in which it was shown that the reactive forms of carcinogens are highly reactive electrophiles, has been a critical element in providing a basis for alerting scientists to the possibility that a particular compound might be carcinogenic (17,18). Mutagenicity screening systems of the type developed by Ames have recently provided an important additional technique in the search for carcinogenic substances (1). To a much lesser extent than the finding of increasing numbers of chemical carcinogens has been the demonstration of a growing number of compounds that have the capacity to inhibit chemical carcinogenesis when given prior to or simultaneously with exposure to the carcinogen (34,40,42,43). The mechanisms of inhibition of these compounds have not been established in most instances which makes their classification difficult. Some are antioxidants. Others have as a common property the ability to induce increased mixed-function oxidase activity. In addition, there are a variety of compounds for which no common features are apparent.

The diversity of chemical structures of inhibitors of chemical carcinogenesis suggests very strongly that others exist which have yet to be identified. If, as anticipated, there is a wide range of inhibitors, the possibility exists that these may provide a protection against carcinogens occurring in the environment. Thus the neoplastic response could be determined by the relative amounts of carcinogen(s) and inhibitor(s) that individuals are exposed to. At the present time, information is clear that carcinogens cause cancer in man. Data as to whether or not inhibitors in the environment truly exert an effect in suppressing neoplasia are lacking. Adequate information is simply not available. Further

85

work on mechanisms of inhibition and the range of compounds having carcinogen-inhibiting properties is necessary for an evaluation of the role that inhibitors play.

This chapter deals with the inhibitory effects of compounds that have as a common characteristic their ability to function as antioxidants. The use of antioxidants as possible inhibitors of the chemical carcinogens has been based in general on the concept that these compounds may exert a scavenging effect on the reactive species of carcinogens, thus protecting cellular constituents from attack. In early studies, wheat germ oil and α-tocopherol were employed. Experiments showing positive and negative results have been published. Confirmatory reports on the positive experiments have not appeared so that the implications of this work are not clear. These investigations, as well as our own experience with α-tocopherol which has not shown it to be inhibitory, have been summarized previously (35). However, it is possible that under some appropriate conditions suppression of neoplasia does occur. In the following sections, the inhibitory effects of various antioxidants will be presented. Since only limited experience exists with animal procedures for demonstrating inhibition of carcinogens, an initial discussion of such procedures will be given.

ANIMAL TEST SYSTEMS FOR THE STUDY OF INHIBITORS
OF CHEMICAL CARCINOGENESIS

Test systems for detecting inhibitors of chemical carcinogenesis have characteristics that are quite distinctive from the more familiar reverse pursuit of determining whether or not a particular compound is a carcinogen. In the latter case, high doses of the test material are generally used. For studies aimed at evaluating the carcinogen-inhibiting capacity of a particular compound, the dose or doses of the carcinogen employed in the test system must be on a portion of the dose-response curve sensitive to alterations in the dose of the carcinogen. Inhibitors of carcinogen, in essence, reduce the effective dose of the carcinogen. Thus, they may not be detected if excessive doses of carcinogen are given. Let us suppose that a dose schedule of carcinogen administration is being employed such that a reduction of the concentration of the carcinogen of 50% produces a decrease in tumor incidence of only 5 or 10%. Under these conditions, an inhibitor producing an effective reduction of carcinogen dose of 50% could easily be missed. On the other hand, the inhibitor would be readily detected if the dose of carcinogen employed were on a linear portion of the dose-response curve so that a reduction of the effective carcinogen dose of 50% would produce a 50% decrease in tumor incidence. The systems can be made more sensitive to inhibitors by reducing the dose of carcinogen and prolonging the period that the experimental animals are allowed to survive. This may be warranted when an inhibitor is showing uncertain results or where it is desirable to use low doses of the inhibitor. Human exposures to carcinogen and inhibitor are of low dose and long duration. Animal systems that reflect these conditions are indicated in later stages of inhibitor studies in which evaluations are being made of conditions under which inhibitors will exert their effects.

A considerable number of experimental procedures have been employed to evaluate the carcinogen-inhibiting capacities of test compounds as will be noted from Tables 1 and 2. Several of these test compounds have the desirable attributes discussed above and will be described briefly. A very simple test system entails the use of strains of mice that are highly sensitive to carcinogen-induced pulmonary adenoma formation. Pulmonary adenomas are produced by a wide variety of carcinogens and the dose-response relationships have been extensively studied (28,29). The usefulness of this system for studying inhibitors of a number of carcinogens has been demonstrated by several investigators as will be noted in Tables 1 and 2. A typical testing procedure is to administer 2 or 3 doses of a polycyclic aromatic hydrocarbon carcinogen such as benzo*(a)*pyrene (BP) or 7,12-dimethylbenz*(a)*anthracene (DMBA) with an interval of 2 weeks between the administrations. The substance being tested for its inhibitory capacities can be given either in the diet or as discrete single administrations at some specific time interval prior to carcinogen administration. Approximately 24 weeks after the initial administration of carcinogen, the animals are sacrificed and pulmonary adenomas counted. A comparable type of procedure can be used for urethane, uracil mustard, diethylnitrosamine, and a number of other carcinogens (36,37). The precise dose level and number of doses vary with the particular carcinogen employed. In some instances, as with urethane, only a single administration is required to give a large enough number of pulmonary adenomas for a valid

TABLE 1. *Inhibition of carcinogen-induced neoplasia by BHA, BHT, and Ethoxyquin*

Carcinogen	Antioxidant	Species	Site of neoplasm inhibited	Ref.
BP	BHA, ethoxyquin[a]	Mouse	Lung	37
BP	BHA, BHT	Mouse	Forestomach	35
DMBA	BHA, ethoxyquin	Mouse	Forestomach	35
DMBA	BHA, BHT	Mouse	Skin	30
DMBA	BHA, BHT, ethoxyquin	Rat	Breast	35
DMBA	BHA	Mouse	Lung	37
7-Hydroxymethyl-12-methyl-benz(*a*)anthracene	BHA	Mouse	Lung	37
Dibenz(*a,h*)anthracene	BHA	Mouse	Lung	37
DENA	BHA, ethoxyquin	Mouse	Lung	36
4-Nitroquinoline-*N*-oxide	BHA, ethoxyquin	Mouse	Lung	36
Uracil mustard	BHA	Mouse	Lung	37
Urethane	BHA	Mouse	Lung	37
FAA	BHT	Rat	Liver	33
N-OH-FAA	BHT	Rat	Liver, breast	33
Azoxymethane	BHT	Rat	Large intestine	45

[a] Unpublished observations.

TABLE 2. *Inhibition of carcinogen-induced neoplasia by sulfur-containing compounds and selenium and selenium salts*

Carcinogen	Inhibitor[a]	Species	Site of neoplasm inhibited	Ref.[a]
BP	Disulfiram[1,2], bis(ethylxanthogen)[3], 2-chloroallyl-diethyldithiocarbamate[3], S-propyl dipropylthiocarbamate[3]	Mouse	Forestomach	3[1],38[2],41[3]
DMBA	Cysteamine[4], disulfiram[5]	Rat	Breast	16[4],38[5]
1,2-Dimethylhydrazine	Sodium selenite[6], disulfiram[7], diethyldithiocarbamate[8], bis(ethylxanthogen)[8], carbon disulfide[9]	Mouse	Large intestine	13[6],39[7],41[7,8], 44[9]
Azoxymethane	Sodium selenite[10], disulfiram[11]	Mouse	Large intestine	13[10],41[11]
FAA	Sodium selenite	Rat	Liver, Breast	9
3'-Methyl-4-dimethylamino-azobenzene	Sodium selenite, selenium	Rat	Liver	8

[a]Superscript numbers refer to the references designated in the last column of this table.

testing. For carcinogens that are less potent in terms of their effects on the mouse lung, a sizable number of administrations may be required.

The forestomach of the mouse is sensitive to a number of carcinogens (2,22). This experimental model has been found to be useful for the study of inhibitors of chemical carcinogens. A typical protocol entails the administration of eight doses of BP by oral intubation. Two doses of the carcinogen are given per week for 4 weeks. Approximately 20 weeks after the initial dose of carcinogen, the experiment is terminated and the number of neoplasms of the forestomach recorded. The substance being tested for its inhibitory capacities can be added to the diet or can be given in the form of discrete administrations at a precise period prior to the carcinogen. Another way in which this model can be employed is to add both the inhibitor and carcinogen to the diet. A number of variations are possible including the use of very low doses of both carcinogen and inhibitor. An additional positive attribute of the model is that the carcinogen and inhibitor both come into direct contact with the target tissue rather than acting at a remote site.

DMBA-induced mammary tumor formation in the female rat is another experimental system that is readily employed to evaluate potential inhibitors of chemical carcinogenesis. This model has been extensively developed by Huggins *et al.* (10,11). It is very simple in that a single oral administration of DMBA will induce mammary tumors in a large percentage of animals within a period of 3 to 6 months, depending upon the particular strain of Sprague Dawley rat or other sensitive strain of rat employed. A single dose of DMBA is usually given. The system can be made more sensitive to inhibitors by using several smaller doses of carcinogen. Compounds being studied for carcinogen-inhibiting properties can be administered either as discrete administrations or they can be added to the diet of animals subsequently subjected to carcinogen challenge. A limitation of the system is that the hormonal status of the animal affects the tumor incidence. If an investigation is directed toward inhibitors that act by virtue of alteration of detoxification mechanisms or some direct interaction with carcinogen metabolites, inadvertant changes that are produced in the hormonal balance might give spurious results.

During the past several years, 1,2-dimethylhydrazine (DMH) and some related compounds have been found to be highly effective in inducing neoplasia of the large bowel in a number of rodent species. The morphology and biology of these neoplasms closely resemble their human counterpart. Since cancer of the large bowel is an important neoplasm in man, an experimental model simulating that of the human disease is of considerable interest. A simple procedure for obtaining large bowel neoplasms has been worked out in the mouse. This entails subcutaneous administration of DMH given at weekly intervals (32,39). In studies of inhibitors of DMH-induced large bowel neoplasia, the compound under investigation, generally is added to the diet. However, it would also be possible to give the test substance as discrete administrations at some designated time prior to the carcinogen administration. Within a period of 6 to 9 months following the initial dose of DMH, neoplasms of the large intestine are present in a large proportion of the animals subjected to this regime. In the mouse, the vast majority of the tumors occur in the rectum and adjacent portion of the distal colon. A number of variations of this experimental procedure are possible. In place of DMH, two of its oxidative metabolites which are carcinogenic have been employed. These are azoxymethane and methylazoxymethanol (MAM) administered as the acetate (45). A further variation is to use a direct-acting carcinogen, i.e., one not requiring metabolic activation, and to administer it by the intrarectal route (19,21).

An additional experimental model that can be employed for the study of inhibitors is carcinogen-induced epidermal neoplasia in the mouse. Both the carcinogen and the inhibitor can be administered topically. This experimental system has several advantages. The materials under investigation can be applied directly to the target tissue and the neoplastic response followed readily by visualization. However, there are some disadvantages. One of these is that the carcinogen reaches the target tissue abruptly at a high concentration and generally dissolves in a solvent which itself might have some effect on the response of the system. Factors such as hair cycle and licking of the skin can alter the results obtained, although these factors can be controlled if care is taken. An additional problem is that some detoxification systems have weak activity in the epidermis so that only low doses of carcinogen can be employed if their capacities are not to be exceeded. In addition to the test systems presented, many other possibilities exist. Their selection would be dependent on factors such as a particular interest in a specific target tissue and/or carcinogen. Some of the considerations discussed in the models described above may serve as guides for constructing effective new test procedures.

INHIBITION OF CARCINOGENESIS BY ANTIOXIDANTS

Butylated Hydroxyanisole, Butylated Hydroxytoluene, and Ethoxyquin

Several antioxidants have been found to inhibit the effects of a substantial variety of chemical carcinogens (Fig. 1). The most extensive work of this type has been done with phenolic antioxidants, in particular, butylated hydroxyanisole (BHA) and butylated hydroxytoluene (BHT) (Table 1). Inhibition occurs under a number of experimental conditions (30,33,35–37,44). It has been found in situations where the route of carcinogen administration results in direct contact of carcinogen with the target tissue. A number of experiments have been carried out in which BHA or BHT were added to diets and polycyclic aromatic hydrocarbon carcinogens such as BP and DMBA were given either in the diet or by oral intubation. In these studies the target tissue in which neoplasia occurred was the forestomach. Those animals that received BHA or BHT in the diet showed pronounced suppression of neoplasia at this site (Table 1). Comparable levels of inhibition under the same conditions have also been obtained with

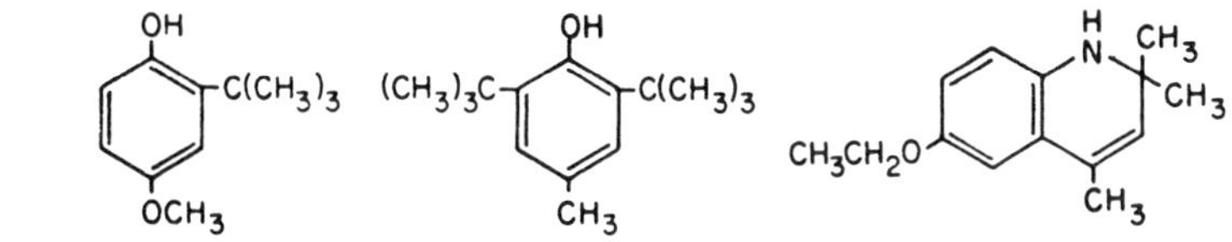

Butylated hydroxyanisole — Butylated hydroxytoluene — Ethoxyquin

$(C_2H_5)_2NC(=S)\text{-}SS\text{-}C(=S)N(C_2H_5)_2$ — Disulfiram

$CH_3CH_2OC(=S)\text{-}SS\text{-}C(=S)\text{-}OCH_2CH_3$ — Bis(ethylxanthogen)

CS_2 — Carbon disulfide

$H_2NCH_2CH_2SH$ — Cysteamine

Na_2Se — Sodium selenide

FIG. 1. Some compounds inhibiting chemical carcinogenesis.

ethoxyquin (Fig. 1), an antioxidant widely used in commercial animal diets but only rarely for human food. Suppression of neoplasia is also obtained in experiments in which the carcinogen is acting at a site remote from that of administration, i.e., inhibition of pulmonary neoplasia in experiments in which the carcinogen is given by oral intubation (37).

BHA and BHT are of interest because of their extensive use as additives in food for human consumption. Of the two compounds, BHA is preferable because it is considerably less toxic than BHT. Studies in mice have been carried out in which BHA and BHT were added to the diet along with BP, a carcinogen widely encountered in the environment. At a concentration of either antioxidant of 5 mg/g diet, inhibition of the carcinogenic effect on the forestomach of the mouse of a concentration of BP of 1 mg/g diet occurs (35). In the United States, the human consumption of phenolic antioxidants is of the order of magnitude of several milligrams a day. Assuming that the results of the animal experiments hold for man, this amount of the antioxidants could be of importance in inhibiting the effects of chronic exposure to low doses of carcinogens, the type of exposure which is most likely to occur in human populations.

In an early investigation, BHT was found to inhibit the carcinogenic effects of *N*-2-fluorenylacetamide (FAA) and *N*-hydroxy-*N*-2-fluorenylacetamide (N-OH-FAA) (33). It was found that administration of BHT in the diet led to an excretion in the urine of a larger percentage of each carcinogen. This higher level of excretion was accounted for chiefly by glucuronic acid conjugates. Animals receiving BHT showed lower levels of radioactivity in blood, liver, and liver DNA 48 hr after injection with labeled carcinogen. It was concluded that BHT increases detoxification of FAA and N-OH-FAA, thus lowering the amount available for activation reactions.

More recently, work has been carried out to determine the mechanism of inhibition of BP-induced carcinogenesis by BHA. Several possibilities were considered which can be divided into two major categories. The first involves direct chemical interaction between antioxidant and reactive species of carcinogen. The second possibility is that the antioxidant is acting in an indirect manner. Of primary interest in the latter regard is alteration of enzyme activity. Both types of mechanisms have been under investigation. Data obtained thus far show that BHA administration produces enzyme alterations that appear to be consistent with its inhibitory effects.

BP is metabolized by the microsomal mixed function oxidase system which acts upon a wide variety of xenobiotic compounds including polycyclic aromatic hydrocarbons. Reactive metabolites as well as detoxification products are produced. The effects of dietary administration of BHA on microsomal metabolism of BP have been studied, employing experimental conditions similar to those in which BHA inhibits neoplasia caused by this carcinogen. Incubation of BP and DNA with liver microsomes from the BHA-fed mice results in approximately one-half the binding of BP metabolites to DNA as compared to that found employing microsomes from control mice (31). Studies of a comparable nature have been carried out by Slaga and Bracken (30) employing mouse skin. In this work, BHA or BHT was applied topically. The animals were sacrificed 3 or 5 hr later, and the binding of [³H]BP or [³H]DMBA to DNA determined in epidermal homogenates. Both carcinogens showed approximately one-half as much binding to DNA in homogenates from mice which had received BHA or BHT 3 hr before death than in homogenates from control mice. The inhibition of binding was still apparent at 12 hr but of a lesser order of magnitude.

Investigations have been undertaken to determine if differences in metabolites of BP are formed when this carcinogen is incubated with liver microsomes prepared from BHA-fed and control female A/HeJ mice. The metabolites were extracted from the incubation mixture and analyzed by high-pressure liquid chromatography. Of major interest were the effects of BHA feeding on epoxide formation. BP-4,5-oxide was isolated and identified. It was present in both the BHA-fed and control microsomal incubations but was substantially reduced in the former. Because of instability, BP-9,10-oxide and BP-7,8-oxide cannot be determined directly. However, data based on summation of diols and phenols resulting respectively from the enzymatic and spontaneous conversions of these oxides indicate that they are present in reduced amounts in the microsomal incubations from BHA-fed mice. 3-Hydroxybenzo(a)pyrene (3-HOBP) was the major metabolite in microsomal incubations from BHA-fed and control mice. This metabolite constituted a significantly higher percentage of the total metabolites formed on incubating BP with microsomes from BHA-fed as compared to control mice. Thus BHA administration causes two metabolic alterations which could result in its exerting an inhibitory effect on BP-induced carcinogenesis. The first is a decrease in epoxidation, which is an activation process, and the second is an increase in 3-HOBP, a metabolite of detoxification (15).

Disulfiram and Related Compounds

Experimental studies of the capacity of disulfiram (Antabuse, tetraethylthiuram disulfide) (Fig. 1) and some related compounds to inhibit chemical carcinogenesis have been carried out using the same experimental models employed for the phenolic antioxidants. Like the phenolic antioxidants and ethoxyquin, disulfiram in the diet will inhibit neoplasia under conditions where the route of administration of the carcinogen results in direct contact with the target tissue. It is a potent inhibitor of BP-induced neoplasia of the forestomach (Table 2). This experimental model is being used in studies of mechanism of inhibition. Work carried out thus far has shown that administration of disulfiram in the diet results in an inhibition of binding of [^{3}H]BP and [^{14}C]BP to DNA, RNA, and protein of the forestomach (3). Inhibition of carcinogenesis occurring at a site remote from that of administration of the carcinogen is brought about by disulfiram. Thus, this compound will inhibit mammary tumor formation in the rat resulting from oral administration of DMBA (38). However, unlike BHA, BP-induced pulmonary neoplasia in the mouse is not inhibited by disulfiram.

Disulfiram and its reduction product, diethyldithiocarbamate, are exceedingly interesting in their effects on carcinogen-induced neoplasia of the large intestine. In experiments of this nature, both disulfiram and diethyldithiocarbamate profoundly inhibit large bowel neoplasia resulting from subcutaneous administration of DMH (39,41). Work has been carried out with azoxymethane, an oxidative metabolite of DMH. This compound also produces neoplasia of the large intestine. Under experimental conditions comparable to those used for DMH, addition of disulfiram to the diet inhibits azoxymethane-induced neoplasia of the large intestine but to a considerably lesser extent than it inhibits DMH (41).

Studies bearing on the mechanism of inhibition of DMH-induced neoplasia of the large bowel have shown that both disulfiram and diethyldithiocarbamate inhibit the oxidation of this carcinogen *in vivo* (5–7). Work has been carried out bearing on the question as to whether the intact molecule of disulfiram is the inhibitor or if a metabolite of this compound is the active species. These investigations have demonstrated that carbon disulfide (CS_2) (Fig. 1), a metabolite of disulfiram, inhibits the oxidation of DMH (5–7). Likewise, it was found that oral administration of CS_2, 4 hr prior to subcutaneous injection of DMH, inhibits neoplasia of the large bowel (L. W. Wattenberg and E. S. Fiala, *unpublished data*). The data obtained suggest that CS_2 may be the chemical species responsible for the inhibitory action of disulfiram and diethyldithiocarbamate on DMH-induced large bowel neoplasia. In work carried out by others, it has been reported that incubation of microsomes with CS_2 in the presence of reduced nicotinamide adenine dinucleotide phosphate (NADPH) results in covalent binding of the sulfur to the microsomes. There is an accompanying decrease in cytochrome P-450 as measured spectroscopically (4,12,20). Several thionosulfur-containing compounds, including disulfiram and diethyldithiocarbamate, produce a similar decrease in cytochrome P-450 when incubated with microsomes under comparable conditions (12). This raises the possibility that thionosulfur-containing compounds as a group may have the capacity to modify cytochrome P-450 so as to alter the microsomal metabolism of DMH and possibly other carcinogens in a manner that decreases their carcinogenicity.

The carcinogen-inhibiting effects brought about by disulfiram and diethyldithiocarbamate have drawn attention to the possibility that a number of widely used pesticides having dithiocarbamate or thiocarbamate groups might have similar properties. Several have been tested for their capacity to inhibit chemical carcinogenesis. Two of these when added to the diet were found to inhibit BP-induced neoplasia of the forestomach of the mouse. These are S-propyl dipropyl thiocarbamate (Vernolate) and 2-chloroallyl diethyldithiocarbamate (CDEC). An additional pesticide, bis(ethylxanthogen) (Bexide), was also found to exert an inhibitory effect in this test system. Bis(ethylxanthogen) is the only one of these pesticides studied thus far for its effects on DMH-induced neoplasia of the large bowel. When added to the diet at a level of 5 mg/g, it completely inhibited DMH-induced large bowel neoplasia and at a level of 1 mg/g it reduced the number of animals bearing large bowel tumors to approximately one-half that occurring in the control group. Its inhibitory potency is of a similar order of magnitude to that of disulfiram (41).

Bis(ethylxanthogen) has a feature that makes it of particular interest. The molecule does not contain nitrogen (Fig. 1). This is of importance since structurally similar dithiocarbamate pesticides have been shown to form nitrosamines representing a hazard not occurring with bis(ethylxanthogen). A second relationship between disulfiram and nitrosamines has been reported recently (23). These investigators have found that disulfiram influences the organotropy of diethylnitrosamine (DENA) and dimethylnitrosamine (DMNA). In the case of DENA, disulfiram added to the diet inhibits liver tumor formation but enhances neoplasia of the esophagus. With DMNA, suppression of neoplasia of the liver is again found but there is an increase in tumors of the paranasal sinuses.

Selenium and Selenium Salts

Inhibition of chemical carcinogenesis by selenium salts (Table 2) has been reported. In an initial paper, the experimental system employed consisted of initiation of epidermal neoplasia with DMBA, followed by promotion with croton oil. Sodium selenide (Fig. 1) added to the croton oil suppressed the development of skin tumors (24). In a subsequent paper, repeated applications of 3-methylcholanthrene (MC) to the skin were carried out. Again, addition of sodium selenide inhibited epidermal neoplasia. In a further experiment, mice were placed on a selenium-deficient diet (Torula yeast) without supplements or with added sodium selenide or sodium selenite. BP was applied to the skin daily to produce epidermal neoplasia. Under these conditions a slight inhibition was found with both of the selenium salts (25). In other investigations, experiments were performed in which rats were placed on a selenium-deficient diet without supplement or with added amounts of selenite. The various groups of rats were given FAA in the diet and the neoplastic response recorded. Animals given selenite showed a partial inhibition of FAA-induced neoplasia of the liver and breast (9). In further work, it has been shown that addition of sodium selenite to the drinking water will inhibit large-bowel neoplasia in the rat resulting from administration of DMH or MAM acetate (13). In these experiments, the rats were fed a conventional diet rather than one deficient in selenium as in the previous work cited. In addition, inhibition of 3′-methyl-4-dimethylaminoazobenzene-induced neoplasia of the liver also has been reported to be brought about by addition of sodium selenite to the drinking water or addition of selenium itself to the diet. In these experiments the rats were fed a commercial diet (8). *In vitro* studies have shown that selenium salts will inhibit mutagenic effect of FAA and its derivatives and carcinogen-induced chromosomal breakage (14,27).

Evidence has been presented showing that there was an inverse relationship between selenium content of the soil and of forage crops and human cancer death rates in the United States and Canada in 1965. Likewise, an inverse relationship between human blood levels of selenium and human cancer death rates in several cities was found (26).

Cysteamine-HCl

Cysteamine-HCl (Fig. 1) has been shown to inhibit DMBA-induced mammary tumor formation in experiments in which the carcinogen was administered intravenously and the antioxidant i.p. In further work, the effects of this compound were studied on mouse fibroblasts (M2 line) in culture. Addition of cysteamine-HCl prior to or after addition of DMBA did not affect toxicity; however, this compound did reduce the number of transformed foci (16).

DISCUSSION

The information on the mechanisms whereby various inhibitors exert their effects is incomplete. Some data are available. In the case of BHA inhibition of BP-induced neoplasia, the antioxidant alters microsomal mixed-function oxidase activity. Likewise, the inhibition of DMH oxidation by disulfiram and related compounds is probably due to an effect on microsomal enzyme activity. Studies of inhibition of FAA-induced neoplasia by BHT indicate that increased conjugation may be the mechanism of inhibition in this instance. Thus, the data that are available implicate altered enzyme activity as one general category of inhibitory mechanism. Obviously, considerable additional work is required and is very critical. With an understanding of mechanisms, it is likely that predictions could be made as to which compounds might be inhibitors. Thus identification of additional environmental constituents having the capacity to inhibit chemical carcinogenesis would be facilitated. Furthermore, an understanding of mechanisms might provide a means of directly assessing the susceptibility of individuals as opposed to efforts at such assessment on the basis of estimates of their intake of inhibitors. Finally, a knowledge of mechanisms would provide a basis for possibly developing effective means of stimulating increased host defense against chemical carcinogens.

One of the important problems that exists with regard to inhibitors of chemical carcinogenesis is toxicity. Inhibitors range from compounds that are very toxic to compounds such as BHA with low toxicity. At least some noxious properties can be separated away from those required for inhibition. Thus, amongst phenolic antioxidants BHA is considerably less toxic than BHT and is a more effective inhibitor. As more is learned about the basic requirements for inhibition, it is likely that compounds with increasing inhibitory potency and fewer side effects can be found. It is important to stress this point since the inhibitors that are currently available are a first-generation group. Many have been discovered by chance. If a particular mechanism was being explored, compounds that were readily available were used. With more complete information it should be possible to design inhibitors in which unnecessary biological activities are peeled away providing less toxic and more effective compounds.

ACKNOWLEDGMENTS

Work cited from the author's laboratory was supported by Contract CP-33364 and Research Grants CA-14146, CA-09599, and CA-15638 all from the National Cancer Institute.

REFERENCES

1. Ames, B. N., McCann, J., and Yamasaki, E. (1975): Methods for detecting carcinogens and mutagens with the salmonella/mammalian-microsomes mutagenicity test. *Mutat. Res.,* 31:347–364.
2. Berenblum, I., and Haran, N. (1955): The influence of dose of carcinogen, emptiness of the stomach, and other factors on tumor induction in the forestomach of the mouse. *Cancer Res.,* 15:504–509.
3. Borchert, P., and Wattenberg, L. W. (1976): Inhibition of macromolecular binding of benzo(a)pyrene and inhibition of neoplasia by disulfiram in the mouse forestomach. *J. Natl. Cancer Inst.,* 57:173–179.
4. DeMatteis, F. (1974): Covalent binding of sulfur to microsomes and loss of cytochrome P-450 during the oxidative desulfuration of several chemicals. *Mol. Pharmacol.,* 10:849–854.
5. Fiala, E. S., and Weisburger, J. H. (1976): In vivo metabolism of the colon carcinogen 1,2-dimethylhydrazine and the effects of disulfiram. *Proc. Am. Assoc. Cancer Res.,* 17:58.
6. Fiala, E. S., Bobotas, G., Kulakis, C., and Weisburger, J. H. (1976): Inhibition of 1,2-dimethylhydrazine metabolism by disulfiram. *Xenobiotica,* 7:5.

7. Fiala, E. S., Bobotas, G., Kulakis, C., Wattenberg, L. W., and Weisburger, J. H. (1977): The effects of disulfiram and related compounds on the *in vivo* metabolism of the colon carcinogen 1,2-dimethylhydrazine. *Biochem. Pharmacol.,* 26:1763–1768.

8. Griffin, A. C., and Jacobs, M. M. (1977): Effects of selenium on azo dye hepatocarcinogenesis. *Cancer Lett.,* 3:177–181.

9. Harr, J. R., Exon, J. H., Whanger, P. D., and Weswig, P. H. (1972): Effects of dietary selenium on N-2-fluorenylacetamide (FAA)-induced cancer in vitamin E supplemented, selenium depleted rats. *Clin. Toxicol.,* 5:187–194.

10. Huggins, C., Grand, L. C., and Brillantes, F. P. (1961): Mammary cancer induced by a single feeding of polynuclear hydrocarbons, and its suppression. *Nature,* 189:204–207.

11. Huggins, C., Lorraine, G., and Fukunishi, R. (1964): Aromatic influences on the yields of mammary cancers following administration of 7,12-dimethylbenz(a)anthracene. *Proc. Natl. Acad. Sci. USA,* 51:737–741.

12. Hunter, A. L., and Neal, R. A. (1975): Inhibition of hepatic mixed-function oxidase activity in vitro and in vivo by various thiono-sulfur-containing compounds. *Biomed. Pharmacol.,* 24:2199–2205.

13. Jacobs, M. N., Jansson, B., and Griffin, A. C. (1977): Inhibitory effects of selenium on 1,2-dimethylhydrazine and methylazoxymethanol acetate induction of colon tumors. *Cancers Lett.,* 2:133–138.

14. Jacobs, M. M., Matney, T. S., and Griffin, A. C. (1977): Inhibitory effects of selenium on the mutagenicity of 2-acetylaminofluorene (AFF) and AFF derivatives. *Cancer Lett.,* 2:319–322.

15. Lam, L. K. T., and Wattenberg, L. (1977): Effects of butylated hydroxyanisole on the metabolism of benzo(a)pyrene by mouse liver microsomes. *J. Natl. Cancer Inst.,* 58:413–417.

16. Marquardt, H., Sapozink, M., and Zedeck, M. (1974): Inhibition by cysteamine-HCl on oncogenesis induced by 7,12-dimethylbenz(a)anthracene without affecting toxicity. *Cancer Res.,* 34:3387–3390.

17. Miller, E. C., and Miller, J. A. (1974): Biochemical mechanisms of chemical carcinogenesis. In: *The Molecular Biology of Cancer,* edited by H. Busch, pp. 377–402. Academic Press, New York.

18. Miller, J. A., and Miller, E. C. (1974): Some current thresholds of research in chemical carcinogenesis. In: *Chemical Carcinogenesis,* edited by P. O. Ts'o and J. A. Dipaolo, pp. 61–85. Marcel Dekker, Inc., New York.

19. Narisawa, T., Wong, C. Q., Maronpot, R. R., and Weisburger, J. H. (1976): Large bowel carcinogenesis in mice and rats by several intrarectal doses of methylnitrosourea and negative effects of nitrite plus methylurea. *Cancer Res.,* 36:505–510.

20. Norman, B. J., Poore, R. E., and Neal, R. A. (1974): Studies of the binding of sulfur released in the mixed-function oxidase-catalyzed metabolism of diethyl p-nitrophenyl phosphorothionate (Parathion) to diethyl p-nitrophenyl phosphate (Paraoxon). *Biochem. Pharmacol.,* 23:1733–1744.

21. Reddy, B. S., Weisburger, J. H., Narisawa, T., and Wynder, E. H. (1974): Colon carcinogenesis in germfree rats with 1,2-dimethylhydrazine and N-methyl-N'-nitro-N-nitrosoguanidine. *Cancer Res.,* 34:2368–2372.

22. Rigdon, R. H., and Neal, J. (1966): Gastric carcinomas and pulmonary adenomas in mice fed benzo(a)pyrene. *Tex. Rep. Biol. Med.,* 24:195–207.

23. Schmähl, D., Krüger, F. W., Habs, M., and Diehl, B. (1976): Influence of disulfiram on the organotropy of the carcinogenic effect of dimethylnitrosamine and diethylnitrosamine in rats. *Z. Krebsforsch.,* 85:271–276.

24. Shamberger, R. J. (1966): Protection against cocarcinogenesis by antioxidants. *Experientia,* 22:116.

25. Shamberger, R. J. (1970): Relationship of selenium to cancer. I. Inhibitory effect of selenium on carcinogenesis. *J. Natl. Cancer Inst.,* 44:931–936.

26. Shamberger, R., and Willis, C. (1971): Selenium distribution and human cancer mortality. *Clin. Lab. Sci.,* 2:211–221.

27. Shamberger, R. M., Baughman, F. F., Kalchert, S. L., Willis, C. E., and Hoffman, G. C. (1973): Carcinogen-induced chromosomal breakage decreased by antioxidants. *Proc. Natl. Acad. Sci. USA,* 70:1461–1463.

28. Shimkin, M. B. (1940): Induced pulmonary tumors in mice. II. Reaction of lungs of strain A mice to carcinogenic hydrocarbons. *Arch. Pathol.,* 29:239 255.

29. Shimkin, M. B. (1955): Pulmonary tumors in experimental animals. *Adv. Cancer Res.,* 3:223–267.

30. Slaga, T. J., and Bracken, W. M. (1977): The effects of antioxidants on skin tumor initiation and aryl hydrocarbon hydroxylase. *Cancer Res.*, 37:1631–1635.
31. Speier, J., and Wattenberg, L. (1975): Alteration in microsomal metabolism of benzo(a)pyrene in mice fed butylated hydroxyanisole. *J. Natl. Cancer Inst.*, 55:469–472.
32. Thurnherr, N., Deschner, E. E., Stonehill, E. H., and Lipkin, M. (1973): Induction of adenocarcinomas of the colon in mice by weekly injections of 1,2-dimethylhydrazine. *Cancer Res.*, 33:940–945.
33. Ulland, B., Weisburger, J., Yammamoto, R., and Weisburger, E. (1973): Antioxidants and carcinogenesis: Butylated hydroxytoluene, but not diphenyl-p-phenylene diamine, inhibits cancer induction by N-2-fluorenylacetamide and by N-hydroxy-N-2-fluorenylacetamide in rats. *Food Cosmet. Toxicol.*, 11:199.
34. Wattenberg, L. W. (1966): Chemoprophylaxis of carcinogenesis: A review. *Cancer Res.*, 26:1520–1526.
35. Wattenberg, L. W. (1972): Inhibition of carcinogenic and toxic effects of polycyclic hydrocarbons by phenolic antioxidants and ethoxyquin. *J. Natl. Cancer Inst.*, 48:1425–1430.
36. Wattenberg, L. W. (1972): Inhibition of carcinogenic effects of diethylnitrosamine and 4-nitroquinoline-N-oxide by antioxidants. *Fed. Proc.*, 31:633.
37. Wattenberg, L. W. (1973): Inhibition of chemical carcinogen-induced pulmonary neoplasia by butylated hydroxyanisole. *J. Natl. Cancer Inst.*, 50:1541–1544.
38. Wattenberg, L. W. (1974): Inhibition of carcinogenic and toxic effects of polycyclic hydrocarbons by several sulfur-containing compounds. *J. Natl. Cancer Inst.*, 52:1583–1587.
39. Wattenberg, L. W. (1975): Inhibition of dimethylhydrazine-induced neoplasia of the large intestine by disulfiram. *J. Natl. Cancer Inst.*, 54:1005–1006.
40. Wattenberg, L. W. (1976): Inhibition of chemical carcinogenesis by antioxidants and some additional compounds. In: *Fundamentals in Cancer Prevention,* edited by P. N. Magee, S. Takayama, T. Sugimura, and T. Matsushima, pp. 153–166. University Park Press, Baltimore.
41. Wattenberg, L. W., Lam, L. K. T., Fladmoe, A., and Borchert, P. (1977): Inhibitors of colon carcinogenesis. *Cancer,* 40:2435–2445.
42. Wattenberg, L. W. (1978): Inhibitors of chemical carcinogenesis. *Adv. Cancer Res.,* 26:197–223.
43. Wattenberg, L. W. (1978): Inhibition of chemical carcinogenesis. *J. Natl. Cancer Inst.,* 60:11–18.
44. Weisburger, E. K., Evarts, R. P., and Wenk, M. L. (1977): Inhibitory effect of butylated hydroxytoluene (BHT) on intestinal carcinogenesis in rats by azoxymethane. *Food Cosmet. Toxicol.,* 15:139–141.
45. Zedeck, M. S., Sternberg, S. S., McGowan, J., and Poynter, R. W. (1972): Methylazoxymethanol acetate: Induction of tumors and early effects on RNA synthesis. *Fed. Proc.,* 31:1485–1492.

Carcinogenesis, Vol. 5: Modifiers of Chemical Carcinogenesis, edited by T. J. Slaga. Raven Press, New York, 1980.

5

Retinoids and Cancer Prevention

Michael B. Sporn

National Cancer Institute, Bethesda, Maryland 20205

In spite of the widespread occurrence of carcinogens in our environment and the endemic exposure of our population to these carcinogens, most people do not develop invasive malignant disease during their lifetime. Even among the population of heavy cigarette smokers who effectively expose their respiratory epithelium to a potent mixture of carcinogens and promoting agents, the lifetime expectancy of developing invasive lung cancer is less than 10% (9). It is apparent that the body possesses innate, physiological defense mechanisms that protect it from carcinogenesis (4) and that the final practical result, namely whether one does or does not develop invasive malignancy during one's lifetime, is the result of two opposing vectors, the carcinogenic and the anticarcinogenic. Although there may be many physiological contributions to anticarcinogenesis, the innate forces that control normal cell differentiation in target cells would appear to play a particularly important role. Since most malignancy is epithelial in origin, the control of epithelial cell differentiation is a key problem, and one class of substances, the retinoids, have a special role in this area.

The retinoids comprise the class of molecules that include vitamin A alcohol (retinol), vitamin A esters (retinyl acetate and retinyl palmitate), vitamin A aldehyde (retinal), vitamin A acid (retinoic acid), and their various physiological metabolites, as well as synthetic analogs of these substances. They are of unique importance because they are required for maintenance of normal epithelial cell differentiation (31); in their absence proper differentiation of stem cells in epithelia does not occur. This article will cover some recent advances in the use of retinoids for prevention of epithelial cancer; it is not intended to be a comprehensive review. We will discuss the following topics: (a) the rationale for the use of retinoids in cancer prevention, including their role as antipromoting agents; (b) long-term animal studies relating to cancer prevention with retinoids; and (c) the problem of synthesis and evaluation of new retinoids for cancer prevention.

EPITHELIAL TARGET SITES OF RETINOIDS

Since essentially all epithelia require retinoids for normal cell differentiation to occur (17), the anticarcinogenic action of retinoids is germane to most human cancers which include malignancies of the following organ sites: bronchus and trachea, breast, intestine, stomach, esophagus, pancreas, uterus, testis, kidney, bladder, prostate, skin, vagina, and bile ducts. The mechanism of action of retinoids in controlling cell differentiation in these epithelial sites is not well understood at present, although the action of retinoids has a striking resemblance to the control of prostatic cell differentiation by androgenic steroid hormones or to control of uterine cell differentiation by estrogenic steroid hormones. The recent description, isolation, and characterization of several retinoid-binding proteins (2,7,19–21), which are similar to the well-known steroid binding proteins, has further strengthened the hypothesis that retinoids act in a manner resembling the steroids.

The cellular locus of action of retinoids within epithelia is also poorly understood, although the site of action is presumably on stem-cell differentiation. In the absence of retinoids, normal mature epithelial cells are not formed. For example, the highly specialized ciliated and mucus cells of the bronchial epithelium or the transitional cells of the bladder epithelium disappear from their respective epithelia during retinoid deficiency and an alternative pathway of cellular differentiation is seen, namely, the production of flattened squamous cells that produce keratin (11,12). Such keratinized squamous metaplastic lesions are easily reversible by administration of retinoids; the process of reversal of keratinization by retinoids is readily measured *in vitro* in hamster tracheal organ cultures (8,24) or chick embryo skin organ cultures (30) and forms the basis of a quantitative bioassay of potency of retinoids.

The biological effectiveness of retinoids in controlling cell differentiation is not limited to the problem of normal cell differentiation, since retinoids have also been shown to be highly active in reversing the effects of carcinogens in appropriate target epithelia. This has been particularly well documented in studies of mouse prostate organ cultures that have been exposed to carcinogens. The types of carcinogens which have been used include polycyclic hydrocarbons (5,15,16) requiring metabolic activation, as well as direct-acting nitrosamides (5,6). The retinoids are effective even if they are applied after cellular lesions have been caused by the carcinogen; application of retinoids to cultures pretreated with carcinogen results in a disappearance of abnormal, atypical cells and a return to a more normal cellular morphology.

Numerous retinoids have been evaluated in this prostatic organ culture system, and there is a good correlation between the activity of retinoids in controlling cell differentiation in a system that has not been exposed to carcinogens (such as hamster tracheal or chick skin organ cultures) and the activity that is measured in the prostatic system, in which there has been obvious DNA damage caused by a carcinogenic agent. These results strongly suggest that the anticarcinogenic effects of retinoids are related to their fundamental ability to control cell differentiation. Furthermore, the potent activity of retinoids in several organ culture systems also establishes that some of their effects do not need to be mediated through indirect mechanisms, such as the endocrine or immune systems. This is not to state that there may not be synergistic effects between retinoids and endocrine or immune mechanisms in the living animal. However, it is certainly well established by now that the direct effects of retinoids on epithelial target cells may be meaningfully evaluated in defined, isolated, *in vitro* systems in which such synergistic mechanisms play a minimal role.

RETINOIDS AS ANTIPROMOTING AGENTS

The problems of tumor progression and tumor promotion have been intensively studied during the past 30 years and there is an immense literature in this field (22). Particular advances have been made in the elucidation of the structure and activity of the phorbol esters, which are among the most potent tumor-promoting substances known (1). It has been shown that active phorbol esters, such as 12-*O*-tetradecanoyl-phorbol-13-acetate (TPA), cause an immense increase in the activity of ornithine decarboxylase (ODC) in mouse skin, and this increased enzyme activity is believed to be intimately related to the tumor-promoting activity of TPA (18). Recently, the important observation has been made that many retinoids are capable of inhibiting the increase in ODC activity caused by TPA in mouse skin (27). The retinoids are extremely potent in this *in vivo* system; activity can be measured with fractions of 1 nmol retinoic acid (27). A large series of both active and inactive retinoids have been investigated (28), and their activity in mouse skin correlates well with their *in vitro* activity that has been measured in the hamster tracheal organ culture system (reversal of keratinization). Furthermore, a correlation appears to exist between the ability of retinoids to inhibit the biochemical effects of phorbol esters on mouse skin and their ability to inhibit the tumor-promoting effects of phorbol esters in the whole animal (3,28).

Recently, still another system has been described in which retinoids have been shown to inhibit the biological effects of phorbol esters, namely a lymphocyte system in which a mitogenic response initiated by phytohemagglutinin and TPA is blocked by retinoic acid (14). In all of these studies of antagonism of retinoids and phorbol esters, the ultimate biochemical mechanism of retinoid inhibition of tumor promotion is unclear. It has recently been suggested that phorbol esters act as reversible inhibitors of terminal cell differentiation (29). Considering that the retinoids are intrinsic mediators of cell differentiation, one may raise the hypothesis that the phorbol esters exert their promoting activity in epithelial tissues by interfering with the normal biological activity of the retinoids. This does not necessarily imply a direct molecular competition between retinoids and phorbol esters. However, administration of retinoids concomitantly with phorbol esters would appear to stabilize a state of normal cell differentiation and thus block the tumor-promoting effects of the phorbol esters. In this context, the retinoids can truly be considered to be antipromoting agents. The elucidation of the mechanism of antipromoting activity of retinoids and the mechanism of their control of cell differentiation would thus appear to involve similar, if not identical, considerations.

PREVENTION OF EPITHELIAL CANCER IN EXPERIMENTAL ANIMALS WITH RETINOIDS

It has already been shown that retinoids may be used effectively to prevent cancer of the skin, lung, bladder, and breast in experimental animals. Since this literature has been reviewed recently (23,26), it will not be surveyed again here. However, several generalizations should be made, which are illustrated in Fig. 1, which shows the inhibitory effects of retinyl acetate and retinyl methyl ether on the development of mammary cancer in rats that have been pretreated with a single dose of the polycyclic hydrocarbon, 7,12-dimethylbenz*(a)*anthracene (DMBA) (10). First of all, the retinoids are effective in preventing the development of cancer even if they are administered after the process of initiation has been completed. In the experiment shown in Fig. 1, treatment with retinoids

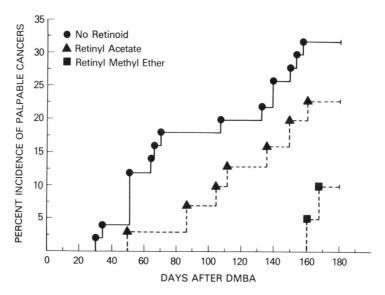

FIG. 1. Effect of retinyl methyl ether and retinyl acetate on time of appearance of palpable mammary cancers confirmed histologically at autopsy. Rats were placed on the various retinoid diets 1 week after the intragastric instillation of 5 mg DMBA. They were palpated for mammary tumors twice weekly for the duration of the experiment, which was terminated at the end of 180 days. The retinoids were fed at the level of 1 mmol/kg of diet. Reprinted with permission from (10).

was not begun until 1 week after the single initiating oral dose of DMBA had been given. By this time there was essentially no free DMBA left in the rat, and the process of initiation had been completed (13). Second, the tumor latency curves shown in Fig. 1 clearly illustrate the antipromoting activity of the retinoids. The retinoids are shown to extend the latency period for development of observable malignancy. If this type of antipromoting activity could be applied in a practical manner to inhibition of human cancer development, it would be of obvious benefit. Extension of latency is a meaningful approach to the human cancer problem; if the latency period for the development of epithelial cancers in man could be doubled, there would be an immense extension of useful, symptom-free life in the human population. Third, the data in Fig. 1 clearly show the superiority of a synthetic retinoid (retinyl methyl ether), as compared to retinyl acetate. There is a definite experimental basis for this finding, since greater effective levels of retinyl methyl ether than of retinyl acetate have been found in the mammary gland, after oral dosing of equivalent molar amounts of these two substances (25). Furthermore, retinyl methyl ether is less toxic than retinyl acetate and can be fed safely in higher doses (32).

By now, it is well established that natural retinoids such as retinyl esters have limited usefulness for cancer prevention because of two critical limitations: (a) natural retinoids may not reach a desired epithelial target site in high enough concentration because of special mechanisms for transport of retinol in the blood and for storage of retinyl esters in the liver, and (b) natural retinoids may cause toxicity if fed chronically in high doses, because of these special mechanisms for storage of retinyl esters in the liver. It is thus clear that the future practical use of retinoids for cancer prevention will depend on the synthesis of new retinoids with better pharmacodynamic, pharmacokinetic, and toxicologic properties. We will conclude this review with a brief consideration of some new advances in this area.

SYNTHESIS AND EVALUATION OF NEW RETINOIDS
FOR CANCER PREVENTION

An immense number of retinoids can theoretically be considered as possible molecules for the organic chemist to synthesize, since it has already been shown that variations in the ring, side chain, or polar terminal group of retinoids all can lead to molecules with useful biological activity (25). The problem then is to develop a logical approach to the question of structure–function relationships, which will enable the most rapid and meaningful evaluation of activity to be made on each new molecule. Although it is obvious that the ultimate utility of any retinoid depends on its properties in the living animal, *in vivo* evaluation is a very expensive and time-consuming method for initial screening of new compounds. For this purpose, we have preferred to take an alternative approach, using *in vitro* methods which are much more rapid, require much less material, and are therefore much less expensive. Accordingly, we have developed new organ culture assays, that have been used to measure desired effects of retinoids on control of cell differentiation, as well as their undesirable toxic effects.

The most practical assay for measurement of the relationship between structure of retinoids and their ability to control normal cell differentiation utilizes tracheal organ cultures (25). Hamster tracheas, maintained *in vitro* in chemically defined, serum-free, retinoid-free medium, undergo epithelial squamous metaplasia and keratinization, which is reversible upon addition of retinoids to the medium. Many retinoids (Fig. 2) have been evaluated in this system for their ability to reverse keratinization (Table 1). Both assays, for desired activity on cell differentiation, and for undesired toxic activity leading to lysis of cartilage, allow construction of quantitative dose-response curves (Fig. 3 and 4), and the relative potencies of different retinoids can be ranked (25). From these assays several conclusions may be drawn:

1. although other ring systems may be substituted for the natural trimethyl-β-cyclohexenyl ring, none has shown greater effectiveness in control of cell differentiation;

2. the presence of a highly polar terminal group, such as a carboxylic acid function, may confer relatively toxic properties on the molecule; and

3. modification of the polar terminal group may be a useful way to diminish toxicity without causing major loss of activity. Since alteration of the polar terminal group also can markedly change the pharmacokinetic properties of a retinoid (25), this would be a particularly useful area of further exploration in synthetic retinoid chemistry.

It is obvious that *in vitro* methods have their intrinsic limitations for assay of activity and toxicity of retinoids. Nevertheless, this type of screening would still appear to offer the best approach for the initial evaluation of milligram amounts of a new molecule. False negatives are extremely rare, since the retinoid is applied directly to the test system, and tracheal epithelium possesses the appropriate enzyme systems which might be required for metabolic activation

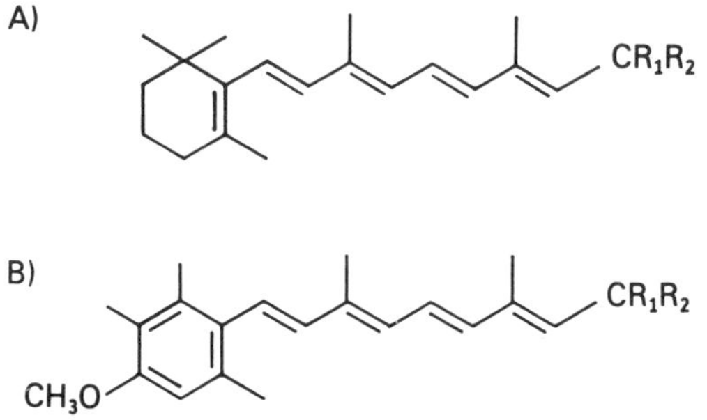

FIG. 2. Structures of retinoids. See Table 1 for activities.

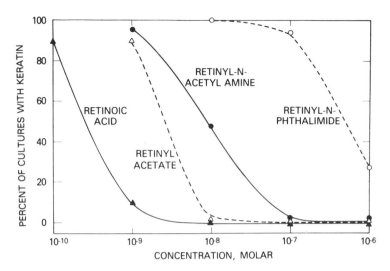

FIG. 3. Dose-response curves for reversal of keratinization in organ cultures of retinoid-deficient tracheal epithelium by application of retinoids. Tracheas (one per culture dish) were treated with retinoids for 7 days before scoring for the presence of both keratin and keratohyaline granules. Similar curves were obtained for all retinoids reported in Table 1, and the ED_{50} was derived from these plots. Numbers of tracheas used in these experiments are shown in Table 1. Reprinted, with permission, from ref. 25.

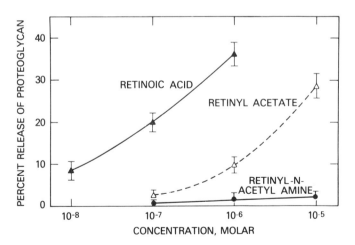

FIG. 4. Dose-response curves for toxic effects of retinoids to tracheal organ culture. Tracheas (one per culture dish) were treated with retinoids for 3 days before measuring both proteoglycan released into the culture medium, and that remaining in the cartilage. Standard error of the mean of measurements is shown. Numbers of tracheas used in these experiments are shown in Table 1. Reprinted, with permission, from ref. 25.

TABLE 1. *Activity of retinoids in tracheal organ culture*[a]

Structure, $R_1 =$, $R_2 =$	Trivial name	Reversal of keratinization, tracheal organ culture, ED_{50} (M) [b]	Toxicity to cartilage, tracheal organ culture, TD_{20} (M) [c]
Figure 2A			
$-H_2$, $-OH$	Retinol	2×10^{-9} (54)[d]	2×10^{-6} (67)
$-H_2$, $-OCH_3$	Retinyl methyl ether	3×10^{-9} (122)	1×10^{-5} (103)
$-H_2$, $-OC_4H_9$	Retinyl butyl ether	3×10^{-8} (55)	Not toxic at 1×10^{-5} (42)
$-H_2$, $-OCOCH_3$	Retinyl acetate	3×10^{-9} (123)	6×10^{-6} (63)
$-H_2$, $-NHCOCH_3$	Retinyl N-acetyl amine	9×10^{-9} (113)	Not toxic at 1×10^{-5} (50)
$-H_2$, $-N(CO)_2C_6H_4$	Retinyl N-phthalimide	5×10^{-7} (49)	Not toxic at 1×10^{-5} (10)
$-H$, $=O$	Retinal	3×10^{-10} (98)	5×10^{-7} (49)
$-H$, $=NNHCOCH_3$	Retinal acetylhydrazone	4×10^{-10} (54)	7×10^{-7} (25)
$-H$, $=NOH$	Retinal oxime	1×10^{-8} (61)	2×10^{-6} (25)
$=O$, $-OH$	Retinoic acid	3×10^{-10} (337)	1×10^{-7} (116)
$=O$, $-OC_2H_5$	Retinoic acid ethyl ester	5×10^{-10} (119)	2×10^{-7} (18)
$=O$, $-NHC_2H_5$	Retinoic acid ethyl amide	2×10^{-9} (52)	9×10^{-7} (32)

		ED_{50}[b]	TD_{20}[c]
—H_2, —OH	TMMP analogue of retinol	2×10^{-8} (48)	9×10^{-7} (34)
—H_2, —OCH_3	TMMP analogue of retinyl methyl ether	3×10^{-8} (70)	4×10^{-6} (57)
=O, —OH	TMMP analogue of retinoic acid	6×10^{-9} (187)	6×10^{-8} (88)
=O, —OC_2H_5	TMMP analogue of retinoic acid ethyl ester	2×10^{-8} (53)	2×10^{-7} (63)
=O, —NHC_2H_5	TMMP analogue of retinoic acid ethyl amide	3×10^{-8} (66)	1×10^{-6} (52)

[a] Reprinted, with permission, from ref. 25.

[b] ED_{50} (M) for reversal of keratinization in tracheal organ culture is the dose for reversal of keratinization in epithelium of 50% of retinoid-deficient hamster tracheas using standard assay conditions (25).

[c] TD_{20} (M) for toxicity to tracheal organ culture is the dose for release of 20% of total proteoglycan from hamster tracheal cartilage into culture medium using standard assay conditions (25).

[d] Numbers of organ cultures used for evaluating each retinoid are shown in parentheses.

of a retinoid. Once compounds have shown desirable properties in these *in vitro* systems, they can then be rationally selected for further evaluation of potentially useful activity in the living animal. Practical application for purposes of cancer prevention can, of course, be determined only in an *in vivo* experimental situation. However, the combination of *in vitro* and *in vivo* testing offers the best approach to development of a useful agent for cancer prevention in man.

ACKNOWLEDGMENTS

I am indebted to my colleagues Nancy Dunlop, Clinton Grubbs, Richard Moon, Dianne Newton, and Joseph Smith for their many contributions to the work reported here. Our collaboration with Hoffmann-La Roche Inc., Nutley, New Jersey, and F. Hoffmann-La Roche and Co., A. G. Basel, Switzerland, has afforded not only the retinoids used in these studies, but also many useful discussions with members of their staff. I also thank Doris Little for valuable secretarial assistance.

REFERENCES

1. Baird, W. M., and Boutwell, R. K. (1971): Tumor promoting activity of phorbol and four diesters of phorbol in mouse skin. *Cancer Res.,* 31:1074–1079.
2. Bashor, M. M., Toft, D. O., and Chytil, F. (1973): *In vitro* binding of retinol to rat-tissue components. *Proc. Natl. Acad. Sci. USA,* 70:3483–3487.
3. Bollag, W. (1972): Prophylaxis of chemically induced benign and malignant epithelial tumors by vitamin A acid (retinoic acid). *Eur. J. Cancer,* 8:689–693.
4. Cairns, J. (1975): Mutation selection and the natural history of cancer. *Nature,* 255:197–200.
5. Chopra, D. P., and Wilkoff, L. J. (1976): Inhibition and reversal by β-retinoic acid of hyperplasia induced in cultured mouse prostate tissue by 3-methylcholanthrene or *N*-methyl-*N'*-nitro-*N*-nitrosoguanidine. *J. Natl. Cancer Inst.,* 56:583–589.
6. Chopra, D. P., and Wilkoff, L. J. (1977): Reversal by vitamin A analogues (retinoids) of hyperplasia induced by *N*-methyl-*N'*-nitro-*N*-nitrosoguanidine in mouse prostate organ cultures. *J. Natl. Cancer Inst.,* 58:923–930.
7. Chytil, F., and Ong, D. E. (1976): Mediation of retinoic acid-induced growth and anti-tumor activity. *Nature,* 260:49–51.
8. Clamon, G. H., Sporn, M. B., Smith, J. M., and Saffiotti, U. (1974): Alpha- and beta-retinyl acetate reverse metaplasias of vitamin A deficiency in hamster trachea in organ culture. *Nature,* 250:64–66.
9. Cutler, S. J., and Loveland, D. B. (1954): The risk of developing lung cancer and its relationship to smoking. *J. Natl. Cancer Inst.,* 15:201–211.
10. Grubbs, C. J., Moon, R. C., Sporn, M. B., and Newton, D. L. (1977): Inhibition of mammary cancer by retinyl methyl ether. *Cancer Res.,* 37:599–602.
11. Harris, C. C., Sporn, M. B., Kaufman, D. G., Smith, J. M., Jackson, F. E., and Saffiotti, U. (1972): Histogenesis of squamous metaplasia in the hamster tracheal epithelium caused by vitamin A deficiency or benzo(a)pyrene-ferric oxide. *J. Natl. Cancer Inst.,* 48:743–761.
12. Hicks, R. M. (1975): The mammalian urinary bladder: An accommodating organ. *Biol. Rev.,* 50:215–246.
13. Janss, D. H., and Moon, R. C. (1970): Uptake and clearance of 9,10-dimethyl-1,2-benzanthracene-9-^{14}C by mammary parenchymal cells of the rat. *Cancer Res.,* 30:473–479.
14. Kensler, T. W., Kajiwara, K., and Mueller, G. C. (1977): Retinoid effects on the phorbol ester-mediated mitogenic response of bovine lymphocytes. *Proc. Am. Assoc. Cancer Res.,* 18:74.
15. Lasnitzki, I. (1955): The influence of A hypervitaminosis on the effect of 20-methylcholanthrene on mouse prostate glands grown *in vitro. Br. J. Cancer,* 9:434–441.

16. Lasnitzki, I., and Goodman, D. S. (1974): Inhibition of the effects of methylcholanthrene on mouse prostate in organ culture by vitamin A and its analogs. *Cancer Res.,* 34:1564–1571.
17. Moore, T. (1967): Effects of vitamin A deficiency in animals. In: *The Vitamins,* 2nd Ed., Vol. 1, edited by W. H. Sebrell and R. S. Harris, pp. 245–266. Academic Press, New York.
18. O'Brien, T. G. (1976): The induction of ornithine decarboxylase as an early, possibly obligatory, event in mouse skin carcinogenesis. *Cancer Res.,* 36:2644–2653.
19. Ong, D. E., and Chytil, F. (1975): Retinoic acid-binding protein in rat tissue: Partial purification and comparison to rat tissue retinol-binding protein. *J. Biol. Chem.,* 250:6113–6117.
20. Sani, B. P., and Hill, D. L. (1976): A retinoic acid-binding protein from chick embryo skin. *Cancer Res.,* 36:409–413.
21. Sani, B. P., and Hill, D. L. (1974): Retinoic acid: A binding protein in chick embryo metatarsal skin. *Biochem. Biophys. Res. Commun.,* 61:1276–1282.
22. Slaga, T. J., Boutwell, R. K., and Sivak, A., editors (1978): *Mechanism of Tumor Promotion and Co-Carcinogenesis.* Raven Press, New York.
23. Sporn, M. B. (1977): Retinoids and carcinogenesis. *Nutr. Rev.,* 35:65–69.
24. Sporn, M. B., Clamon, G. H., Dunlop, N. M., Newton, D. L., Smith, J. M., and Saffiotti, U. (1975): Activity of vitamin A analogs in cell cultures of mouse epidermis and organ cultures of hamster trachea. *Nature,* 253:47–50.
25. Sporn, M. B., Dunlop, N. M., Newton, D. L., and Henderson, W. R. (1976): Relationships between structure and activity of retinoids. *Nature,* 263:110–113.
26. Sporn, M. B., Dunlop, N. M., Newton, D. L., and Smith, J. M. (1976): Prevention of chemical carcinogenesis by vitamin A and its synthetic analogs (retinoids). *Fed. Proc.,* 35:1332–1338.
27. Verma, A. K., and Boutwell, R. K. (1977): Vitamin A acid (retinoic acid), a potent inhibitor of 12-*O*-tetradecanoyl-phorbol-13-acetate-induced ornithine decarboxylase activity in mouse epidermis. *Cancer Res.,* 37:2196–2201.
28. Verma, A. K., Rice, H. M., Shapas, B. G., and Boutwell, R. K. (1978): Inhibition of 12-*O*-tetradecanoylphorbol-13-acetate-induced ornithine decarboxylase activity in mouse epidermis by vitamin A analogs (retinoids). *Cancer Res.,* 38:793–801.
29. Weinstein, I. B., and Wigler, M. (1977): Cell culture studies provide new information on tumour promotors. *Nature,* 270:659–660.
30. Wilkoff, L. J., Peckham, J. C., Dulmadge, E. A., Mowry, R. W., and Chopra, D. P. (1976): Evaluation of vitamin A analogs in modulating epithelial differentiation of 13-day chick embryo metatarsal skin explants. *Cancer Res.,* 36:964–972.
31. Wolbach, S. B., and Howe, P. R. (1925): Tissue changes following deprivation of fat-soluble A vitamin. *J. Exp. Med.,* 42:753–777.
32. Wolbach, S. B., and Maddock, C. L. (1951): Hypervitaminosis A. An adjunct to present methods of vitamin A identification. *Proc. Soc. Exp. Biol. Med.,* 77:825–829.

Carcinogenesis, Vol. 5: Modifiers of Chemical
Carcinogenesis, edited by T. J. Slaga.
Raven Press, New York, 1980.

6

Antiinflammatory Steroids: Potent Inhibitors of Tumor Promotion

Thomas J. Slaga

Cancer and Toxicology Program, Biology Division, Oak Ridge National Laboratory, Oak Ridge, Tennessee 37830

Carcinogenesis studies historically have often considered the induction of neoplastic lesions by single chemicals. Although such studies are valuable for the identification of agents that may have the potential for inducing tumors in man, the actual risk to man from chemicals in his environment is usually the result of multiple exposures to a wide variety of agents. Some of these may not be carcinogenic themselves, but rather act as tumor initiators, cocarcinogens, or modifiers of the carcinogenic process, as in tumor promotion. Table 1 summarizes these various aspects of carcinogenesis. One of the best studied multistep models is the two-stage carcinogenesis system using mouse skin. Skin tumors in mice can be induced by the sequential application of a subthreshold dose of a carcinogen (initiation phase), followed by repetitive treatment with a noncarcinogenic tumor promoter. The initiation phase requires only a single application of either a direct or indirect carcinogen and is essentially irreversible, whereas the promotion phase is initially reversible, later becoming irreversible (55). This system has not only provided an important model for studying carcinogenesis and for bioassaying carcinogenic agents, but is also one of the best

TABLE 1. *Carcinogenesis in man and experimental animals*

Complete carcinogenesis
Cocarcinogenesis
Tumor initiation
Tumor promotion
Additive effects of carcinogens, tumor
  initiators, and tumor promoters
Coinitiating and copromoting agents
Anticarcinogenesis
Antiinitiating and antipromoting agents

systems to investigate the effects of inhibitors of chemical carcinogenesis. One can specifically study the effects of potential inhibitors on both the initiation and promotion phases. This chapter will mainly deal with the effects of inhibitory agents on tumor promotion with emphasis on the potent antiinflammatory steroids. See DiGiovanni, et al., *this volume,* for studies related to modifiers of skin tumor initiation.

INFLAMMATION AND TUMOR PROMOTION

The role of inflammation and cellular proliferation in tumor promotion has been extensively investigated but still remains unclear (4,9,18,21,40,41,44,52). Although most promoters appear to be irritants that induce epidermal hyperplasia (2,5,6,15,21,33,38), not all irritants or inflammatory-hyperplastic agents are promoters (6,21,34,38). There have been several reports concerning the effects of croton oil or phorbol esters on the incorporation of precursors into mouse skin DNA (deoxyribonucleic acid), RNA (ribonucleic acid), and protein (2,33). The tumor-promoting abilities of a series of phorbol esters correlated with their ability to induce a sustained stimulation of RNA, protein, and DNA synthesis in mouse epidermis (1,2). Acetic acid (42) and ethylphenylpropiolate (31,34) were both weak tumor promoters at doses that were able to induce an ordered sequence of metabolic and morphologic changes very similar to those caused by the potent promoter, TPA (1). The above results lead one to conclude that there is no obvious correlation between stimulated macromolecular synthesis or hyperplasia and tumor promotion when the phorbol esters are compared to other hyperplastic agents such as acetic acid and ethylphenylpropiolate.

However, some recent data from this laboratory indicate that a correlation does exist between the saturation of the promoting effect of $P.diC_8$ and the maximum induction of epidermal hyperplasia, as well as between failure to observe promotion and failure to observe hyperplasia (43). When other phorbol esters were compared, our results revealed a strong correlation between the promoting ability of a series of phorbol esters and their ability to induce epidermal hyperplasia: TPA $>$ $P.diC_8$ $\geqslant$ $P.DiC_{10}$ $>$ HPA $\geqslant$ P.dibenz $\geqslant$ $P.diC_{14}$. Furthermore, $P.diC_2$ and phorbol are nonpromoting and do not cause epidermal hyperplasia in female Charles River CD-1 mice.

BIOLOGICAL EFFECTS OF PHORBOL ESTER TUMOR PROMOTERS

In addition to causing epidermal hyperplasia and inflammation, the phorbol esters have several other biological effects. They have been found to alter cell morphology (32) and permeability (59) and to increase phospholipid synthesis (35,49,50), sugar transport (14), ornithine decarboxylase (ODC) activity (28,62), cell transformation by chemical carcinogens in cell culture (26), protease activity in skin (52), and plasminogen activator production in cultured cells (58,61).

The phorbol esters have also been shown to reversibly induce the neoplastic phenotype of normal cells (58) and to enhance mammalian mutagenesis (53). In addition, they decrease cyclic AMP (adenosine-3′,5′-monophosphate) levels and histidase activity in the skin of mice (3,10), decrease large, external, transformation-sensitive (LETS) protein in chicken embryo fibroblast cells (7) and inhibit differentiation in a number of cell systems (12). See Colburn, *this volume,* for details concerning the biological effects of tumor promoters.

INHIBITION OF TUMOR PROMOTION BY STEROIDAL ANTIINFLAMMATORY AGENTS

Belman and Troll (4) showed that a series of steroidal antiinflammatory agents inhibited tumor promotion by croton oil in mouse skin in a dose-dependent manner. The relative potency of these compounds (dexamethasone > Schering No. 11572 > prednisolone > hydrocortisone > cortisone) correlated with their antiinflammatory activities in mouse skin. These investigators also showed that dexamethasone-inhibited croton oil induced epidermal hyperplasia. Cortisone has also been shown to inhibit complete carcinogenesis in mouse skin (16). In separate studies, Nakai (27) demonstrated that the induction of subcutaneous sarcomas in mice by 3-methylcholanthrene was also inhibited by steroids in the following order: dexamethasone > triamcinolone > methylprednesolone > hydrocortisone > cortisone. This effect also correlated with the antiinflammatory potencies of the steroids. Subsequent studies by Scribner and Slaga (41) showed that appropriate doses of dexamethasone completely suppressed tumor promotion in mouse skin by TPA for at least 6 months. Dexamethasone was further found to reduce tumor initiation in mouse skin and carcinogenesis induced by 3-methylcholanthrene alone (51,52).

The antiinflammatory steroids FA, F, and FCA, were later found to be extremely potent inhibitors of tumor promotion in mouse skin (39,56). Table 2 compares the effectiveness of several antiinflammatory steroids in inhibiting tumor promotion. As is quite evident, FA, FCA, and F are much more potent than dexamethasone in inhibiting skin tumor promotion. It is of interest to point out that their antipromoting activity parallels their antiinflammatory activity.

Figure 1 compares the structures of F, FA, FCA, dexamethasone, and cortisol. With the exception that FCA has 9α-fluoro and 11β-dichloro groups, FA and FCA are very similar in structure. The only difference between F and FA is that F has an acetate group on C-21. The major differences observed when comparing the two with dexamethasone are the increased halogenation and the 16,17-acetonide group.

The effects on tumor incidence of five different dosages of FA are shown in Table 3. Simultaneous doses of either 10, 1 or 0.1 μg FA and 2 μg TPA resulted in an almost complete inhibition of tumor promotion both in terms of the number of papillomas per mouse and the percentage of mice with tumors. Follow-

TABLE 2. *Inhibition of TPA tumor promotion in mouse skin by topical treatment with various antiinflammatory steroids*[a]

Modifier	Dose µg	Time to first tumor, weeks	Papillomas per mouse at 30 weeks	% of mice with papillomas at 30 weeks
Acetone	—	6	8.2	88
Tetrahydrocortisol	100	6	8.1	86
Cortisol	100	8	2.4	52
Cortisol	10	6	7.8	84
Dexamethasone	10	8	1.2	36
FA	10	40	0.1	7
F	10	10	0.3	16
FCA	10	17	0.2	10

[a] All mice were treated once with 200 nmol DMBA followed by twice weekly treatments with 2 µg TPA. The steroids were applied simultaneously with TPA at the dose indicated. The percent standard deviation (SD) was less than 20% for all groups.

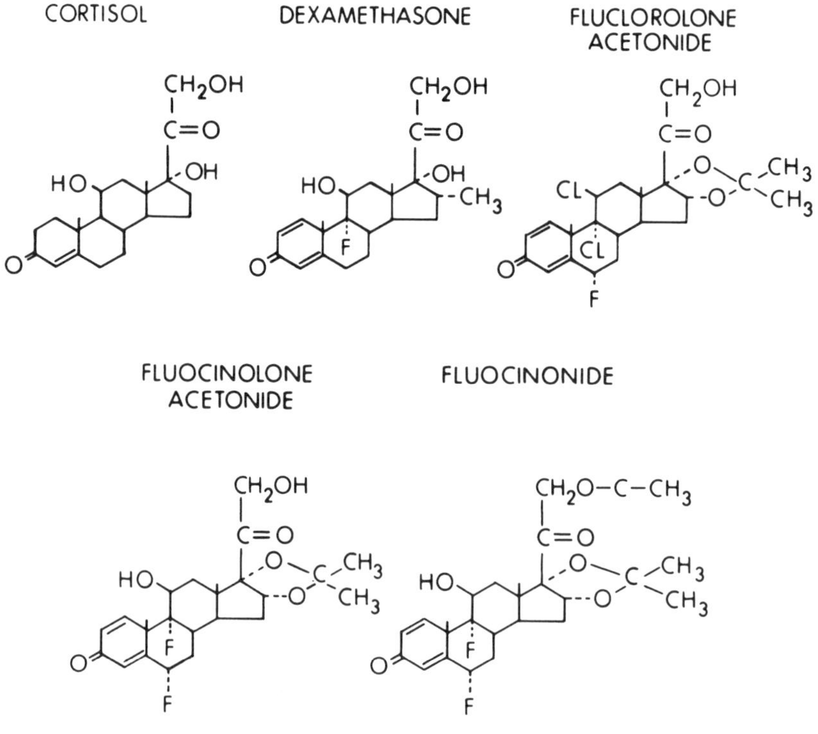

FIG. 1. A comparison of the structures of cortisol, dexamethasone, FCA, F and FA.

TABLE 3. *Dose-response studies on the inhibitory effect of FA on skin tumor promotion in mice[a]*

FA dosage, μg	Time to first tumor[b], weeks	Papillomas per mouse at 30 weeks	% of mice with papillomas at 30 weeks
None (control)	8	6.60	86
0.001	8	6.10	73
0.01	10	1.40	20
0.10	20	0.16	14
1.00	> 40	0.00	0
10.00	24	0.07	10

[a]All mice were treated once with 200 nmol DMBA followed by twice weekly treatments with 2 μg TPA. Various doses of FA were applied simultaneously with TPA. The percent SD was less than 18% for all groups.
[b]Time until > 0.1 papilloma per mouse was observed.

ing the above doses, no carcinomas were found for the duration of the experiment (40 weeks). The 1 μg dose of FA was the most effective in which it completely suppressed tumor promotion. Dose levels of 0.01 and 0.001 μg FA resulted in inhibitions of 82 and 15%, respectively, with respect to the TPA control. Little extension of the latency period was observed at these two lower doses. It is well known that treatment with glucocorticoids can cause weight loss and that caloric restriction itself can inhibit tumor promotion (9). Dexamethasone can produce significant nitrogen catabolism and loss of weight (13). It has also been reported that mice treated with dexamethasone and TPA weighed markedly less than those receiving TPA alone (41), which indicated that this influence may contribute to the antipromoting ability of dexamethasone. In the studies related to the data reported in Table 3, 10 μg FA had a significant effect on body weight; however, this effect was neutralized at dose levels that still had a profound inhibitory effect on tumor promotion.

It is also of interest to point out that an effort was made to determine whether the inhibitory effect of FA was reversible or irreversible. To determine this, mice were initiated with DMBA and promoted simultaneously with TPA and FA for 30 weeks and then the mice received only TPA. The results suggested that the effect of FA was truly reversible (39,56).

Table 4 shows the effect of FA when given topically one day prior to promoter treatment. In addition, a completely saturating initiation dose of DMBA and in some cases a saturating dose of TPA were given in order to determine the effect of FA under these extreme test conditions. FA was found to be an effective inhibitor when given one day prior to each TPA treatment and under saturating initiator-promoter treatment.

Another class of chemicals that have profound inhibitory action on skin tumor promotion and chemical carcinogenesis in general are the vitamin A derivatives (8,48,55,57). Sporn and co-workers have found that certain retinoids are potent

TABLE 4. *Effect of giving FA one day before TPA on skin tumor promotion in mice*[a]

Dose of TPA, µg	Dose of FA, µg	Papillomas per mouse at 16 weeks	% of mice with papillomas at 16 weeks
5	0	20.2	100
5	5	1.6	35
5	1	9.8	75
1	0	14.0	100
1	5	0.4	15
1	1	0.7	18

[a]The mice were initiated with 400 nmol DMBA and promoted twice weekly with either 1 or 5 µg TPA or TPA plus FA. FA was given one day before TPA treatment. The maximum percentage SD for all groups was 22%.

inhibitors of lung, mammary, bladder, and colon carcinogenesis as detailed in Chapter 5 of this volume. Data presented in Table 5 show the effect of varied doses of FA and the vitamin A derivative RO 10–9359 given alone or in combination on two-stage skin tumorigenesis in mice. Both the retinoid and FA provided a dose-dependent inhibition of papilloma formation with FA being more potent in this respect. As can be seen, a combination of FA and the retinoid produced an inhibitory effect on skin tumor promotion greater than that produced by each separately. Such combinations of agents at very low doses (nontoxic doses) may be a rational approach to the chemoprevention of cancer.

TABLE 5. *Effects of FA, vitamin A derivative RO 10–9359 and both FA plus RO 10–9359 on TPA skin tumor promotion in Charles River CD-1 mice*[a]

Experiment	Modifier	Dose µg	Papillomas per mouse at 30 weeks	Percent of control[b]
1	None	—	6.4 ± 1.02	100
2	FA	1.0	0 ± 0	0
3	FA	0.1	0.1 ± 0.12	1
4	FA	0.01	1.3 ± 0.20	18
5	RO 10–9359	100.0	0.4 ± 0.24	6
6	RO 10–9359	10.0	3.1 ± 0.60	48
7	RO 10–9359	1.0	4.3 ± 0.71	67
8	RO 10–9359	0.1	4.9 ± 0.74	76
9	FA + RO 10–9359	0.1 + 1	0 ± 0	0
10	FA + RO 10–9359	0.01 + 1	0.5 ± 0.14	10

[a]The mice were initiated with 200 nmol DMBA and promoted twice weekly with 2 µg TPA plus modifier for 30 weeks. Modifier was given the same time as TPA treatment.
[b]Expressed as a percentage of the DMBA-TPA control.

TABLE 6. *Effects of antiinflammatory steroids on epidermal DNA synthesis*[a]

Antiinflammatory steroid	Dose, μg	Specific activity of DNA (% of controls) at the following times (hr) after treatment [b]			
		12	18	24	48
Tetrahydrocortisol	100	104	97	108	98
Cortisol	100	62	57	76	96
Cortisol	10	90	95	110	107
Dexamethasone	10	45	56	71	102
FA	10	25	14	5	6
F	10	18	6	4	7
FCA	10	29	20	15	12

[a] [³H]thymidine 30 μCi (6 Ci/mmol) was injected 30 min before animals were killed. Each value represents three separate experiments with pooled skins of four mice per experiment.
[b] Specific activity was calculated as dpm/μg DNA and expressed as percent of the value obtained with control mice. The average specific activity for the acetone control was 22.2 dpm/μg DNA. The percent standard deviation was less than 16% in all experiments.

EFFECTS OF ANTIINFLAMMATORY STEROIDS ON EPIDERMAL DNA SYNTHESIS

The steroidal antiinflammatory agents were found to be potent inhibitors of epidermal DNA synthesis (39,46,56). These data are summarized in Table 6. It is apparent that FA, F, and FCA were all very potent inhibitors of epidermal DNA synthesis. The ability of the various steroids shown in Table 6 to inhibit epidermal DNA synthesis correlates with their antiinflammatory ability as well as their ability to inhibit skin tumor promotion.

Table 7 shows the effect of various doses of FA, such as those administered in the tumor experiments, on the incorporation of [³H]thymidine into epidermal DNA. Both the duration and maximum inhibition of DNA synthesis increased with the level of FA applied. Although not shown in Table 7, at the highest two levels of 10 μg and 1 μg FA, inhibition of DNA synthesis was observed 3 hr after treatment, and continued for several days after treatment. In all cases, the inhibition of DNA synthesis caused by FA was followed by a stimulation of DNA synthesis. It is of interest to point out that there appears to be a good dose-response relationship between the ability of FA to inhibit epidermal DNA synthesis and its ability to inhibit skin tumor promotion.

The ability of FA to inhibit epidermal DNA synthesis after the skin was pretreated with 10 μg TPA as a stimulant of DNA synthesis is shown in Table 8. DNA synthesis was 275 and 430% of control levels 24 and 33 hr, respectively, after 10 μg TPA. Administration of 10 μg FA 24 hr after TPA treatment resulted in an inhibition of stimulated DNA synthesis within 6 hr. A 65% inhibition relative to stimulated DNA synthesis was observed 24 hr after FA

TABLE 7. *Effect of a single topical application of various dose levels of FA on epidermal DNA synthesis*[a]

FA dosage, μg	Effect on DNA synthesis	
	Duration, hr[b]	Maximum inhibition, %[c]
None (control)	—	—
0.001	0	29
0.01	9	54
0.10	54	93
1.00	66	95
10.00	150	98

[a][³H]thymidine 30 μCi (6 Ci/mmol) was injected 30 min before animals were killed. Each value represents three separate experiments with pooled skins of four mice per experiment.

[b]Time during which DNA synthesis was 50% or less of control.

[c]DNA synthesis expressed as percent inhibition. The percent SD was less than 14% for all experiments.

treatment as compared to the 98% inhibition seen after 24 hr when 10 μg FA were administered to unstimulated animals. That is, FA was not quite as effective on S-phase as on G-1 cells.

Liver DNA synthesis has also been reported to be inhibited by glucocorticoids (20). However, if the liver is given a potent stimulus to regenerate, as occurs after a partial hepatectomy, glucocorticoids induce only a partial suppression of cell proliferation (20). What causes the liver and epidermis to lose some of their sensitivity to glucocorticoids when given the stimulus to regenerate is unknown.

TABLE 8. *Effect of a single topical application of 10 μg FA on TPA-stimulated epidermal DNA synthesis*[a]

Treatment	Specific activity of DNA (% of controls) at the following times (hr) after treatment[b]				
	27	30	33	36	48
TPA	260	330	440	310	295
TPA + FA	265	125	150	120	100

[a]The FA was administered 24 hr after TPA treatment. [³H]thymidine 30 μCi (6 Ci/mmol) was injected 30 min before animals were killed.

[b]Specific activity was calculated as dpm/μg DNA and expressed as percent of the value obtained with control mice. The percent SD was less than 17% for all experiments.

EFFECTS OF ANTIINFLAMMATORY STEROIDS ON TPA-INDUCED INFLAMMATION AND HYPERPLASIA

The results of topical applications of various antiinflammatory steroids on TPA-induced inflammation and epidermal cell proliferation are shown in Table 9. When FA, FCA, or F were applied simultaneously with TPA in 10 μg doses, they completely counteracted the TPA-induced increase in nucleated IFE (interfollicular epidermal) cell layers, inflammation, and edema, whereas a 10 μg dose of dexamethasone partially counteracted and cortisol and tetrahydrocortisol had no effect at a 10 μg dose level.

The results of topical application at various dose levels of FA on TPA-induced inflammation and epidermal-cell proliferation are shown in Table 10. When FA was applied simultaneously with 10 μg TPA in 10- and 5-μg doses, they completely counteracted the TPA-induced increase in nucleated IFE cell layers, inflammation, and edema. FA was still notably effective at 1 and 0.5 μg but only partially effective at a 0.1 μg dose level. The antiinflammatory steroid fluocinonide, which has the same structure as FA except that it has an acetate group in the 21 position, had similar activity in inhibiting inflammation and hyperplasia as did FA, whereas FCA was slightly less active. Dexamethasone

TABLE 9. *Effects of various topically applied antiinflammatory agents on TPA-induced inflammation and epidermal cellular proliferation* [a]

Secondary treatment [b] antiinflammatory agent	Dose, μg	Nucleated IFE cell layers		Inflammatory index [c]		Edema index [e]
		3 [d]	4 [d]	1 [d]	2 [d]	
None (control)	—	1.5	1.3	0	0	0
None	—	4.6	5.5	4	4	4
FA	10	1.4	1.2	0	0	0
FCA	10	1.7	1.5	1	0	0
F	10	1.6	1.3	0	0	0
Dexamethasone	10	2.2	2.4	1	1	1
Cortisol	10	4.4	5.3	4	4	4
Tetrahydrocortisol	10	4.7	5.6	4	4	4

[a] The number of nucleated IFE cell layers and the inflammatory and edematous indices were determined in 5-μ sections of skin. Each value represents the mean of seven observations. The SD was less than 20% of each value.

A primary treatment of 10 μg TPA was given to induce inflammation and epidermal cellular proliferation in all cases except for the first (control) entry for which acetone, instead of TPA, was used.

[b] Secondary treatment refers to application of the antiinflammatory agent simultaneous with TPA.

[c] The degree of inflammation was classified from 1 to 4, with grade 4 indicating maximal response and zero indicating no effect.

[d] Days posttreatment.

[e] The degree of edema was classified (1 day after treatment) from 1 to 4, with grade 4 representing maximal response and 0 representing no effect.

TABLE 10. *Effects of various dose levels of topically applied FA on TPA-induced inflammation and cellular proliferation*[a]

Secondary treatment		Nucleated IFE cell layers after posttreatment day			Inflammatory index[b] on day 1	Edematous index[b] on day 1
Steroid given	Dose, μg	2	3	4		
None (*)	—	1.3	1.5	1.4	0	0
None	—	3.6	4.7	5.5	4	4
FA	10	1.2	1.4	1.2	0	0
	5	1.4	1.6	1.4	0	0
	1	1.3	1.9	2.1	1	0
	0.5	2.3	2.2	2.4	2	1
	0.1	2.8	2.6	3.0	4	3

[a] The number of nucleated IFE cell layers, and the inflammatory and edematous indices, were determined in 5-μ sections of skin. Each value represents the mean of seven observations. The SD was less than 21% of each value. Primary treatment was TPA in all cases except for the first (*), which was acetone; 10 μg TPA were used to induce inflammation and epidermal cellular proliferation. The secondary treatment refers to application of the steroid simultaneously with the TPA.

[b] The degrees of inflammation and edema were classified from 1 to 4, with grade 4 indicating maximal inflammatory (or edematous) response, and zero indicating no inflammation (or edema).

was less active than FCA. The doses of FA and FCA (0.01 and 0.1 μg, respectively) that were still fairly effective in inhibiting tumor promotion by 2 μg TPA were also fairly effective in counteracting the inflammation and hyperplasia induced by 2 μg TPA.

Table 11 shows the results of applying FA (10 μg) either before, during, or after TPA treatment on TPA-induced epidermal cell proliferation. When FA was given 48, 24, or 4 hr before TPA treatment, FA effectively counteracted the TPA-induced cellular proliferation, whereas, when FA was given 72 hr before, it was without effect. Furthermore, FA was effective when given either simultaneously with or at 4 and 24 hr after TPA treatment; however, it had little effect 48 hr after TPA treatment.

These results support the view that the mechanism by which the steroidal antiinflammatory agents inhibit mouse skin tumor promotion and complete carcinogenesis may be related to their ability to inhibit DNA synthesis. Consequently, this counteracts the induction of inflammation and hyperplasia by tumor promoters and complete carcinogens. Furthermore, based on the results summarized in this chapter as well as other results (4,34,41,56), the antiinflammatory ability of a series of steroids was found to correlate with their ability to inhibit mouse skin tumor promotion by TPA and their ability to counteract TPA-induced hyperplasia (F $\geq$ FA > FCA > dexamethasone > cortisol and tetrahydrocortisol was inactive).

Other glucocorticoids have been shown to inhibit both epidermal mitosis (11,17,22) and DNA synthesis (22,23). Inhibition by glucocorticoids of incorpo-

TABLE 11. *Effect of FA application time (before, during, or after TPA treatment) on TPA-induced epidermal cell proliferation*[a]

Primary treatment	Time of FA treatment in relation to primary treatment	Nucleated IFE cell layers after primary treatment, days		
		2	3	4
Acetone	NA[c]	1.3	1.5	1.5
TPA[b]	NA	3.5	4.6	5.4
	72 hr before	2.5	3.5	4.3
	48 hr before	1.5	2.0	2.3
	24 hr before	1.5	1.7	1.8
	4 hr before	1.4	1.8	1.5
	Same time	1.2	1.4	1.5
	4 hr after	1.8	1.6	1.9
	24 hr after	2.3	2.8	2.8
	48 hr after	—	3.8	4.6

[a] The number of nucleated IFE cell layers was determined in 5-μ sections of skin. Each value represents the mean of seven observations. The SD was less than 18% of each value.
[b] 10 μg of TPA was used to induce epidermal cellular proliferation.
[c] NA = not applicable; no FA treatment given.

ration of radioactive precursors into DNA has also been observed in rat liver (19,30), fibroblasts in culture (29), solid Ehrlich tumor (24), and hepatoma cells in culture (25). The effects of both natural and synthetic steroids on the growth of mouse fibroblasts *in vitro* were studied by Ruhmann and Berliner (36,37). These investigators found that the antiinflammatory ability of a series of steroids correlated with their growth-inhibiting activity (FA $\simeq$ fluocinonide > dexamethasone > prednisolone > cortisol > 11-deoxycortisol, and tetrahydrocortisol was inactive).

EFFECTS OF ANTIINFLAMMATORY STEROIDS ON TPA METABOLISM, CELLULAR BINDING, AND VARIOUS TPA-INDUCED BIOCHEMICAL PARAMETERS

The antiinflammatory steroids have become useful tools in understanding the biochemical mechanism of tumor promotion and chemical carcinogenesis in general. Dexamethasone, FA, F, and FCA were not only found to be potent inhibitors of epidermal DNA synthesis and TPA-induced hyperplasia (39,46,56) but also were found to reduce the levels of several protein fractions on polyacrylamide gels, which were greatly enhanced after TPA treatment (41,45). The binding of phorbol ester tumor promoters to epidermal cytosol receptor protein and chromatin was markedly suppressed by simultaneous treatment with dexamethasone *in vivo* (45). Wigler et al. (60) have found that extremely low concentrations of FA, FCA, F, and dexamethasone were found to markedly inhibit plasminogen-activator production in certain tumor cell cultures (56,60).

On the other hand, TPA proved to be a potent inducer of plasminogen activator in certain cell cultures (61).

When tritiated TPA was applied to mouse skin, the majority of the tritiated product recovered was TPA (98%), indicating only minimal metabolism of TPA and no need for metabolic activation for tumor promotion (47). Slaga et al. (47) reported that FA was without effect on TPA metabolism in mouse skin. *In vitro* metabolism of TPA by epidermal homogenates was likewise unaffected by the addition of FA (47).

CONCLUSION

The information in this review indicates that the antiinflammatory steroids are extremely active inhibitors of the tumor-promoting phorbol esters. The relative antiinflammatory potencies of a series of synthetic fluorinated glucocorticoids have been shown to correlate with their ability: (a) to inhibit mouse skin-tumor promotion by TPA; (b) to counteract TPA-induced skin hyperplasia; and (c) to inhibit epidermal DNA synthesis. The relative potencies of the steroids tested followed the order F > FA > FCA > dexamethasone > cortisol and tetrahydrocortisol was inactive. It is remarkable that the compounds F, FA, and FCA were active on mouse skin at dosages as low as a fraction of a microgram.

Since the precise mechanism of action of TPA and related promoting agents is not known, any discussion of the mechanism of inhibition of tumor promotion by steroidal agents must at the present time be largely speculative. It has recently been emphasized that phorbol ester promoters induce several biological effects in mouse skin or in cell cultures that mimic the phenotype of cells transformed by viral or chemical carcinogens (59). These include: (a) epidermal hyperplasia in mouse skin and increased saturation density of certain cell cultures (43,59); (b) altered cell morphology and membrane permeability (31,60); (c) increased phospholipid synthesis and sugar transport (14,35,49,50); (d) induction of ornithine decarboxylase (28,63); (e) induction of DNA synthesis (63); (f) decreased cellular cyclic AMP, histidase, and LETS levels (3,7,10); (g) induction of plasminogen-activator production (62); (h) cell transformation by chemical carcinogens in cell culture (26); and (i) inhibit terminal differentiation in a number of cell systems (12).

The mechanism by which fluocinolone acetonide and other glucocorticoids inhibit mouse skin tumor promotion and complete carcinogenesis may be related to their ability to inhibit DNA synthesis, which consequently counteracts the induction of hyperplasia induced by tumor promoters and carcinogens.

The antiinflammatory agents definitely do not have an effect on the metabolism of TPA. These agents may also have an effect on the specific cellular binding of TPA. Table 12 summarizes some of the known effects of antiinflammatory steroids. Regardless of the precise underlying mechanism, the results obtained with highly potent synthetic steroids lend encouragement to further explorations of the important area of inhibition of specific stages in the process of carcinogen-

TABLE 12. *Summary: effects of the antiinflammatory steroids*

1. Inhibit tumor promotion
2. Inhibit DNA synthesis
3. Inhibit inflammation induced by phorbol esters
4. Inhibit cell proliferation induced by phorbol esters
5. Inhibit TPA-induced DNA, RNA, and protein synthesis
6. Inhibit *in vivo* binding of phorbol esters to cytosol and chromatin
7. Inhibit induction of certain cytosol proteins by phorbol esters
8. Inhibit plasminogen-activator production
9. Does not counteract the ODC and S-adenyl methionine decarboxylase induced by phorbol esters
10. Does not alter the metabolism of TPA
11. Does not inhibit *in vitro* binding of TPA to cytosol receptor protein
12. Highest specific activity of dexamethasone binding is to chromatin
13. Inhibit TPA induced comitogenesis in lymphocytes
14. Inhibit TPA enhanced comutagenesis

esis. The results of the extremely potent inhibitory effect on tumor promotion of a combination of an antiinflammatory steroid and vitamin A derivative at very low, nontoxic doses are very encouraging in that this may be a rational approach to the prevention of human cancer.

ACKNOWLEDGMENTS

This research was supported in part by NIH Grant CA 20076 and by the Division of Biomedical and Environmental Research, U.S. Department of Energy under contract W-7405-eng-26 with the Union Carbide Corporation.

REFERENCES

1. Baird, W. M., and Boutwell, R. D. (1971): Tumor promoting activity of phorbol and four diesters of phorbol in mouse skin. *Cancer Res.,* 31:1074–1079.
2. Baird, W. M., Sedgwick, J. A., and Boutwell, R. D. (1971): Effects of phorbol and four diesters of phorbol on the incorporation of tritiated precursors into DNA, RNA and protein in mouse epidermis. *Cancer Res.,* 31:1434–1439.
3. Belman, S., and Troll, W. (1974): Phorbol-12-myristate-13-acetate effect on cyclic adenosine-3′,5′-monophosphate levels in mouse skin and inhibition of phorbol-myristate acetate-promoted tumorigenesis. *Cancer Res.,* 34:3446–3455.
4. Belman, S., and Troll, W. (1972): The inhibition of croton oil-promoted mouse skin tumorigenesis by steroid hormones. *Cancer Res.,* 32:450–454.
5. Berenblum, I. (1954): A speculative review: The probable nature of promoting action and its

NOTE: Abbreviations used in this chapter are: TPA, 12-*O*-tetradecanoylphorbol-13-acetate; P.DiC$_8$, phorbol-12,13-dioctanoate; P.diC$_{10}$, phorbol-12,13-didecanoate; HPA, 12-*O*-hexadecanoyl-phorbol-13-acetate; P.diBenz, phorbol-12,13-dibenzoate; P.diC$_{14}$, phorbol-12,13-dimyristate; P.diC$_2$, phorbol-12,13-diacetate; DMBA, 7,12-dimethylbenz*(a)*anthracene; F, fluocinonide, 6α,9α-difluoro-11β,16α,17,21-tetrahydroxypregnan-1,4-diene-3,20-dione, cyclic 16,17-acetal, 21 acetate; FA, fluocinolone acetonide, 6α,9α-difluoro-11β,16α,17,21-tetrahydroxy-pregnan-1,4-diene-3,20-dione, cyclic 16–17-acetal; FCA, fluclorolone acetonide-6α-fluoro-9α,11β-dichloro-16α,17α,21-triolpregnan-1,4-diene-3,20-dione, cyclic 16,17 acetal; IFE, interfollicular epidermis.

significance in the understanding of the mechanism of carcinogenesis. *Cancer Res.,* 14:471–477.

6. Berenblum, I. (1944): Irritation and carcinogenesis. *Arch. Pathol.,* 38:233–244.
7. Blumberg, P. M., Driedger, P. E., and Rossow, P. W. (1976): Effect of phorbol ester on a transformation sensitive surface protein of chick fibroblasts. *Nature,* 264:446–447.
8. Bollag, W., (1975): Prophylaxis of chemically induced epithelial tumors with an aromatic retinoic acid analog (RO 10–9359) *Eur. J. Cancer,* 11:721–724.
9. Boutwell, R., (1964): Some biological aspects of skin carcinogenesis. *Prog. Exp. Tumor Res.,* 4:207–250.
10. Colburn, N. H., Lau, S., and Head, R. (1975): Decrease of epidermal histadase activity by tumor-promoting phorbol esters. *Cancer Res.,* 35:3154–3159.
11. Davis, J. C. (1964): The effect of cortisol on mitosis in the skin of the mouse. *J. Pathol. Bacteriol.,* 88:247–254.
12. Diamond, L., O'Brien, T., and Rovera, G. (1978): Tumor promoters inhibit terminal cell differentiation in culture. In: *Carcinogenesis, Vol. 2, Mechanisms of Tumor Promotion and Cocarcinogenesis,* edited by T. J. Slaga, A. Sivak, and R. K. Boutwell, pp. 335–341. Raven Press, New York.
13. K. Diem, editor (1962): *Geigy Scientific Tables,* 6th Ed., pp. 487–493. Geigy Pharmaceuticals, Ardsley, New York.
14. Driedger, P. E., and Blumberg, P. M. (1977): The effect of phorbol diesters on chicken embryo fibroblasts. *Cancer Res.,* 37:3257–3265.
15. Frei, J. V., and Stephens, P. (1968): The correlation of promotion of tumor growth and of induction of hyperplasia in epidermal two-stage carcinogenesis. *Br. J. Cancer,* 22:83–92.
16. Ghadially, R. N., and Green, H. N. (1954): The effect of cortisone on chemical carcinogenesis in the mouse skin. *Br. J. Cancer,* 8:291–295.
17. Green, H. N., and Ghadially, F. H. (1951): Relation of shock, carbohydrate utilization and cortisone to mitotic activity in the epidermis of the adult male mouse. *Br. Med. J.,* 1:496–498.
18. Gwynn, R. H., and Salamon, N. H. (1953): Studies on cocarcinogenesis. SH-reactors and other substances tested for co-carcinogenic action in mouse skin. *Br. J. Cancer,* 7:482–489.
19. Henderson, I. C., Fischel, R. E., and Loeb, J. N. (1971): Suppression of liver DNA synthesis by cortisone, *Endocrinology,* 88:1471–1476.
20. Henderson, I. C., and Loeb, J. N. (1974): Hormone-induced changes in liver DNA synthesis: Effects of glucocorticoids and growth hormone on liver growth and DNA polymerase activity. *Endocrinology,* 94:1637–1643.
21. Hennings, H., and Boutwell, R. K. (1970): Studies on the mechanism of skin tumor promotion. *Cancer Res.,* 30:312–320.
22. Hennings, H., and Elgjo, K. (1971): Hydrocortisone: Inhibition of DNA synthesis and mitotic rate after local application to mouse epidermis. *Virchows Arch. B,* 8:42–49.
23. Kalkoff, K. W., and Born, W. (1965): Zur Wirkung von Fluocinolonacetonid auf die DNA-synthese in der Epidermis. *Klin. Wochenschr.,* 43:1335–1337.
24. Kodama, M., and Kodama, T. (1970): Effect of steroid hormones on the *in vitro* incorporation of glycine-2-^{14}C into solid Ehrlich tumors, kidney and liver, *Cancer Res.,* 30:228–235.
25. Loeb, J. N., Corek, C., and Young, L. L. (1973): Suppression of DNA synthesis in hepatoma cells exposed to glucocorticoid hormones *in vitro. Proc. Natl. Acad. Sci. USA,* 70:3852–3856.
26. Mondal, S., Brankow, D. W., and Heidelberger, C. (1976): Two-stage chemical oncogenesis in cultures of C3H/10T1/2 cells. *Cancer Res.,* 36:2254–2260.
27. Nakai, T. (1961): Influences of small doses of various corticosteroids on the incidence of chemically induced subcutaneous sarcomas in mice. *Cancer Res.,* 21:221–227.
28. O'Brien, T. G., Simsiman, R. C., and Boutwell, R. K. (1975): Induction of the polyamine biosynthetic enzymes in mouse epidermis by tumor-promoting agents. *Cancer Res.,* 35:1662–1670.
29. Pratt, W. B., and Aronow, L. (1966): The effect of glucocorticoid on protein and nucleic acid synthesis in mouse fibroblast *in vitro. J. Biol. Chem.,* 241:5244–5250.
30. Raab, K. H., and Webb, T. E. (1969): Inhibition of DNA synthesis in regenerating rat liver by hydrocortisone, *Experientia,* 25:1240–1242.
31. Raick, A. N. (1974): Cell proliferation and promoting action in skin carcinogenesis. *Cancer Res.,* 34:920–926.

32. Raick, A. N. (1974): Cell differentiation and tumor-promoting action in skin carcinogenesis. *Cancer Res.,* 34:2915–2925.
33. Raick, A. N. (1973): Ultrastructural, histological and biochemical alterations produced by 12-*O*-tetradecanoyl-phorbol-13-acetate on mouse epidermis and their relevance to skin tumor promotion. *Cancer Res.,* 33:269–286.
34. Raick, A. N., and Burdzy, K. (1973): Ultrastructural and biochemical changes induced in mouse epidermis by a hyperplastic agent, ethylphenylpropiolate. *Cancer Res.,* 33:2221–2230.
35. Rohrschneider, L. R., O'Brien, D. H., and Boutwell, R. K. (1972): The stimulation of phospholipid metabolism in mouse skin following phorbol ester treatment. *Biochim. Biophys. Acta,* 280:57–70.
36. Ruhmann, A. G., and Berliner, D. L. (1965): Effect of steroids on growth of mouse fibroblasts *in vitro. Endocrinology,* 76:916–927.
37. Ruhmann, A. B., and Berliner, D. L. (1967): Influence of steroids on fibroblasts. II. The fibroblast as an assay system for topical anti-inflammatory potency of corticosteroids. *J. Invest. Dermatol.,* 49:123–130.
38. Saffiotti, U., and Shubik, P. (1963): Studies on promoting action of skin carcinogenesis. *Natl. Cancer Inst. Monogr.,* 10:489–507.
39. Schwarz, J. A., Viaje, A., Slaga, T. J., Yuspa, S. H., Hennings, H., and Lichti, U. (1977): Fluocinolone acetonide: A potent inhibitor of mouse skin tumor promotion and epidermal DNA synthesis. *Chem. Biol. Interact.,* 17:331–347.
40. Scribner, J. D., and Boutwell, R. K. (1972): Inflammation and tumor promotion: Selective protein induction in mouse skin by tumor promoters. *Eur. J. Cancer,* 8:617–621.
41. Scribner, J. D., and Slaga, T. J. (1973): Multiple effects of dexamethasone on protein synthesis and hyperplasia caused by a tumor promoter. *Cancer Res.,* 33:542–546.
42. Slaga, T. J., Bowden, G. T., and Boutwell, R. K. (1975): Acetic acid, a potent stimulator of mouse epidermal macromolecular synthesis and hyperplasia but with weak tumor-promoting ability. *J. Natl. Cancer Inst.,* 55:983–987.
43. Slaga, T. J., Scribner, J. D., Thompson, S., and Viaje, A. (1976): Epidermal cell proliferation and promoting ability of phorbol esters. *J. Natl. Cancer Inst.,* 57:1145–1149.
44. Slaga, T. J., and Scribner, J. D. (1973): Inhibition of tumor initiation and promotion by anti-inflammatory agents. *J. Natl. Cancer Inst.,* 51:1723–1725.
45. Slaga, T. J., Scribner, J. D., Rice, J. M., Das, S. B., and Thompson, S. (1974): Inhibition by dexamethasone of intracellular binding of phorbol esters to mouse skin. *J. Natl. Cancer Inst.,* 52:1611–1618.
46. Slaga, T. J., Thompson, S., and Smuckler, E. A. (1975): Prolonged inhibition of mouse epidermal DNA synthesis by dexamethasone. *J. Natl. Cancer Inst.,* 54:931–936.
47. Slaga, T. J., Fischer, S. M., Viaje, A., Berry, D. L., Bracken, W. M., LeClerc, S., and Miller, D. L. (1978): Inhibition of tumor promotion by anti-inflammatory agents: An approach to the biochemical mechanism of promotion. In: *Carcinogenesis, Vol. 2, Mechanisms of Tumor Promotion and Cocarcinogenesis,* edited by T. J. Slaga, A. Sivak, and R. K. Boutwell, pp. 173–195. Raven Press, New York.
48. Sporn, M. B., Dunlop, N. M., Newton, D. L., and Smith, J. M. (1976): Prevention of chemical carcinogenesis by vitamin A and its synthetic analogs (retinoids). *Fed. Proc.,* 35:1332–1338.
49. Suss, R., Kinzel, V., and Kreibich, G. (1971): Cocarcinogenic croton oil factor A stimulates lipid synthesis in cell cultures. *Experientia,* 27:46–47.
50. Suss, R., Kreibich, G., and Kinzel, V. (1972): Phorbol esters as a tool in cell research. *Eur. J. Cancer,* 8:299–304.
51. Thompson, S., and Slaga, T. J. (1976): The effects of dexamethasone on mouse skin initiation and aryl hydrocarbon hydroxylase. *Eur. J. Cancer,* 12:363–370.
52. Troll, W., Klassen, A., and Janoff, A. (1970): Tumorigenesis in mouse skin. Inhibition by synthetic inhibitors of proteases. *Science,* 169:1211–1213.
53. Trosko, J. E., Chang, C. C., Yotti, L. P., and Chu, E. H. (1977): Effect of phorbol myristate acetate on the recovery of spontaneous and ultraviolet light-induced 6-thioguanine and ouabain-resistant chinese hamster cells. *Cancer Res.,* 37:188–193.
54. Van Duuren, B. L., Sivak, A., Katz, C., Seidman, I., and Melchionne. (1975): The effect of aging and interval between primary and secondary treatment in two-stage carcinogenesis on mouse skin. *Cancer Res.,* 35:502–505.
55. Verma, A. K., Rice, H. M., Shapas, B. F., and Boutwell, R. K. (1978): Inhibition of 12-*O*-

tetradecanoylphorbol-13-acetate induced ornithine decarboxylase activity in mouse epidermis by vitamin A analogs (retinoids). *Cancer Res.,* 38:793–801.

56. Viaje, A., Slaga, T. J., Wigler, M., and Weinstein, I. B. (1977): The effects of anti-inflammatory agents on mouse skin promotion, epidermal DNA synthesis, phorbol ester-induced cellular proliferation and production of plasminogen activator. *Cancer Res.,* 37:1530–1536.

57. Weeks, C. E., Slaga, T. J., Hennings, H., Gleason, G. L., and Bracken. W. M. (1979): Inhibition of phorbol ester-induced tumor promotion by vitamin A analog and anti-inflammatory steroid. *J. Natl. Cancer Inst. (in press).*

58. Weinstein, I. B., Wigler, M., Fisher, P. B., Sisskin, E., and Pietropaolo, C. (1978): Cell culture studies on the biologic effects of tumor promoters. In: *Carcinogenesis, Vol. 2, Mechanisms of Tumor Promotion and Cocarcinogenesis,* edited by T. J. Slaga, A. Sivak, and R. K. Boutwell, pp. 313–333. Raven Press, New York.

59. Wenner, C. E., Moroney, J., and Porter, C. W. (1978): Early membrane effects of phorbol esters in 3T3 cells. In: *Carcinogenesis, Vol. 2, Mechanisms of Tumor Promotion and Cocarcinogenesis,* edited by T. J. Slaga, A. Sivak, and R. K. Boutwell, pp. 363–378. Raven Press, New York.

60. Wigler, M., Ford, J. P., and Weinstein, I. B. (1975): Glucocorticoid inhibition of the fibrinolytic activity of tumor cells, In: *Proteases and Biological Control,* edited by E. Reich, D. B. Rifkin, and E. Shaw, pp. 849–856. Cold Spring Harbor Laboratory, New York.

61. Wigler, M., and Weinstein, I. B. (1976): Tumour promoter induces plasminogen activator. *Nature,* 259:232–233.

62. Yuspa, S. H. Lichti, U., Ben, T., Patterson, E., Hennings, H., Slaga, T. J., Colburn, N., and Kelsey, W. (1976): Phorbol-ester tumor promoters stimulate DNA synthesis and ornithine decarboxylase activity in mouse epidermal cell cultures. *Nature,* 262:402–404.

Carcinogenesis, Vol. 5: Modifiers of Chemical Carcinogenesis, edited by T. J. Slaga. Raven Press, New York © 1980.

7

Protease Inhibitors in Carcinogenesis: Possible Sites of Action

Toby G. Rossman and Walter Troll

New York University Medical Center, Department of Environmental Medicine, New York, New York 10016

Proteases are enzymes that catalyze the hydrolysis of peptide bonds. The pancreatic digestive enzymes are proteases that break down food proteins into small oligopeptides. There is, however, another type of protease that is involved not in digestion but in control mechanisms. These proteases engage in limited proteolysis, cleaving only at very specific sites rather than digesting the whole protein molecule (49). Both types of proteases may be involved in tumorigenesis, and protease inhibitors may be able to block tumorigenesis at any number of sites.

We will give a brief review of what has been accomplished in the field of experimental tumorigenesis using a variety of protease inhibitors administered by various routes. Following this, we will suggest possible sites of action for protease inhibitors. These include the inhibition of (a) proteases induced by tumor promoters and malignant transformation, (b) proteases that are required for inflammation, (c) proteases involved in invasiveness and metastasis, (d) proteases that cause membrane changes, including alterations of cyclic nucleotide levels, and (e) mitogenic (growth stimulating) proteases.

Many of these proteases work on extracellular sites, e.g., the digestion of connective tissue, the formation of chemotactic peptides in inflammation, and the alteration of surface proteins. We end this chapter with the suggestion that an important site of action of proteases may be an intracellular one, i.e., the removal of protein repressors from DNA in the derepression of genes.

EFFECTS OF PROTEASE INHIBITORS IN EXPERIMENTAL TUMORIGENESIS

The earliest experiments on the effects of protease inhibitors on tumorigenesis were stimulated by the discovery that the tumor promoter 12-*O*-tetradecanoyl-phorbol-13-acetate (TPA) caused the appearance of a trypsin-like protease in mouse skin (72,74). In order to determine whether this protease is a necessary factor in tumor promotion, protease inhibitors were tested as antipromoting agents in two-stage carcinogenesis in mouse skin.

Briefly, two-stage carcinogenesis involves painting a subcarcinogenic dose of a carcinogen (the "initiator") on mouse skin, followed by repeated applications of a promoting agent without which tumors would not appear. Initiators are carcinogens. Most carcinogens or their metabolites have been shown to react with DNA (47,73) and to cause mutations in bacterial systems (1). The promoter (TPA is the most commonly used) is not itself a carcinogen or a mutagen. The induction of a protease by TPA gave one of the earliest clues as to its mechanism of action.

The protease inhibitors tosyl lysine chloromethyl ketone (TLCK), tosyl phenylalanine chloromethyl ketone (TPCK), and tosyl alanine methyl ester (TAME) (Table 1) were used in a two-stage carcinogenesis study where DMBA was the initiator and croton oil (in which the active ingredient is TPA) was the promoter. Results presented in Table 2 show that all three protease inhibitors are effective antitumorigenic agents, with TPCK being the best inhibitor on a weight basis (72,76).

A word of caution must be injected here concerning TLCK and TPCK: chloromethyl ketones are also sulfhydryl-reacting agents. We have found, for example, that TLCK reacts very quickly with glutathione as well as with proteases in *E. coli,* and that at least some of its biological action can be ascribed to the former reaction (63). One might argue that the inhibition of tumorigenesis by TLCK and TPCK is due to the sulfhydryl reactions of these compounds and not to their action as protease inhibitors although the sulfhydryl agent iodoacetamide has been shown to act as a tumor promoter (27). The same argument cannot be made for TAME which is not a sulfhydryl agent. TAME is a substrate for trypsin-like proteases and therefore acts as a competitive inhib-

TABLE 1. *Protease inhibitors*

Compound	Type of inhibition	Enzymes inhibited
TLCK	Noncompetitive alkylation	Trypsin-like serine proteases, sulfhydryl proteases
TPCK	Noncompetitive alkylation	Chymotrypsin sulfhydryl proteases
TAME	Competitive	Trypsin-like proteases
NPGB	Forms slowly dissociating complex	Trypsin-like proteases
SBTI	Forms macromolecular complex	Trypsin, chymotrypsin
Leupeptin	Competitive	Plasmin, trypsin, cathepsin B, papain
Antipain	Competitive	Papain, trypsin cathepsin A and B
Elastatinal	Competitive	Elastase

TABLE 2. *Inhibition of tumorigenesis by proteinase inhibitors*

Weeks on promotion	Control		TPCK		TLCK		TAME	
	T	S	T	S	T	S	T	S
10	8	19	0	21	0	21	0	21
12	10	19	0	21	0	21	0	21
14	11	19	0	21	1	21	3	21
16	11	19	0	21	4	21	5	21
18	11	19	0	21	4	21	5	21
20	11	19	0	21	4	21	5	21
22	11	19	0	21	5	21	5	21
24	11	19	1	21	5	21	5	21
30	11	19	1	21	5	21	5	21

All animals were given 10 μg of DMBA as initiator, and then 5.0 μg of croton oil in acetone was applied three times weekly as promoter. The proteinase inhibitors TLCK, TPCK, and TAME were applied in DMSO three times weekly in 1.0 μg doses, 1–2 hr after applications of croton oil. All treatments were applied to ear skin of mice (the controls received DMSO alone). The average times of appearance of tumors in all three experimental groups are significantly different from the controls at $P < 0.005$; T indicates the number of tumor-bearing mice; S indicates the number of survivors, DMSO = dimethyl sulfoxide. (Data from Troll, Klassen, and Janoff 1970.)

itor. In order to delineate the role of proteases in tumorigenesis, protease inhibitors without side effects must be used. Fortunately, a new class of compounds has recently been isolated from Actinomycetes (77). These are small peptide inhibitors with aldehyde end groups. They do not alkylate sulfhydryl groups, and they have very low toxicity. For example, the LD_{50} of leupeptin (subcut) in mice is 1450 mg/kg (45).

The inhibition of mouse skin tumorigenesis by protease inhibitors was confirmed by Hozumi et al. (33) using the protease inhibitor leupeptin (Table 1), one of the new peptide inhibitors. Leupeptin inhibited tumor formation in mouse skin initiated by DMBA (dimethylbenz(a)anthracene) and promoted by croton oil.

A series of experiments were performed by feeding rats and mice pellets containing 0.1% leupeptin. This diet had no effect on weight gain of the animals. The results are summarized in Table 3. Leupeptin in the diet inhibited tumorigenesis in a number of cases (rat colon, esophagus, and mammary gland; mouse skin and leukemia), had no effect in other cases (rat liver and forestomach; mouse lung) and enhanced tumor growth in two cases (rat glandular stomach and bladder).

Some reasons for these different effects in different tissues may be:

1. The inhibitor may not get to the tissue in question or may be metabolized to an inactive product in some organs.

2. Proteases may differ in different tissues so leupeptin may not be equally effective against proteases in different tissues.

TABLE 3. *Effect of feeding leupeptin on tumorigenesis in various organs*[a]

Carcinogen	Site of tumors	Effect of leupeptin
In rats		
Azoxymethane	Colon	Decreased number of tumors per rat
Butylnitrosourethan	Esophagus	Decreased squamous cell carcinoma
DMBA	Mammary gland	Decreased number of tumors per rat
Diethylnitrosamine	Liver	No effect
Butylnitrosourethane	Forestomach	No effect
MNNG	Glandular stomach	Enhanced tumor growth but not yield
Butyl-(4-hydroxybutyl)nitrosamine	Bladder	Increased weight of bladder with tumor
In mice		
DMBA [b]	Skin	Decreased incidence and number of tumors per mouse
n-Nitrosobutylurea	Leukemia	Extended induction time
Urethan	Lung	No effect

[a] Data from Matsushima (45).
[b] Promoted with croton oil.

3. In cases where metabolic activation is required, leupeptin may inhibit the induction of microsomal enzymes, although neither TPCK nor TLCK inhibits induction of benzo (a)pyrene hydroxylase in mouse skin (A. Klassen, *unpublished data*).

One natural source of protease inhibitors is in seed foods, such as soybeans and lima beans. Injections of soybean trypsin inhibitor (SBTI) into mice daily for 5 days after mice were innoculated with Ehrlich ascites tumor cells "cured" 70% of the mice. If the SBTI injections were started on day 7, 30% of the mice were cured (82).

Soybeans are a major protein source in many vegetarian and low meat diets. Breast, prostatic, colon, and bladder cancer incidences are lower in populations eating such diets (e.g., Japanese and Seventh Day Adventists), perhaps owing to the presence of protease inhibitors in the diet. Stable proteins, soybean protease inhibitors capable of inhibiting trypsin, chymotrypsin, plasmin, and elastase have been described (3,36).

We have fed mice diets containing 50% raw soybeans and the same diet heated to 120° for 6 hr. Inhibitors against trypsin were 90% destroyed by the heat treatment. The mice were initiated with 200 mg nitroquinoline-N-oxide (NQO) followed by promotion three times a week with 5 μg TPA. Compared with the heated diet, the raw diet delayed the appearance of tumors by 45 days and decreased the number of tumors 50% after 200 days. Confirmation of this type of feeding experiment in other experimental carcinogenesis systems is required before the epidemiological data in man can be ascribed only to the consumption of protease inhibitors.

THE INDUCTION OF PROTEASES BY TPA
AND MALIGNANT TRANSFORMATION

In vivo studies on mouse skin established that TPA induces one or more proteases (72,74). The original studies used three substrates: [^{3}H]TAME, [^{3}H]ALME (N-α-acetyl-L-lysine methyl ester) and protamine. Increased hydrolysis of all three substrates was seen in mouse ears treated with TPA. TPCK and TLCK inhibited the hydrolysis of TAME only partially, and TLCK but not TPCK inhibited the hydrolysis of protamine completely. Hozumi *et al.* (33), using the substrate N-α-benzoyl-L-arginine ethyl ester, also found increased hydrolysis in mouse skin treated with TPA (croton oil). Leupeptin was found to inhibit this activity. Painting leupeptin on mouse skin also resulted in an inhibition of the TPA-induced protease activity. The nature and number of proteases induced in mouse skin by TPA have not yet been established. However, because the substrates used involve the hydrolysis of lysine- and arginine-containing bonds, and because TLCK and leupeptin are trypsin inhibitors, it seemed likely that at least one of the proteases induced is a trypsin-like protease.

The discovery by Reich and co-workers (52) that, in general, tumor cells contain more plasminogen activator than their normal counterpart resulted in an upsurge of interest in proteases involved in malignant transformation. Plasminogen activators produced by malignant cells are trypsin-like serine proteases, i.e., they contain an essential serine at their active site and can be inhibited by DFP. Most normal fibroblasts contain low levels of plasminogen activator, but after transformation by viruses or chemical carcinogens, the amount of plasminogen activator produced and released is increased. Intracellular plasminogen activator appears to be associated with the membrane fraction (57). Other proteases may also be produced and excreted. For example, following transformation by mouse sarcoma virus, at least five serine enzymes accumulate in mouse fibroblast culture fluids. Four of these enzymes are proteases, two of which are plasminogen activators (58). A plasminogen-independent fibrinolytic activity produced by chick embryo fibroblasts transformed by Rous sarcoma virus (RSV-CEF), but not by normal chick embryo fibroblasts (CEF) has been reported (11).

A few nonmalignant cells also produce plasminogen activator, including "activated" macrophages (80). However, for fibroblasts, tumorigenicity and plasminogen activator activity are usually coordinately expressed. When chick embryo fibroblasts are infected with a temperature-sensitive mutant of RSV, ta 68, growth at 41°C results in normal cells (nontransformed) by morphological and biochemical criteria. Growth at 36°C, however, results in a transformed phenotype, typical of RSV transformed cells. When cells grown at 41°C are shifted to 36°C increases in plasminogen activator activity can be seen within 3 hr. Conversely, when cells grown at 36°C are shifted to 41°C a loss in plasminogen activator activity occurs (60,79).

A second example of coordinate expression of plasminogen activator activity and tumorigenicity is found in a mouse melanoma line B16, clone B_5 (59). When these cells are grown in the presence of 5-bromodeoxyuridine (BrdU), they change from highly melanotic, piled-up cells to flat, amelanotic fibroblast-like cells that have lost their tumorigenic potential. These effects are reversible upon removal of the BrdU. Along with altered morphology and loss of tumorigenicity, BrdU also causes a decrease in the production of plasminogen activator (16).

A significant advance was made in this area by the discovery that TPA induces plasminogen activator in tissue culture cells (90). Using CEF, it was found that as little as 5×10^{-9}M TPA was effective, with a maximum effect at 1.5×10^{-8}M. The increase in plasminogen activator by TPA could be blocked by actinomycin D, suggesting that a new messenger RNA is required and that the increase is an induction in the classical sense of the word. When TPA is removed, plasminogen activator levels return to normal within 12 hr. TPA is also able to enhance the level of plasminogen activator in transformed cells that already have high levels (87). Using a variety of phorbol compounds, it was found that the ability to induce plasminogen activator in CEF correlates with tumor-promoting activity in mouse skin. Some other diterpene esters also induce plasminogen activator, but promoting agents and cocarcinogens of different chemical type (e.g., anthralin, cantharidin, and tween 60) failed to induce, suggesting a different mode of action (86).

INFLAMMATION AND PROTEASES

Although tumor promoters cause inflammation and epidermal hyperplasia, evidence suggests that inflammation and hyperplasia may be necessary but not sufficient for promotion (28,68). The locus of inflammation usually shows the gradual accumulation of polymorphonuclear leukocytes caused by local production and diffusion of chemotactic factors. TPA causes such an infiltration (37). The cleavage products of several complement components have chemotactic properties. These may be produced by plasmin (67). Since TPA induces protease(s), its inflammatory effects might be due to the local production of plasmin which would result in chemotactic factors. Protease inhibitors inhibit the inflammatory response due to TPA (37) probably by inhibiting the formation of chemotactic factors.

Recently, a protease has been purified from human skin which induces leukocyte infiltration upon injection into skin. This enzyme is a serine protease but not a plasminogen activator (71). It would be of interest to know whether this protease is also induced by TPA.

The relationship between inflammation and tumor promotion led to the investigation of antiinflammatory steroids as possible inhibitors of tumor promotion. Glucocorticoids were found to inhibit tumor promotion in roughly the same order as their abilities to inhibit inflammation: dexamethasone > Schering No. 11572 > prednisolone > hydrocortisone > cortisone (2). In rat hepatoma cultures, dexamethasone causes morphological changes, inhibition of the synthesis of plasminogen activator, and growth in soft agar (89). Growth in semisolid medium is a property that correlates well with tumorigenicity (55). A structural similarity between TPA and cortisol has led to the suggestion that these compounds share the same receptors (91). The suppression of plasminogen activator production is specific for glucocorticoids and does not occur with other steroids (89). Other more powerful antiinflammatory steroids, such as fluocinonide acetonide, inhibit both tumor promotion and the production of plasminogen activator better than dexamethasone (81).

A protease inhibitor in human urine is under the influence of the adrenal hypophyseal system (21). The decrease in plasminogen activator activity caused by dexamethasone is dependent upon *de novo* RNA synthesis (89). The induction of a protease inhibitor by dexamethasone would be consistent with this finding. This hypothesis was tested by measuring plasminogen activator in lysates from dexamethasone-treated and control rat hepatoma cells, using a new fluorometric assay (40). As expected, lysates from dexamethasone-treated cells did not activate plasminogen, whereas lysates from control cells did. However, mixing lysates from treated and control cells abolished the plasminogen activator activity in the latter, suggesting the presence of an inhibitor in the treated cells. The lysates from treated cells also inhibited trypsin, whereas lysates from control cells showed increased proteolytic activity when mixed with trypsin (39).

Thus, it is possible that the inhibition of tumorigenesis by antiinflammatory agents is a result of the inhibition of proteases. Since nonsteroid, antiinflammatory agents were not very active either in suppressing plasminogen activator production in culture or in inhibiting tumor promotion in mouse skin (81), it seems likely that only an antiproteolytic mode of inhibition of inflammation results in inhibition of tumor promotion.

PROTEASES IN TUMOR INVASION AND METASTASIS

In order for a tumor to grow into an area where other tissue already exists, some method of creating space for the tumor may be necessary. Proteases should be ideally suited for this role. Besides plasminogen activator, tumors also contain higher collagenase activity than normal cells (19). Reich (58) has suggested that circulating plasminogen is a reservoir of protease activity that can be tapped for local protease action. Tumor cells secreting plasminogen activator in an uncontrolled and continuous fashion may activate plasmin which, along with collagenase, could degrade surrounding connective tissue. A protease excreted by macrophages has been found to activate collagenase (31).

It has been suggested that the high concentration of proteases in the interstitial fluids of solid tumors may also be responsible for metastasis (70). Support for this idea comes from studies in tissue culture using plasminogen-free serum. It was found that although plasminogen (which is converted to the protease plasmin by cells secreting plasminogen activator) is not required for the growth of cells, it is required for cell migration (52). A naturally occurring protease inhibitor from pig leukocytes is able to inhibit metastases of a lung carcinoma in mice (24).

One phenomenon which has often been noted is the lack of tumor invasion into cartilage. Osteosarcomas erode and replace bone tissues whose major organic component is collagen. Cartilage, which also contains collagen (of a slightly different type) is found adjacent to many bones but is rarely invaded. Bony metastases from mammary carcinomas also do not invade cartilage. Osteosarcoma and mammary carcinoma cells in culture secrete collagenase and other proteases. A small protein from cartilage, purified by affinity chromatography on immobilized trypsin, is able to inhibit the breakdown of cartilage by enzymes secreted from these cells (42). A similar (or identical) protein from cartilage, also purified on a trypsin affinity column, has been shown to inhibit tumor-induced neovascularization (43). A protease inhibitor which is part of the normal cartilage matrix thus appears to be responsible for the lack of both tumor invasion and vascularization of cartilage.

PROTEASES AND GROWTH

Brief treatment with proteases has been found to cause changes in the surface of normal cells similar to those occurring in chemical or viral transformation. Tumor cells are often more agglutinable by plant lectins than their normal counterparts. Protease treatment increases the agglutinability of normal cells (9). The protease inhibitors TLCK and nitrophenyl guanido benzoate (NPGB) render tumor cells less agglutinable (9,25). A surface glycoprotein called LETS (large, external, transformation-sensitive) is present on normal cells but absent after transformation. Proteases can also remove this protein (35). Proteases can also increase the rate of glucose transport, alter cyclic nucleotide metabolism, and reduce cell to substrate adhesion (62). Normal cells also contain actin cables, whereas transformed cells contain few. Proteases can remove the cables from normal cells (54). Proteases have been reported to cause normal cells to assume a more transformed morphology, whereas protease inhibitors added to tumor cells cause a morphological change in the direction of normalcy (62).

Schnebli and Burger (66) initially reported that five protease inhibitors, including TLCK and TPCK had a selective inhibitory effect on the growth of spontaneous or virally transformed cells. Other workers, however, report that normal and transformed cells are equally effected by protease inhibitors (13). As we have pointed out above, the chloromethyl ketone protease inhibitors react with sulfhydryl groups. Protein and RNA synthesis are inhibited by these compounds in *E. coli* (63) and in normal and transformed animal cells (13,51,56). Thus, experiments using these compounds must be interpreted with caution. In an attempt to circumvent the problem of nonspecific effects of chloromethyl ketones, Goldberg and co-workers (25) compared the tripeptide chloromethyl ketones, L-alanine-L-phenyl-D-lysine-COCH$_2$Cl and L-alamine-L-phenyl-L-lysine-COCH$_2$Cl. The latter inhibits plasmin 100 times better than the former and also inhibited the growth of SV3T3 cells at a lower concentration. TLCK was found to cause RSV-CEF to behave like normal CEF (loss of microvilli, decrease in 2-deoxyglucose transport, flatter morphology), whereas cyclohexamide, an inhibitor of protein synthesis, had no effect on the morphology of these cells (84). Other protease inhibitors were examined for their abilities to cause flattening of RSV-CEF, and only inhibitors of trypsin-like proteases gave this effect (84).

Many cell surface changes are correlated with growth rate or stages of the cell cycle, as well as with transformation. Cells in G$_1$ have the highest levels of LETS protein. During mitosis, the level drops to that characteristic of virus-transformed cells (34). Untransformed cells in mitosis are also more agglutinable than are interphase cells; the differences are less striking for transformed cells (69). These findings suggest that the membrane changes that occur during mitosis of normal cells may be a more permanent feature of cells after transformation.

The secretion of plasminogen activator is also correlated with the state of growth in Swiss 3T3 cells, being higher in growing cells and decreasing in confluency (14). High CA^{2+} or calcium ionophore A23187, when added to confluent 3T3 cells, both induce DNA synthesis (mitogenic response) and increase the secretion of plasminogen activator (15). There was no effect on SV_{40} virus-transformed 3T3 cells. The TPA-induced DNA synthesis and proliferation of thymic lymphoblasts is also calcium dependent (88). It is of interest that a Ca^{2+}-activated protease capable of degrading myofibrils has been purified from muscle (18).

Although there are correlations between production of plasminogen activator (or addition of exogenous proteases), surface membrane changes, and growth or transformation, sorting out the causal relationships between these phenomena has been difficult. Is the production of plasminogen activator by transformed cells and cells exposed to TPA the cause of the mitogenic and proliferative response? When proteases are added externally to normal cells, do they achieve their effects solely by altering surface proteins and, if so, which proteins are the important ones for growth control? Various hypotheses have been put forth based on the assumption that proteases affect growth control via the cell surface. Burger (8) has suggested that (a) proteases may cause cells to become less firmly attached to their substration and to other cells, providing them with the necessary mobility for cytokinesis, (b) surface changes prevent the exchange between cells of a "message" for contract inhibition, (c) surface changes may cause an increased uptake of nutrients or growth factors, or (d) proteases may be involved in the formation of mediators (e.g., cyclic nucleotides) or other enzyme reactions. It has also been suggested that proteases may bind to or cleave receptors for more specific growth factors and thus mimic their actions (30).

The idea that enhanced proteolytic activity in transformed cells could be responsible for some of their altered phenotypic characteristics by cleaving proteins on the cell surface has been tested in a number of ways. When cells are grown in plasminogen-free serum, plasmin cannot be formed by plasminogen activator, although this does not eliminate the possibility of direct proteolytic action by plasminogen activator and other proteases excreted from cells. It was found that plasmin may be responsible for the morphology of transformed cells in culture, their ability to grow in agar, and their migration (52), but is not involved in the expression of LETS (35), the rate of 2-deoxyglucose transport (11), or the growth rate and final cell density of normal or transformed hamster cells (52).

There is also a lack of correlation between cell surface effects of exogenous proteases and their growth stimulatory ability when examined more carefully. The protease-mediated cell surface change measured by agglutinability with the plant lectin concanavalin A (Con A) was not sufficient to lead to cell division in density-inhibited 3T3 cells (17). Thrombin was found to stimulate DNA synthesis and cell division in resting CEF without removing Z (similar to LETS) protein (4,12).

One possible mechanism whereby proteolytic action on the cell surface might influence growth is via an alteration in cyclic nucleotide levels. Virus transformed fibroblasts generally have lower cAMP (adenosine 3′,5′-cyclic monophosphate) levels than confluent normal fibroblasts. Although low concentrations of several nucleotides have been reported to enhance the growth rate of some cells, higher concentrations of cAMP or its analogs usually depress the growth rate (53).

In the case of 3T3 cells, it was found that as confluence is reached, the level of cGMP (guanosine 3′,5′-cyclic monophosphate) is reduced but cAMP levels are not changed (48). Often, cAMP and cGMP levels fluctuate in opposite directions, agents which stimulate growth causing increases in cGMP levels (26). It has been suggested that growth control may be maintained by the ratio of cGMP/cAMP, a high ratio corresponding to high growth rate (26,65). Increases in intracellular levels of cGMP are among the earliest changes caused by mitogens. A greater than 20-fold increase in the cGMP level was reported shortly after the addition of TPA to 3T3 cells (20). We have found an increase in cGMP levels and no change in cAMP levels in mouse epidermis after treatment with TPA *in vivo* (23).

Trypsin has been found to activate adenylate cyclase in fibroblasts (83). A variety of protease inhibitors block the activation of adenyl cyclase by proteases as well as by hormones, suggesting that a membrane protease may be involved in these activations (59). Since the effect of trypsin is to decrease the cAMP level in mammalian cells (10), or to increase slightly the cGMP level in chick cells (32), there are probably effects on other enzymes as well. Fibroblasts growth factor has been reported to activate guanyl cyclase (65). In mammalian cells, a variety of proteases are able to cause a drop in the cAMP level, and exogenous dibutryl cAMP is able to block the growth stimulation by proteases or by serum. However, the increased agglutinability after protease treatment is not inhibited by dibutryl cAMP (6).

Alterations in the cAMP level may result in a variety of membrane effects. High levels of cAMP seem to be associated with a higher percentage of tubulin present as microtubules (64). Lowering the cAMP level should therefore be associated with increased lateral mobility of membranes, a feature thought to be responsible for the clustered distribution of Con A binding sites characteristic of transformed cells (50).

AN INTRACELLULAR ROLE FOR PROTEASES?

Although it seems likely that at least some of the effect of proteases on cells are mediated either by direct cleavage of surface proteins or as a result of alterations in cyclic nucleotide levels, evidence has been accumulating that at least some of the action of proteases might be intracellular. For example, although a 10-min treatment with low concentrations of proteases can increase the agglutinability of CEF, at least a 2-hr treatment is required in order to induce cell division (17). These results suggest that the mitogenic effect of proteases may involve more than the cleavage of surface proteins.

Originally, the concept of mitogenic action via the cell surface had been supported by the finding that trypsin bound to sepharose beads, which are too large to enter cells, was still mitogenic (9). This conclusion is based on the assumption that sepharose-trypsin is stable. However, it has been shown that insulin leaks from sepharose-insulin beads, and that this leakage is enough to account for the total biological activity of the preparation (41). The same is true for growth hormone bound to sepharose (5). Thus, it is still an open question whether or not the mitogenic action of proteases is accomplished by cleavage of surface proteins. This question might be answered using immobilized enzymes that have a stronger linkage to their support (22).

If there is an intracellular role for protease action, it must be shown that exogenous proteases can enter cells. This was first demonstrated for trypsin which is taken up by cells in a temperature-dependent fashion (29). More recently, [^{125}I]thrombin was shown to be internalized by normal CEF at three times the rate of RSV-transformed CEF (93). Thrombin is mitogenic to the former but not to the latter. Autoradiography revealed that most of the label was in the cytoplasm. The internalization of thrombin by CEF approaches its maximum level after 8 to 12 hr. Chymotrypsin, which is not mitogenic, has very low levels of internalization (44). Cell fractionation studies suggest that much of the thrombin may reach the nucleus (44). The discrepancy between the autoradiography and cell fractionation studies remains to be explained. The thrombin that enters the cell appears to be enzymatically active (44).

A new role in the intracellular action of proteases is suggested by the discovery that during the induction of lambda prophage in *E. coli,* the lambda repressor is proteolytically cleaved (61). This is the first demonstration of genetic derepression by proteolytic action. The induction of lambda prophage in *E. coli* is controlled by the same genes responsible for error-prone DNA repair after UV irradiation (see review by Witkin, Ref. 92). The Ames test for chemical carcinogens (1) is also dependent upon this system. We have shown that the protease inhibitor antipain is able to inhibit UV mutagenesis (46), and Umezawa *et al.* (78) have shown that elastatinal inhibits N-methyl-N'-nitro-N-nitrosoguanidine (MNNG) and N-ethyl-N'-nitro-N-nitrosoguanidine (ENNG) mutagenesis in *Salmonella.*

It was suggested by Boutwell (7) that the function of tumor promoters is to cause gene activation. The induction of proteases(s) by TPA might be a mechanism for the subsequent derepression of other genes, including those for error-prone DNA repair. A more detailed molecular model has been presented elsewhere (75).

In rodents, estradiol induces a protease in the uterus of ovariectomized animals (38,76). The protease first appears to be associated with the plasma membrane and later appears in the nucleus (38,76). Antipain and leupeptin inhibit this protease and also inhibit uterine DNA synthesis and function (38). These results support the concept of a nuclear involvement of proteases as a control mechanism.

One might speculate that in animal cells growth control is accomplished by derepression of particular genes whose products initiate DNA synthesis and subsequent mitosis. The derepression of these genes might require proteolytic cleavage of repressors analogous to the situation in *E. coli* mentioned above. Perhaps the inhibition by phorbol ester of terminal differentiation (85) is accomplished by the continuous cleavage of growth repressors that would normally prevent growth in cells which were about to differentiate.

REFERENCES

1. Ames, B. N., Dunston, W. E., Yamanski, F., and Lee, F. D. (1973): Carcinogens are mutagens: A simple test system combining liver homogenates for activation and bacterial detection. *Proc. Natl. Acad. Sci. USA,* 70:2281–2285.
2. Belman, S., and Troll, W. (1972): The inhibition of croton oil-promoted mouse skin tumorigenesis by steroid hormones. *Cancer Res.,* 32:450–454.
3. Bieth, J., and Frechin, J. C. (1974): Elastase inhibitors as impurities in commercial preparations of soybean trypsin inhibitor (Kunitz). In: *Proteinase Inhibitors,* edited by H. Fritz, H. Tschesche, L. J. Greene, and E. Truscheit, pp. 291–304. Springer-Verlag, New York.
4. Blumberg, P. M., and Robbins, P. W. (1975): Relation of protease action on the cell surface to growth control and adhesion. In: *Proteases and Biological Control,* edited by E. Reich, D. Rifkin, and E. Shaw, pp. 945–956. Cold Spring Harbor Laboratories, Cold Spring Harbor, New York.
5. Balander, F. K., and Fellows, R. E. (1975): Growth hormone covalent bound to sepharose or glass: analysis of ligand release rates and characterization of soluble radiolabeled products. *Biochemistry,* 14:2938–2943.
6. Bombik, B. M., and Burger, M. M. (1973): cAMP and the cell cycle: inhibition of growth stimulation. *Exp. Cell Res.,* 80:88–94.
7. Boutwell, R. K. (1974): The function and mechanism of promoters of carcinogenesis. *CRC Crit. Rev. Toxicol.,* 2:419–442.
8. Burger, M. M. (1970): Proteolytic enzymes initiating cell division and escape from contact inhibition of growth. *Nature,* 227:170.
9. Burger, M. M. (1973): Surface changes in transformed cells detected by lectens. *Fed. Proc.,* 32:91–101.
10. Burger, M. M., Bombik, B. M., Breckenridge, B. M., and Sheppard, J. R. (1972): Growth control and cyclic alterations of cyclic AMP in the cell cycle. *Nature [New Biol.],* 239:161–163.
11. Chen, L. B., and Buchanan, J. M. (1975): Plasminogen-independent fibrinolysis by proteases produced by transformed chick embryo fibroblasts. *Proc. Natl. Acad. Sci. USA,* 72:1132–1136.
12. Chen, L. B., Teng, N. N. H., and Buchanan, J. M. (1975): The mitogenic activity and related effects of thrombin on chick embryo fibroblasts. In: *Proteases and Biological Control,* edited by E. Reich, D. Rifkin, and E. Shaw, pp. 957–965. Cold Spring Harbor Laboratory, Cold Spring Harbor, New York.
13. Chou, I. N., Black, P. H., and Roblin, R. (1974): Non-selective inhibition of transformed cell growth by protease inhibitors. *Proc. Natl. Acad. Sci. USA,* 71:1748–1752.
14. Chow, I. N., O'Donnell, S. P., Black, P. H., and Roblin, R. O. (1977): Cell density dependent secretion of plasminogen activator by 3T3 cells. *J. Cell Physiol.,* 91:31–38.
15. Chou, I. N., Roblin, R. O., and Black, P. H. (1977): Calcium stimulation of plasminogen activator secretion/production by Swiss 3T3 cells. *J. Biol. Chem.,* 252:6256–6259.
16. Christman, J. K., Acs, G., Silagi, S., and Silverstein, S. C. (1975): Plasminogen activator: Biochemical characterization and correlation with tumorigenicity. In: *Proteases and Biological Control* edited by E. Reich, D. B. Rifkin, and E. Shaw, pp. 827–839. Cold Spring Harbor Laboratory, Cold Spring Harbor, New York.
17. Cunningham, D. D., and Ho, T. S. (1975): Effects of added proteases on concanavalin A— specific agglutinability and proliferation of quiescent fibroblasts. In: *Proteases and Biological Control* edited by E. Reich, D. Rifkin, and E. Shaw, pp. 795–806. Cold Spring Harbor Laboratory, Cold Spring Harbor, New York.
18. Dayton, W. R., Soll, D. E., Stromer, M. H., Reville, W. J., Zeece, M. G., and Robson,

R. M. (1975): Some properties of a Ca^{++}-activated protease that may be involved in myofibrillar protein turnover. In: *Proteases and Biological Control,* edited by E. Reich, D. B. Rifkin, and E. Shaw, pp. 551–577. Cold Spring Harbor Laboratory, Cold Spring Harbor, New York.

19. Dresden, M. H., Heilman, S. A., and Schmidt, J. D. (1972): Collagenolytic enzymes in human neoplasms. *Cancer Res.,* 32:933–996.

20. Estensen, R. D., Hadden, J. W., Hadden, E. M., Touraine, F., Touraine, J. L., Haddox, M. K., and Goldberg, N. D. (1974): Phorbol myristate acetate: Effects of a tumor promoter on intracellular cyclic GMP in mouse fibroblasts and as a mitogen on human lymphocytes. In: *Control of Proliferation in Animal Cells,* edited by B. Clarkson and R. Baserga, pp. 627–634. Cold Spring Harbor Laboratory, Cold Spring Harbor, New York.

21. Faawang, H. J. (1962): The influence of glucocorticosteroids and corticotropic hormone on output of human urinary trypsin inhibitor. *Acta Pharmacol. Toxicol. (Kbh),* 19:293–304.

22. Finlay, T. H., Troll, V. G., Levy, M., Johnson, A. J., and Hodgins, L. T. (1978): New methods for the preparation of biospecific adsorbents and immobilized enzymes utilizing trichloro-s-triazine. *Anal. Biochem.,* 87:77–90.

23. Garte, S. J., Troll, W., and Belman, S. (1978): Effect of phorbol myristate acetate on cyclic nucleotide levels in normal and stimulated mouse epidermis *in vivo. Proc. Am. Assoc. Cancer Res.,* 19:7.

24. Giraldi, T., Kopitar, M., and Sava, G. (1977): Anti metastatic effects of a leukocyte intracellular inhibitor of neutral proteases. *Cancer Res.,* 37:3834–3835.

25. Goldberg, A. R., Walf, B. A., and Lefelve, P. A. (1975): Plasminogen activators of transformed and normal cells. In: *Proteases and Biological Control,* edited by E. Reich, D. B. Rifkin, and E. Shaw, pp. 857–868. Cold Spring Harbor Laboratory, Cold Spring Harbor, New York.

26. Goldberg, N. D., Haddox, M. K., Estensen, R., Lopez, C., and Hadden, J. W. (1973): Evidence for a dualism between cyclic GMP and cyclic AMP in the regulation of cell proliferation and other cellular processes. In: *Cyclic AMP in Immune Response and Tumor Growth,* edited by L. Lichtenstein and C. Parker, pp. 247–262. Springer-Verlag, New York.

27. Gwyn, R. H., and Salaman, M. H. (1953): Studies on cocarcinogenesis: SH-reactors and other substances tested for cocarcinogenic action in mouse skin. *Br. J. Cancer,* 7:428–438.

28. Hennings, H., and Boutwell, R. K. (1970): Studies on the mechanism of skin tumor promotion. *Cancer Res.,* 30:312–320.

29. Hodges, G. M., Livingston, D. C., and Franks, L. M. (1973): The localization of trypsin in cultured mammalian cells. *J. Cell Sci.,* 12:887–902.

30. Holley, R. W. (1973): Control of growth of mammalian cells in cell culture. *Nature,* 258:487–490.

31. Horwitz, A. L., Kelman, J. A., and Crystal, R. G. (1976): Activation of alveolar macrophage collagenase by a neutral protease secreted by the same cell. *Nature,* 264:772–774.

32. Hovi, T., Keski-Oja, J., and Vaheri, A. (1974): Growth control in chick embryo fibroblasts: No evidence for a specific role for cyclic purine nucleotides. *Cell,* 2:235–240.

33. Hozumi, M., Ogawa, M., Sugimura, T., Takeuchi, T., and Umezawa, H. (1972): Inhibition of tumorigenesis in mouse skin by leupeptin, a protease inhibitor from actinomycites. *Cancer Res.,* 32:1725–1728.

34. Hynes, R. O., and Bye, J. M. (1974): Density and cell cycle dependence of cell surface proteins in hamster fibroblasts. *Cell,* 3:113–118.

35. Hynes, R. O., Wyke, J. A., Bye, J. M., Humphryes, K. C., and Pearlstein, E. S. (1975): Are proteases involved in altering surface proteins during viral transformation. In: *Proteases and Biological Control,* edited by E. Reich, D. B. Rifkin, and E. Shaw, pp. 931–944. Cold Spring Harbor Laboratory, Cold Spring Harbor, New York.

36. Ikenaka, T., Odani, S., and Koide, T. (1974): Chemical structure and inhibitory activities of soybean proteinase inhibitors. In: *Proteinase Inhibitors,* edited by J. Fritz, H. Tschesche, L. H. Greene, and E. Truscheit, pp. 325–343. Springer-Verlag, New York.

37. Janoff, A., Klassen, A., and Troll, W. (1970): Local vascular changes induced by the cocarcinogen, phorbol myristates acetate. *Cancer Res.,* 30:2568–2571.

38. Katz, J., Troll, W., Adler, S. W., and Levitz, M. (1977): Antipain and leupeptin restrict uterine DNA synthesis and function in mice. *Proc. Natl. Acad. Sci. USA,* 74:3754–3757.

39. Kessner, A. (1977): Ph.D. thesis, New York University, Dept. of Biochemistry.

40. Kessner, A., and Troll, W. (1976): Fluorometric microassay of plasminogen activators. *Arch. Biochem. Biophys.,* 176:411–416.

41. Kolb, H. J., Renner, R., Hepp, K. D., Weiss, L., and Wieland, O. H. (1975): Re-evaluation of sepharose-insulin as a tool for the study of insulin action. *Proc. Natl. Acad. Sci. USA,* 72:248–252.

42. Kuettner, K. E., Soble, L., Croxen, R. L., Marczynska, B., Hiti, J., and Harper, E. (1977): Tumor cell collagenase and its inhibition by a cartilage-derived protease inhibitor. *Science,* 196:653–654.

43. Langer, R., Brem, H., Talterman, K., Klein, M., and Folkman, J. (1976): Isolation of a cartilage factor that inhibits tumor neovascularization. *Science,* 194:70–72.

44. Martin, B. M., and Quigley, J. P. (1977): Binding and uptake of thrombin: possible role in the thrombin-induced mitogenesis of chick embryo fibroblasts. In: *Chemistry and Biology of Thrombin,* edited by R. L. Lundblad, J. W. Fenton II, and K. G. Nann, pp. 531–544. Ann Arbor Science, Ann Arbor, Michigan.

45. Matsushima, T., Kaziko, T., Kawachi, T., Hara, K., Sugimura, T., Takeuchi, T., and Umezawa, H. (1975): Effects of protease-inhibitors of microbial origin on experimental carcinogenesis. In: *Fundamentals in Cancer Prevention,* edited by P. N. Magee et al., pp. 57–69. University of Tokyo Press, Tokyo/University Park Press, Baltimore.

46. Meyn, M. S., Rossman, T., and Troll, W. (1977): A protease inhibitor blocks SOS functions in *Escherichia coli:* Antipain prevents λ repressor inactivation, ultraviolet mutagenesis and filamentous growth. *Proc. Natl. Acad. Sci. USA,* 74:1152–1156.

47. Miller, E. C., and Miller, J. M. (1971): The mutagenicity of chemical carcinogens: Correlations, problems and interpretations. In: *Chemical Mutagens,* Vol. I, edited by A. Hollaender, pp. 83–119. Plenum Press, New York.

48. Moens, W., Vokaer, A., and Kram, R. (1975): Cyclic AMP and cyclic GMP concentrations in serum and density-restricted fibroblast cultures. *Proc. Natl. Acad. Sci. USA,* 72:1063–1067.

49. Neurath, H. (1975): Limited proteolysis and zymogen activation. In: *Proteases and Biological Control,* edited by E. Reich, D. Rifkin, and E. Shaw, pp. 51–64. Cold Spring Harbor Laboratories, Cold Spring Harbor, New York.

50. Nicolson, G. L. (1972): Topography of membrane concanavalin A sites modified by proteolysis. *Nature [New Biol.],* 239:193–197.

51. Noonan, N. E., and Noonan, K. D. (1977): The effect of TLCK on transcription and its role in modifying cell growth. *J. Cell Physiol.,* 92:137–144.

52. Ossowski, L., Quigley, J. P., Kellerman, G. M., and Reich, E. (1973): Fibrinolysis associated with oncogenic transformation. Requirement of plasminogen for correlated changes in cellular morphology, colony formation in agar and cell migration. *J. Exp. Med.,* 138:1056–1064.

53. Pastan, I. H., Johnson, G. S., and Anderson, W. B. (1975): Role of cyclic nucleotides in growth control. *Ann. Rev. Biochem.,* 44:491–522.

54. Pollack, R., Osborn, M., and Weber, K. (1975): Patterns of organization of actin and myosin in normal and transformed cultured cells. *Proc. Natl. Acad. Sci. USA,* 72:994–998.

55. Pollack, R., Risser, R., Conlon, S., Freedman, V., Shin, S., and Rifkin, D. B. (1975): Production of plasminogen activator and colonial growth in semisolid medium are in vitro correlates of tumorigenicity in the immune-deficient nude mouse. In: *Proteases and Biological Control,* edited by E. Reich, D. Rifkin, and E. Shaw, pp. 885–899. Cold Spring Harbor Laboratory, Cold Spring Harbor, New York.

56. Pong, S. S., Nuss, T. L., and Koch, G. (1975): Inhibition of initiation of protein synthesis in mammalian tissue culture cells by L-1-tosylamide-2-phenylethyl chloromethyl ketone. *J. Biol. Chem.,* 250:240–245.

57. Quigley, J. P. (1976): Association of a protease (plasminogen activator) with a specific membrane fraction isolated from transformed cells. *J. Cell Biol.,* 71:472–486.

58. Reich, E. (1975): Plasminogen activator: Secretion by neoplastic cells and macrophages. In: *Proteases and Biological Control,* edited by E. Reich, D. B. Rifkin, and E. Shaw, pp. 333–342. Cold Spring Harbor Laboratory, Cold Spring Harbor, New York.

59. Richert, N. D., and Ryan, R. J. (1977): Protease inhibitors block hormonal activation of adenylate cyclase. *Biochem. Biophys. Res. Commun.,* 78:799–805.

60. Rifkin, D. B., Beal, L. P., and Reich, E. (1975): Macromolecular determinant of plasminogen activator synthesis. In: *Proteases and Biological Control,* edited by E. Reich, D. B. Rifkin, and E. Shaw, pp. 841–847. Cold Spring Harbor Laboratory, Cold Spring Harbor, New York.

61. Roberts, J. W., and Roberts, C. W. (1975): Proteolytic cleavage of bacteriophage lambda repressor in induction. *Proc. Natl. Acad. Sci. USA,* 72:147–151.

62. Roblin, R., Chou, I., and Black, P. H. (1975): Proteolytic enzymes, cell surface changes, and viral transformation. *Adv. Cancer Res.,* 22:203–260.
63. Rossman, T., Norris, C., and Troll, W. (1974): Inhibition of macromolecular synthesis in *Escherichia coli* by protease inhibitors: Specific reversal by glutathione of the effect of chloromethyl ketones. *J. Biol. Chem.,* 249:1152–1156.
64. Rubin, R. W., and Weiss, G. D. (1975): Direct biochemical measurements of microtubule assembly and disassembly in chinese hamster ovary cells. *J. Cell Biol.,* 64:42–53.
65. Rudland, P. S., Gospodarowicz, D., and Seifert, W. (1974): Activation of guanyl cyclase and intracellular cGMP by fibroblasts growth factor. *Nature,* 250:741–774.
66. Schnebli, H. P., and Burger, M. M. (1972): Selective inhibition of growth of transformed cells by protease inhibitors. *Proc. Natl. Acad. Sci. USA,* 69:3825–3829.
67. Schultz, D. R. (1976): Biological functions of activated complement proteins in normal and disease states. In: *Proteases and Physiological Regulation,* edited by D. W. Ribbons et al., pp. 143–185. Academic Press, New York.
68. Slaga, T. J., Bowden, G. T., and Boutwell, R. K. (1975): Acetic acid, a potent stimulator of mouse epidermal macromolecular synthesis and hyperplasia but with weak tumor-promoting activity. *J. Natl. Cancer Inst.,* 55:983–987.
69. Smets, L. A., and De Ley, L. (1974): Cell cycle dependent modulations of the surface membrane of normal and SV40 virus transformed 3T3 cells. *J. Cell Physiol.,* 84:343–348.
70. Sylven, B. (1973): Biochemical and Enzymatic factors involved in cellular detachment. In: *Chemotherapy of Cancer Dissemination and Mitartases,* edited by S. Garattini and G. Franchi, pp. 129–136. Raven Press, New York.
71. Thomas, C. A., Yost, F. J., Snyderman, R., Hatcher, V. B., and Lazarus, G. S. (1977): Cellular serine proteinase induces chemotaxis by complement activation. *Nature,* 269:521–523.
72. Troll, W. (1976): Blocking tumor promotion by protease inhibitors. In: *Fundamentals of Cancer Prevention,* edited by P. N. Magee et al., pp. 41–53. University of Tokyo Press, Tokyo/University Park Press, Baltimore.
73. Troll, W., Belman, S., and Levine, E. (1963): The effect of metabolites of 2-naphthylamine and the mutagen hydroxylamine on the thermal stability of DNA. *Cancer Res.,* 23:841–846.
74. Troll, W., Klassen, A., and Janoff, A. (1970): Tumorigenesis in mouse skin: Inhibition by synthetic inhibitors of proteases. *Science,* 169:1211–1213.
75. Troll, W., Meyn, M. S., and Rossman, T. G. (1978): Mechanisms of protease action in carcinogenesis. In: *Carcinogenesis, Vol. 2. Mechanisms of Tumor Promotion and Cocarcinogenesis,* edited by T. J. Slaga, A. Sivak, and R. K. Boutwell, pp. 301–312. Raven Press, New York.
76. Troll, W., Rossman, T., Katz, J., Levitz, M., and Sugimura, T. (1975): Proteinases in tumor promotion and hormone action. In: *Proteases and Biological Control,* edited by E. Reich, D. Rifkin, and E. Shaw, pp. 977–987. Cold Spring Harbor Laboratory, Cold Spring Harbor, New York.
77. Umezawa, H. (1972): *Enzyme Inhibitors of Microbial Origin,* pp. 29–32. University of Tokyo Press, Tokyo.
78. Umezawa, K., Matsushima, T., and Sugimura, T. (1977): Antimutagenic effect of elastatinal, a protease inhibitor from actinomycetes. *Proc. Jap. Acad.,* 53 B:30–33.
79. Unkeless, J., Dano, K., Kellerman, G. M., and Reich, E. (1974): Fibrinolysis associated with oncogenic transformation. *J. Biol. Chem.,* 249:4295–4305.
80. Unkeless, J. C., Gordon, S., and Reich, E. (1974): Secretion of plasminogen activator by stimulated macrophages. *J. Exp. Med.,* 139:834.
81. Viaje, A., Slaga, T. J., Wigler, M., and Weinstein, I. B. (1977): Effects of antinflammatory agents on mouse skin tumor promotion, epidermal DNA synthesis, phorbol ester-induced cellular proliferation and production of plasminogen activator. *Cancer Res.,* 37:1530–1536.
82. Verloes, R., and Kanerek, L. (1976): Proteolytic activity associated with tumor growth and metastasis. Influence of trypsin inhibitor (soya bean) on Ehrlich assites tumor growth. *Arch. Int. Physiol. Biochem.,* 84:1119–1120.
83. Wallach, D., Anderson, W., and Pastan, I. (1978): Activation of adenylate cyclase in cultured fibroblasts by trypsin. *J. Biol. Chem.,* 253:24–26.
84. Weber, M. J., Hale, A. H., and Rall, D. E. (1975): Role of protease activity in malignant transformation by Rous sarcoma virus. In: *Proteases and Biological Control,* edited by E. Reich, D. Rifkin, and E. Shaw, pp. 915–930. Cold Spring Harbor Laboratories, Cold Spring Harbor, New York.

85. Weinstein, I. B., and Wigler, M. (1977): Cell culture studies provide new information on tumor promoters. *Nature,* 270:659–660.

86. Weinstein, I. B., Wigler, M., Fisher, P. B., Sisskin, E., and Pietrapaolo, C. (1978): Cell culture studies on the biologic effects of tumor promoters. In: *Carcinogenesis, Vol. 2: Mechanisms of Tumor Promotion and Cocarcinogenesis,* edited by T. J. Slaga, A. Sivak, and R. K. Boutwell, pp. 313–333. Raven Press, New York.

87. Weinstein, I. B., Wigler, M., and Pietrapaolo, C. (1976): The action of tumor promoting agents in cell culture. In: *The Origins of Human Cancer,* Cold Spring Harbor Symposium, edited by H. H. Hiatt, J. D. Watson, and J. A. Winsten, pp. 751–772. Cold Spring Harbor, New York.

88. Whitfield, J. F., Mac Manus, J. P., and Gillan, D. J. (1973): Calcium-dependent stimulation by a phorbol ester (PMA) of thymic lymphoblast DNA synthesis and proliferation. *J. Cell Physiol.,* 82:151–156.

89. Wigler, M., Ford, J. P., and Weinstein, I. B. (1975): Glucocorticoid inhibition of the fibrinolytic activity of tumor cells. In: *Proteases and Biological Control,* edited by E. Reich, D. B. Rifkin, and E. Shaw, pp. 849–856. Cold Spring Harbor Laboratory, Cold Spring Harbor, New York.

90. Wigler, M., and Weinstein, I. B. (1976): Tumor promoter induces plasminogen activator. *Nature,* 259:232–233.

91. Wilson, S. R., and Huffman, J. C. (1976): The structural relationship of phorbol and cortisol: A possible mechanism for the tumor promoting activity of phorbol. *Experientia,* 32:1489.

92. Witkin, E. M. (1976): Ultraviolet mutagenesis and inducible DNA repair in *Escherichia coli. Bact. Rev.,* 40:869–907.

93. Zetter, B. R., Chen, L. B., and Buchanan, J. M. (1977): Binding and internalization of thrombin by normal and transformed chick cells. *Proc. Natl. Acad. Sci. USA,* 74:596–600.

Carcinogenesis, Vol. 5: Modifiers of Chemical Carcinogenesis, edited by T. J. Slaga. Raven Press, New York, 1980.

8

Inhibitory Effects of Environmental Chemicals on Polycyclic Aromatic Hydrocarbon Carcinogenesis

*John DiGiovanni, **Thomas J. Slaga, **D. L. Berry, and †M. R. Juchau

*The McArdle Laboratory for Cancer Research, University of Wisconsin Medical Center, Madison, Wisconsin 53706; **Biology Division, Oak Ridge National Laboratory, Oak Ridge, Tennessee 37830; and †Department of Pharmacology, School of Medicine, University of Washington, Seattle, Washington 98195*

The majority of human cancers, approximately 80 to 90%, are considered to be induced by chemicals present in the environment. The area of epidemiology and geographic pathology has established the most impressive incrimination of chemicals in the environment as a major cause of cancer in man. Many of these environmental chemicals are known to cause cancer in experimental animals. Polycyclic aromatic hydrocarbons (PAH) are widespread contaminants in our environment, occurring primarily as the result of combustion and pyrolysis of organic materials (e.g., cigarette smoke, automobile exhaust, industrial combustion processes, etc.). Concern over the prevalence of PAH arises from evidence that a significant number of these compounds are known to be carcinogenic. It has been estimated that approximately 2,000 tons of benzo(a)pyrene (BP), a widely studied PAH carcinogen, are dumped into the atmosphere in the United States annually (61). Not only PAH, but also a wide variety of other environmentally occurring, structurally diverse chemicals including aromatic amines, nitrosamines, nitrosamides, aflatoxins, and many others are known to be carcinogenic (36).

In addition to the wide variety of *known* carcinogenic chemicals found dispersed in our environment, a large number of noncarcinogenic or weakly carcinogenic foreign substances are also present. Many of these chemicals occur as unwanted contaminants whereas others are present as the result of intentional usage. It has been estimated that approximately 1.06 billion lb of additives are incorporated intentionally into food annually in this country alone. Some of these additives are obviously beneficial to man (e.g., vitamins, minerals) whereas others may be harmful, such as food coloring agents (e.g., red dye #2), nitrites, saccharin, etc. Furthermore, many chemicals known to possess diverse biological activities occur naturally in fruits and vegetables (e.g., flavonoids and indoles). Those chemicals occurring as unwanted contaminants include pesticides, herbicides, industrial chemicals, and mycotoxins as well as PAH. With such a wide variety of chemicals found in the environment, the potential for interaction with two or more compounds (one of which may be a carcinogen) in a biological system is highly probable. The combined effect(s) may be insignificant, but, on the other hand, anticarcinogenic or cocarcinogenic interactions are quite possible. The type of effect ultimately observed depends on the nature of the chemicals, time, dose, and sequence of exposure.

The present chapter deals with the *anticarcinogenic* effects of the following chemicals found in the environment (either as a result of intentional usage or unintentional contamination): flavonoids, antioxidants, PAH, and chlorinated hydrocarbons. Special emphasis will be placed on understanding the mechanisms by which these compounds inhibit PAH carcinogenesis. Understanding the mechanism(s) by which various compounds inhibit chemically induced cancer will not only aid in an understanding of chemical carcinogenesis per se, but also may open potential avenues to a rational approach for chemoprevention.

REQUIREMENT FOR METABOLIC ACTIVATION OF PAH

Biologic activation is presumed to be essential for the observed toxic effects of PAH. The microsomal system of mixed-function oxygenases has been implicated in the activation of PAH to toxic, mutagenic and/or carcinogenic metabolites. Gelboin et al. (31,32) have proposed that the specific enzyme complex aryl hydrocarbon hydroxylase (AHH, E.C. 1.14.14.2) is responsible for activation of PAH to epoxide intermediates. Epoxide intermediates can then undergo spontaneous rearrangement to phenols, be converted enzymatically to trans-dihydrodiols via epoxide hydratase, become conjugated with glutathione, react directly with cellular macromolecules, or, after conversion to trans-dihydrodiols, be subsequently oxidized to diol-epoxides (4,15,21,22,36,46,62,70,76,77,95). As stated previously, a wide structural diversity exists among the various classes of chemical carcinogens. E. C. Miller and J. A. Miller (59) have proposed a general theory of chemical carcinogenesis that represents a unifying concept for this wide diversity of chemical structures. They proposed that: (a) all chemical carcinogens that are not themselves chemically reactive must be converted metabolically into a chemically reactive form; (b) the activated metabolite is an electrophilic reagent; and (c) this activated metabolite reacts with nucleophilic groups in cellular macromolecules to initiate carcinogenesis. The extent of binding of several PAH to mouse skin DNA (deoxyribonucleic acid) (16) and protein (35) *in vivo* has been reported to correlate well with the carcinogenic activity of the hydrocarbon. Furthermore, a positive correlation was found between the tumor-initiating activity of several PAH and their ability to bind to DNA *in vitro* using epidermal homogenates as the source of metabolizing enzymes (18). A positive correlation was also observed with respect to the degree of carcinogenicity and covalent binding of PAH to DNA in hamster embryo cells in culture (41) but not to RNA or protein.

Many of the chemicals to be discussed in this chapter appear to modify PAH carcinogenesis by altering the levels of critical electrophilic intermediates capable of forming covalent bonds with macromolecules. This appears in many cases to be an effect on the enzyme systems responsible for formation or degradation of carcinogenic electrophiles.

THE TWO-STAGE SYSTEM OF MOUSE SKIN CARCINOGENESIS

It is important to utilize a test system appropriate for studying modifiers of carcinogenesis, i.e., one that will allow dissection of the carcinogenic process into component parts. This allows a more critical evaluation of the mechanism of a given modifier. One such system that has been used extensively in our laboratories, as well as others, is the two-stage, initiation-promotion system of mouse skin carcinogenesis. That mouse skin carcinogenesis occurs in at least two stages, initiation and promotion, has been demonstrated clearly by the

1. Modification of Tumor Initiation

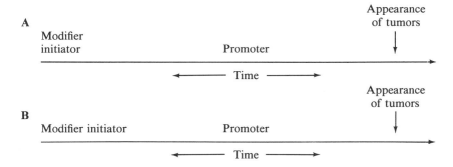

2. Modification of tumor promotion

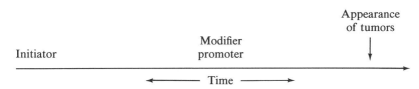

Scheme 1. Methods for studying modifiers of carcinogenesis in the two-stage system of mouse skin carcinogenesis. Each time line depicted above represents a classical initiation-promotion experiment, i.e., application of a subcarcinogenic dose of a carcinogen followed one week later by repeated applications of a promoting substance (e.g., TPA). Modifiers of tumor initiation may be studied by application simultaneously with or prior to the initiator (**A** and **B,** respectively). Modifiers of tumor promotion may be analyzed by administration subsequent to application of the initiator and in conjunction with the promoter.

work of Boutwell (12). Initiation is a rapid, irreversible cellular change accomplished by a single application of a very small, noncarcinogenic dose of a carcinogen, e.g., 7,12-dimethylbenz*(a)*anthracene (DMBA), to the skin of mice. No tumors result from this treatment, but it so affects the skin that the process of tumor development may then be accomplished by repeated applications of a noncarcinogenic agent (promoter). The advantages of using mouse skin as a model system for studying carcinogenesis have been outlined in detail (13). A particular advantage is that systemic metabolism of the carcinogen is not likely to affect the overall response since only very small doses of the carcinogen are applied locally. When carcinogens are given in test systems that measure *complete* carcinogenesis, modifiers may affect the level of carcinogen reaching the target tissue by altering its disposition or metabolism in other tissues such as the liver. In the two-stage system, the effects of modifiers on initiation and/ or promotion can be analyzed, depending upon the time of administration as illustrated in Scheme 1. To determine whether modifiers are likely to alter tumor initiation, they may be applied prior to or simultaneously with the initiator. Agents that inhibit the AHH enzyme system have been tested by concomitant administration with initiator. Compounds that are known to induce the AHH enzyme system are tested by applying them prior to administration of the initiator at a time that allows for maximum enzyme induction. Finally, compounds can be tested for their effects on tumor promotion by administration subsequent to application of the initiator and in conjunction with promoter.

INHIBITORY EFFECT OF FLAVONES ON PAH CARCINOGENESIS

7,8-Benzoflavone (7,8-BF) and 5,6-benzoflavone (5,6-BF), two synthetic derivatives from a large class of naturally occurring flavonoid compounds, have marked inhibitory effects on carcinogenesis by PAH. Wattenberg and Leong (92) reported that intraperitoneal injections of 5,6-BF inhibited formation of pulmonary tumors in mice and mammary tumors in rats resulting from exposure to DMBA. 5,6-BF was found to be an effective inducer of the AHH enzyme complex of liver, lung, and small intestine. A series of naturally occurring flavones were tested for their ability to induce AHH in liver and lung of rats (94). 5,6,7,8,3',4'-Hexamethoxyflavone (nobiletin) was the most potent inducer of AHH in the series of natural flavones followed by 5,6,7,8,4'-pentamethoxyflavone (tangeretin) and 3,3',4',5,7-pentamethoxyflavone (quercetin pentamethyl ether). An extension of the latter study revealed that the feeding of three flavones of varying inducing activity (5,6-BF > quercetin pentamethyl ether > rutin) produced an inhibition of the formation of BP-induced pulmonary adenomas in A/HeJ mice (93). The ability to inhibit tumor formation correlated well with the ability of these flavones to induce lung AHH. 5,6-BF also reduced skin tumor formation by BP under conditions in which prior exposure to the flavone had induced a high level of AHH activity in the target tissue (93).

7,8-BF is an isomer of 5,6-BF and has been shown to inhibit the AHH enzyme system in hepatic tissue preparations from rats pretreated with methylcholan-threne (MCA) (23,32) as well as in mouse epidermal tissue preparations from either untreated or MCA-pretreated animals (14,31). The liver of adult rodents normally is a nontarget tissue for PAH carcinogens. Mouse skin, however, is a known target tissue for PAH and contains a highly inducible AHH enzyme system (17,84,96). 7,8-BF given topically to mice inhibited skin tumor initiation by DMBA (14,31) and also binding of DMBA to epidermal macromolecules (14,49). On the other hand, 7,8-BF was found to enhance the skin tumorigenesis elicited by BP (48). This flavone inhibited binding of DMBA to epidermal DNA, RNA, and protein and, to a lesser degree, the binding of BP to macro-molecules (48). Bowden et al. (14) also reported that 7,8-BF inhibited skin tumor initiation by DMBA and reversed its inhibition of DNA synthesis. In this investigation, 7,8-BF stimulated tumor initiation by dibenz(a,h)anthracene (DB(a,h)A) but had no effect on the covalent binding of DB(a,h)A to epidermal macromolecules. 5,6-BF slightly inhibited tumor initiation and macromolecular binding in the case of either DMBA or DB(a,h)A. 5,6-BF inhibited mouse epidermal AHH *in vitro,* although it was less potent than 7,8-BF (14,31,80).

Table 1 summarizes some results from our laboratories regarding the effects of 7,8-BF on PAH-elicited skin tumor initiation in female CD-1 mice. 7,8-BF was applied topically at the doses indicated 5 min prior to initiation with the hydrocarbon. Under these conditions, 7,8-BF slightly inhibited epidermal AHH (31,80). A 100 μg dose of 7,8-BF produced a marked inhibition in the tumor response to both DMBA and MCA. Initiation with BP also was inhibited but to a lesser degree than with DMBA or MCA as the initiating agents. Interest-

TABLE 1. *Effects of 7,8-BF on DMBA, MCA, BP, and DB(a,h)A tumor initiation*[a]

Initiator	Dose of initiator (nmol)	Modifier 7,8-BF[b] (100 μg)	Number of mice[c]	Papillomas per mouse[d]	Percent of controls
DMBA	10	none	29	4.2	100
DMBA	10	7,8-BF	30	0.8	19
MCA	50	none	28	6.4	100
MCA	50	7,8-BF	29	1.5	23
BP	400	none	30	7.4	100
BP	400	7,8-BF	29	5.4	73
BP	400	7,8-BF[e]	29	5.0	68
DB(a,h)A	180	none	28	5.4	100
DB(a,h)A	180	7,8-BF[f]	29	8.8	163

[a]One week after tumor initiation the mice were treated twice weekly with 10 μg TPA for 30 weeks.
[b]7,8-BF was given 5 min before the tumor initiator.
[c]Number of mice surviving after 30 weeks of promotion.
[d]Total papillomas per total number of surviving mice.
[e]7,8-BF was given at a dose of 200 μg 5 min before BP.
[f]7,8-BF was given at a dose of 1000 μg 5 min before DB(a,h)A.

ingly, initiation with DB(a,h)A was enhanced. The observed inhibitory effect of 7,8-BF on tumor initiation by BP stands in contrast to a previous report (48) and may be related to the doses of both BP and 7,8-BF utilized.

Table 2 summarizes further work from our laboratories on the effects of several other flavones on skin tumor initiation by DMBA and BP. 7,8-BF and 5,6-BF each (when tested in the two-stage system) produced an inhibition of skin tumor initiation by DMBA that correlated most closely with their ability to inhibit the AHH enzyme in homogenates from this target tissue (80). 3,3',4',5,7-Pentahydroxyflavone (quercetin) was the only naturally occurring flavone that produced a reproducible inhibition of skin tumor initiation by both DMBA and BP. 3,3',4',5,5',7-Hexahydroxyflavone (myricetin) and 4',5,7-trihydroxyflavanone (naringenin) enhanced skin tumor initiation by DMBA (26). A previous report (49) also showed 4',5,7-trihydroxyflavone (apigenin) to enhance skin tumor initiation by DMBA. These results reemphasize the complexity of the carcinogenic process and demonstrate the difficulties involved in applying generalizations within a series of inhibitors.

7,8-BF (6,24,71) and 5,6-BF (6,24) have been analyzed for their effects on metabolism *in vitro* of BP and DMBA in adult rat liver and mouse skin utilizing high pressure liquid chromatography (HPLC). These flavones appear to inhibit the initial oxidative attack by monooxygenases present in the tissue. This is demonstrated by a reduced formation of all detectable metabolites appearing in the chromatographic profiles. Furthermore, 7,8-BF and 5,6-BF inhibit the formation *in vitro* of electrophilic intermediates of PAH capable of binding covalently to DNA (80). Finally, a recent study by DiGiovanni et al. (26)

TABLE 2. *Effects of flavones on skin tumor initiation by BP and DMBA[a]*

Initiator	Modifier[b] treatment	Modifier dose/mouse (μg)	Number of mice[c]	Papillomas per mouse[d]	Percent of control
DMBA	none	—	30	3.4	100
DMBA	7,8-BF	25	30	0.9	26
DMBA	7,8-BF	25 (x3)[e]	30	0.4	12
DMBA	5,6-BF	100	29	2.6	76
DMBA	5,6-BF	1,000	26	2.2	65
DMBA	quercetin	100	28	2.6	78
DMBA	myricetin	100	29	5.2	154
DMBA	naringenin	100	30	4.4	129
BP	none	—	30	7.8	100
BP	quercetin	100	28	5.7	72

[a] All mice were initiated with either 10 nmol DMBA or 400 nmoles BP and promoted two times per week with 10 μg TPA starting one week after initiation.
[b] Modifier was given 5 min prior to initiation with hydrocarbon.
[c] Number of surviving mice after 30 weeks of promotion.
[d] Total papillomas/total number of surviving mice.
[e] 7,8-BF was applied topically as three separate 25 μg applications 6 hr prior to, 5 min prior to, and 6 hr after initiation with DMBA.

suggested that 7,8-BF does not inhibit tumor initiation with chemically reactive derivatives of DMBA by a direct chemical interaction with the hydrocarbon.

In summary, there appear to be several possible mechanisms for the inhibition by flavones of PAH-induced carcinogenesis. Wattenberg and co-workers (92,93) have suggested that, under conditions of complete carcinogenesis testing and prior exposure of animals to inducing doses of flavones, inhibition results from an increased AHH activity in the target tissue. The exact mechanism by which increased AHH would bring about a decrease in carcinogenicity is not fully understood. It should be emphasized that other mechanisms could be responsible for the observed inhibitory effects. The flavones could, in fact, reduce carcinogenicity by inducing AHH in nontarget tissues resulting in greater metabolism at these sites and a reduction of carcinogen at the target tissue, i.e., an effective reduction in dose. Investigations with the two-stage, initiation-promotion system of mouse skin carcinogenesis have suggested that the flavones, when applied simultaneously with several PAH, reduce tumor formation at least in part by virtue of their ability to inhibit the enzyme system(s) responsible for generating electrophilic intermediates. Why certain flavones enhance tumor initiation with some PAH is not clear. However, these compounds may affect inactivating as well as activating metabolic pathways and this requires further investigation. It is apparent that the mechanism of inhibition of PAH-induced carcinogenesis by flavones depends on many factors including the test system utilized, dose of carcinogen and flavone, time of exposure, route of exposure and the chemical nature of the flavone and PAH.

INHIBITION OF PAH CARCINOGENESIS BY ANTIOXIDANTS

Butylated hydroxyanisole (BHA), butylated hydroxytoluene (BHT), and propyl gallate are antioxidants that are commonly added to foods to maintain freshness and prevent spoilage by oxidation. They are frequently used in dried cereals, cooking oils, canned goods, and various animal foods. The average daily intake of phenolic antioxidants by man has been estimated at 2 mg (20). They are not readily excreted and tend to accumulate in the body (20). Although the phenolic antioxidants are generally recognized as safe by the FDA, there are varying reports as to the effects of these food additives on organisms. It has been reported that BHT is toxic to developing insect larvae (5) and reduces the growth rate of cultured cells (58). On the other hand, the phenolic antioxidants, selenium and vitamins C and E, each have been shown to exert a protective function in experimental animals against liver damage, aging, carcinogen-induced chromosomal breakage and chemical carcinogenesis (19,34,45,75,87–89).

When added to the diet, BHA, BHT and ethoxyquin inhibited the carcinogenic effect of dietary DMBA or BP on the forestomach of the mouse and the mammary gland of the rat by 50% or greater (87). Addition of BHA to the diet protected against pulmonary neoplasms produced by acute exposures to DMBA, BP, urethan or uracil mustard (89). The addition of BHA to the diets containing

DMBA, 7-hydroxymethyl-12-methylbenz *(a)*anthracene or DB(a,h)A likewise inhibited pulmonary tumor formation (89). Reportedly, the antioxidants selenium (72), vitamin E (74), and ascorbic acid (73), applied to mouse skin, significantly reduced the formation of tumors resulting from DMBA initiation in a two-stage system of tumorigenesis. This topic is covered more fully in Chapter 4.

Table 3 summarizes results from our laboratories regarding the effects of several antioxidants on skin-tumor initiation by DMBA in CD-1 mice. With the conditions utilized, all the antioxidants studied significantly inhibited tumor initiation by DMBA. When 1 mg BHT was applied topically as three separate applications (total 3 mg) at 6 hr and 5 min prior to and 6 hr after DMBA initiation, it inhibited tumorigenesis quite effectively. None of the antioxidants were found to significantly increase epidermal AHH or had any effect on the activity of AHH *in vitro* when epidermal homogenates were utilized as the enzyme source (79). Speier and Wattenberg (81) recently reported that BHA feeding did not change hepatic AHH activity. However, BHA or BHT applied topically to mice inhibited the epidermally mediated, NADPH-dependent covalent binding of [^{3}H]BP and [^{3}H]DMBA to calf thymus DNA *in vitro* (79). In general, BHT was more effective in inhibiting this binding than BHA. It is interesting to note that when added *in vitro,* BHT had no effect on epidermally mediated, NADPH-dependent covalent binding of either BP or DMBA to DNA. Speier and Wattenberg (81) also reported that incubation of radioactive BP with DNA and hepatic microsomes from BHA-fed mice resulted in significantly less covalent binding of BP to DNA when compared with control microsomes.

Other antioxidants have been shown to have a protective action against the development of neoplasms induced by PAH, nitrosamines, or dimethylhydrazine.

TABLE 3. *Effects of several antioxidants on skin tumor initiation by DMBA[a]*

Experiment	Modifier treatment[b]	Number of mice[c]	Papillomas per mouse[d]	Percent of control[e]
1	None	30	3.4	100
2	BHT	30	1.6	47
3	BHT	29	0.9	26
4	BHA	29	2.4	70
5	Vitamin C	30	1.9	56
6	Vitamin E	29	2.1	26

[a] All mice were initiated with 10 nmol DMBA and promoted 1 week later with 10 μg TPA two times per week.

[b] Modifiers were applied 5 min prior to initiation with DMBA as 1 mg topical doses. In experiment 3, mice received BHT as three separate 1 mg applications 6 hr and 5 min prior to and 6 hr after initiation with DMBA.

[c] Number of mice surviving after 30 weeks of promotion.

[d] Total papillomas/total number of surviving mice.

[e] Expressed as a percentage of the papillomas per mouse in the DMBA-initiated, TPA-promoted group (experiment 1).

Disulfiram and dimethyldithiocarbamate, when added to the diet, inhibited the formation of DMBA-induced mammary tumors and adrenal necrosis in female rats (90). In the mouse, disulfiram prevented BP-induced tumors of the forestomach (90).

In general, the antioxidants may protect against PAH carcinogenesis by altering the enzymes responsible for converting hydrocarbons to electrophilic intermediates. The result is a decrease in the amount of active PAH reaching the critical cellular target, in this case presumed to be DNA. However, it must be emphasized that the mechanism of the inhibitory effects of antioxidants may be unrelated to the biotransformation of the carcinogens. Other possibilities remain to be explored and also have been discussed by Wattenberg, *this volume.*

INHIBITORY EFFECTS OF WEAK OR NON-CARCINOGENIC PAH ON PAH CARCINOGENESIS

Combustion processes generate mixtures of PAH with a wide range of carcinogenic activity. Exposure to mixtures of PAH may produce variable effects, depending on the ratios of the various strongly carcinogenic to weakly or noncarcinogenic constituents. As an example, 1,2-benz*(a)*anthracene (BA), a weak carcinogen, when applied simultaneously with DB(a,h)A by subcutaneous injection, inhibited the carcinogenic action of DB(a,h)A (83). Hill et al. (38) investigated the effects of a number of PAH applied simultaneously with DMBA to the skins of mice. Several of these hydrocarbons were structurally quite similar to DMBA. 6,8-Dimethylbenz*(a)*anthracene and 1,2,5,6-dibenzofluorene were found to delay the appearance of tumors as well as reduce tumor yields, whereas 2-, 7-, or 8-methylbenz*(a)*anthracene prolonged the mean latent period but had no effect on the tumor yield. None of the inhibitors had any appreciable carcinogenic activity. 1,2,5,6-Dibenzofluorene also was found to delay the appearance of skin tumors caused by MCA when the two PAH were administered simultaneously (69). As a result of early studies such as these, it was postulated that the tumor-inhibiting actions of hydrocarbons were related to their weak carcinogenicity. However, DBA, BP and MCA also were shown to delay the appearance of DMBA-induced skin tumors when mixtures of these chemicals were applied simultaneously to the backs of mice (39), indicating that moderately strong carcinogens could likewise inhibit the action of strongly carcinogenic PAH.

Various partially hydrogenated derivatives of DB(a,h)A and MCA were found to inhibit the formation of sarcomas elicited by the parent hydrocarbons at the sites of subcutaneous injection (28,50). When tested in the two-stage system of mouse skin carcinogenesis, several hydrogenated derivatives of DB(a,h)A were found to inhibit initiation, whereas others were found to enhance tumor initiation (52). Enhancement or summation effects were noted by other investigators as well (82,83) when various hydrocarbon mixtures were administered simultaneously by subcutaneous injection. It should be pointed out that most of these early studies involved the use of test systems that measured complete carcinogenesis and thus did not discriminate with respect to the stage of carcinogenesis at which inhibition occurred. Furthermore, differences can be noted in the responses observed when complete carcinogenesis in the skin and in the subcutaneous tissues are compared. Huh and McCarter (42) attempted to resolve some of these difficulties by testing the effects of phenanthrene on tumor initiation in mouse skin by DMBA. Phenanthrene appeared to inhibit initiation by DMBA although the experiment was terminated at 20 weeks. Phenanthrene also was found to enhance rather than inhibit the absorption of DMBA into the skin.

The mechanism for the inhibitory effect of weak or noncarcinogenic PAH was proposed to be some type of competitive interaction with the more potent carcinogen, possibly at some critical intracellular target. The effects of BA on the DMBA-induced suppression of DNA synthesis and cytotoxicity in hamster embryo cells in culture have been investigated to further clarify the mechanism of inhibition of tumorigenesis. BA exerted a protective action against the suppressive activity of DMBA on DNA synthesis (1). Notably, the binding of [^{3}H]DMBA to the DNA of hamster embryo cells was almost completely abolished in the presence of equimolar concentrations of BA. BA also protected hamster embryo cells from cytotoxic damage caused by DMBA (2). Two mechanisms were postulated: (a) simultaneous treatment with BA and DMBA induced a high level of the AHH enzyme in the cells and thus a more rapid degradation of DMBA; or (b) competition between DMBA and BA for DNA binding sites resulted in a reduction of DMBA binding. In view of the time required for induction, the first postulate seems unlikely. Competition for a bioactivation process or for a DNA binding site, however, seems entirely possible.

It is important to point out that a number of the inhibitors discussed above possess the ability to induce the AHH enzyme system in a wide variety of tissues. As discussed in the section on flavones and as will be discussed at length in the following section, induction of monooxygenase enzymes may explain the mechanism of inhibition of formation of chemically induced tumors by certain compounds. In analyzing the role of induction, the time and sequence of exposure to the inducer are critical. Falk et al. (28) found that phenanthrene produced maximal inhibition of the production of sarcomas by DB(a,h)A at the site of injection when given 2 days prior to application of the carcinogen. This would be compatible with the suggestion that enzyme induction is an important mechanism of inhibition by phenanthrene. The microsomal enzyme-inducing potency of phenanthrene, however, appears to be extremely low (3).

We have been studying the effects of various weakly or noncarcinogenic PAH on the tumorigenic responses to moderately or strongly carcinogenic PAH. These investigations have utilized the two-stage, initiation-promotion regimen of skin carcinogenesis in mice to aid in an understanding of the mechanism(s) of inhibition produced by those compounds. Table 4 illustrates the effects of the weakly carcinogenic dibenz*(a,c)*anthracene (DB(a,c)A) on initiation of skin tumors by DMBA. When applied topically (at doses of 20 nmoles or greater) 5 min prior to initiation with DMBA, DB(a,c)A was found to be a potent

TABLE 4. *Effects of DB(a,c)A on the initiation of skin tumors by DMBA*

Pretreatment dose of DB(a,c)A (nmol)	Pretreatment time	Initiating dose of DMBA (nmol)[a]	Papillomas per mouse (% of control)[b]
5	5 min	5	103
20	5 min	20	45
100	5 min	100	11
200	5 min	200	4.5
200	5 min	5	6.5
200	1 hr	10	11
200	12 hr	10	17
200	36 hr	10	18

[a] 30 mice were used per experimental group. One week after initiation, tumors were promoted with twice weekly applications of 10 μg TPA.

[b] The average number of papillomas per mouse after 24 weeks of promotion is expressed as a percentage of the DMBA control.

inhibitor of tumor initiation. DB(a,c)A, administered at a 200 nmole dose and followed 1 week later by twice weekly applications of 12-O-tetradecanoylphorbol-13-acetate, did not produce any tumors after 40 weeks of promotion. Also illustrated in Table 4 is the effect of topical *pretreatment* (1, 12, and 36 hr) with 200 nmoles of DB(a,c)A on DMBA tumor initiation. Maximum inhibition was observed with the 5 min pretreatment (i.e., simultaneous application) although pretreatment for 1, 12, or 36 hr produced significant inhibition as well. DB(a,c)A is a potent inducer of mouse epidermal AHH (84) with peak activity at 6 and 36 hr after treatment (78). When applied simultaneously at various doses, DB(a,c)A- and DMBA-induced AHH activity was much less than additive at all but the lowest doses (78). Furthermore, DB(a,c)A was found to inhibit the activity of epidermal AHH *in vitro* when added at concentrations approximately four times that of the substrate BP (78). These observations strongly suggest that induction of the carcinogen biotransforming enzymes are not involved in the mechanism of inhibition and that other mechanisms must be invoked.

Table 5 shows the effects of topical application of either DB(a,c)A, DMBA, or a combination of both on the epidermally mediated covalent binding of radioactive DMBA to DNA *in vitro*. Pretreatment (12 hr) with 200 nmol unlabeled DMBA increased the binding of [^{3}H]DMBA to DNA more than twofold when compared with that observed in acetone-treated controls. Pretreatment with 200 nmole doses of unlabeled DB(a,c)A increased the binding by more than fourfold at 12 to 36 hr after treatment. It should be noted that the covalent binding of [^{3}H]DMBA to DNA *in vitro* was substantially decreased when epidermal homogenates were isolated from mice pretreated with both DMBA and DB(a,c)A (administered concurrently) as compared with pretreatment with DMBA alone.

Table 6 summarizes the effects of several weakly or noncarcinogenic PAH on skin tumor initiation by DMBA and BP. When applied topically 5 min

TABLE 5. *Effect of a topical application of either DB(a,c)A or DMBA on the covalent binding* in vitro *of [³H]DMBA to DNA as effected by epidermal homogenates from pretreated mice*[a]

Time after pretreatment (hr)	Pretreatment	Specific activity[b] ($\times 10^4$)
12	Acetone	3.9
1	DMBA	5.2
12	DMBA	10.4
36	DMBA	4.6
1	DB(a,c)A	7.5
12	DB(a,c)A	17.3
36	DB(a,c)A	19.2
12	DMBA + DB(a,c)A [c]	7.3
12	DMBA + DB(a,c)A [d]	6.9

[a] Mice were treated topically with 200 nmol and killed at the times indicated.
[b] Specific activity is expressed as pmol bound per μg DNA per mg protein per 15 min incubation at 37°C (in the dark). Each value represents two experiments, with duplicate determinations per experiment. The standard deviation for each figure was less than 22%.
[c] DMBA and DB(a,c)A were given in 200 nmol doses simultaneously.
[d] DB(a,c)A was given in a 200 nmol dose 1 hr before a 10 nmol dose of DMBA. The mice were killed 12 hr after treatment with DMBA.

TABLE 6. *Effects of weak or noncarcinogenic PAH on skin tumor initiation by DMBA or BP*[a,b]

Pretreatment	Initiator	Papillomas per mouse (% of control)[c]
None	DMBA	100
Benzo(e)pyrene	DMBA	16
Pyrene	DMBA	50
Fluoranthene	DMBA	66
None	BP	100
Benzo(e)pyrene	BP	130
Pyrene	BP	135
Fluoranthene	BP	120

[a] The mice were initiated with either 10 nmol DMBA or 200 nmol BP and promoted twice weekly with 10 μg TPA. Benzo(e)pyrene, pyrene, and fluoranthene were given 5 min before the initiator at a dose of 100 μg.
[b] 30 mice were used per experimental group.
[c] The average number of papillomas per mouse after 20 weeks of promotion is expressed as a percentage of the DMBA or BP controls.

prior to initiation with DMBA, benzo*(e)*pyrene (BeP), pyrene, and fluoranthene produced varying degrees of inhibition of tumor formation. However, when applied 5 min prior to BP, they did not inhibit but actually may have slightly enhanced tumor initiation with the latter hydrocarbon.

There are several possible mechanisms to explain the inhibitory effects of DB(a,c)A, BeP, pyrene, and fluoranthene on DMBA tumor initiation. The first is induction of monooxygenases (AHH) in the skin. Although this mechanism cannot be ruled out at present, two factors argue against it: (a) the hydrocarbons were applied nearly simultaneously in single doses probably allowing insufficient time for significant enzyme induction by the inhibitor, and (b) several of the inhibitors are very poor inducers of microsomal enzyme activity (e.g., BeP, pyrene, and fluoranthene) (3). An alternate explanation may be that some competition between metabolites of the weak or noncarcinogen and those of the strong carcinogen may exist at the genome level. Finally, the only metabolic explanation that appears reasonable at present is that competition for bioactivation of DMBA takes place. A metabolic mechanism could also explain the apparent enhancing effect of weakly carcinogenic PAH on skin tumorigenesis initiated by BP. In this case, competition for *detoxifying* pathways may be the primary interaction. It is entirely possible that several of the above-mentioned mechanisms could operate simultaneously in addition to other unknown mechanisms. Further study is required to elucidate the exact nature of this interesting inhibitory response.

INHIBITORY EFFECTS OF CHLORINATED HYDROCARBONS ON PAH CARCINOGENESIS

Chlorinated hydrocarbons are recognized as among the most common man-made contaminants in the environment. DDT, for example, has been used extensively as a pesticide and its accumulation and persistence in the food chain is well established. Other organochlorine pesticides also present in the environment include dieldrin, aldrin, heptachlor, and chlordane. Polychlorinated biphenyls (PCBs) and chlorinated dibenzo-*p*-dioxins are two other major classes of chlorinated hydrocarbons with widespread distribution. 2,3,7,8-Tetrachlorodibenzo-*p*-dioxin (TCDD) is an extremely toxic and widely studied dioxin found as a contaminant in the commercial production of the herbicide and defoliant 2,4,5-T, as well as in certain pesticides. PCBs, on the other hand, have received wide usage in industry as plasticizers, and as heat exchange and hydraulic fluids. Other uses include their utilization in the manufacture of adhesives, paints, and in printing inks.

A common feature of these compounds is the capacity to induce microsomal enzyme systems of the liver as well as of other tissues. This section will limit discussion primarily to the PCBs and dioxins, although other pertinent data will be included. The PCBs are effective inducers of hepatic monooxygenase enzyme systems (including AHH) (10,11,86). PCBs were initially suggested to be a new class of inducer since the spectrum of enzyme induction with these compounds exhibited properties similar to both phenobarbital and MCA. However, it is now known that PCBs are mixtures of isomers, each of which possesses inducing properties that fall into one of the two well-established categories (i.e., phenobarbital or MCA type) (33). PCBs are also known to enhance hepatic UDP (uridine-5'-diphosphate) -glucuronosyltransferase (33,55,86) and to increase epoxide hydratase and glutathione-S-transferase activities (55). The dioxin, TCDD, is an extremely potent inducer of hepatic microsomal monooxygenase activity with properties similar to MCA. TCDD was shown to be 30,000 times more potent than MCA in inducing hepatic AHH (67). In addition, TCDD is capable of inducing monooxygenase enzymes transplacentally (8,9,40) and in "nonresponsive" mice (63). Furthermore, TCDD has been shown to enhance UDP-glucuronosyltransferase activity in hepatic (53) and renal (30) preparations from pretreated rats. A remarkable feature of enzyme induction with TCDD is the duration of elevated enzyme activity. AHH, for example, remains elevated for up to 35 days following a single intraperitoneal administration (67).

Microsomal enzyme induction has been suggested as a mechanism for the anticarcinogenic effects of a wide variety of compounds. These include PAH (43,57,60,68), flavones (92–94), coumarins (29), phenothiazines (91), and phenobarbital (56,66). DDT also has been shown to inhibit the formation of DMBA-induced mammary tumors (65) as well as adrenal necrosis in rats (85). The effects of PCBs on carcinogenicity of various chemicals also have been investigated. Administration of Kanechlor-500 (a PCB) in combination with several hepatocarcinogens, including 3'-methyl-4-dimethylaminoazobenzene (3'-Me-DAB), N-2-fluorenylacetamide, and diethylnitrosamine in the diets of rats markedly decreased the incidence of hepatic tumors (54). Kimura et al. (47) reported that inclusion of Kanechlor-400 in the diets of rats 4 months prior to and 2 months during 3'-Me-DAB administration completely protected against the formation of hepatocarcinomas induced by this carcinogen. The time of treatment and sequence of exposure to both compounds were critical in these experiments. When Kanechlor-400 was administered subsequent to exposure to 3'-Me-DAB, the incidence of hepatocarcinomas was significantly enhanced (47). This finding as well as other reports (44,64) suggest that PCBs may have promoting properties in the liver when administered at appropriate times. Aroclor 1254, a widely studied PCB, was found to reduce tumorigenesis by aflatoxin in rainbow trout when incorporated in the diet (37). The inhibitory effects of PCBs in the studies described above were attributed to induction of hepatic microsomal enzymes.

TCDD and Aroclor 1254 were recently shown to possess little or no tumor-initiating properties (27) or tumor-promoting properties (7) in mouse skin using the two-stage, initiation-promotion system of carcinogenesis. These findings suggested the use of these two potent enzyme inducers as tools for studying the effects of enzyme induction on tumor initiation by PAH-carcinogens. We have found that Aroclor 1254 and TCDD each possess remarkable inhibitory actions on skin tumor initiation by PAH (25). The dioxin is extremely potent in this regard. Table 7 illustrates the effects of topical administration of TCDD, at

TABLE 7. *Effects of TCDD on skin tumor initiation by DMBA[a]*

Pretreatment (μg/mouse)	Pretreatment time	Initiator	Number of mice[b]	Papillomas per mouse[c]	Percent of control[d]
None	—	None[e]	30	0.06	1.5
None	—	DMBA[f]	30	0.00	0
None	—	TCDD[g]	21	0.10	2.6
Acetone	5 min	DMBA	30	3.80	100
TCDD (2)	5 min	DMBA	22	3.70	97
TCDD (1)	1 day	DMBA	29	0.53	14
TCDD (1)	3 days	DMBA	28	0.34	9
TCDD (1)	5 days	DMBA	29	0.23	6

[a] Pretreated mice were initiated with 10 nmoles DMBA and promoted with twice weekly applications of 10 μg TPA.
[b] Number of mice surviving after 20 weeks of promotion; 30 mice were used per experimental group.
[c] Average number of papillomas per mouse after 20 weeks of promotion.
[d] Expressed as a percentage of the papillomas per mouse in the DMBA-initiated, TPA-promoted group.
[e] Mice in this group only received twice weekly applications of 10 μg of TPA.
[f] Mice in this group were only initiated with 10 nmoles of DMBA; promoter was not applied.
[g] Mice in this group were initiated with 2 μg of TCDD and promoted twice weekly with 10 μg of TPA for 32 weeks.

various pretreatment times, on skin tumor initiation by DMBA. At doses of 1 μg per mouse, TCDD almost completely abolished tumor initiation by DMBA with pretreatment times of 3 and 5 days. When administered 5 min prior to initiation with DMBA, TCDD had no effect.

Table 8 illustrates a similar inhibitory effect of TCDD on skin tumor initiation by BP; however, the magnitude of the effect was slightly less than that observed with DMBA as the initiating agent. The same dependence on the time of pretreatment was noted with both hydrocarbons. Maximum inhibition of tumor initiation occurred at pretreatment times of 3 to 5 days. Mice in both these experiments appeared normal in terms of weight gain and morphologic appearance of the skin.

Table 9 summarizes the inhibitory effects of Aroclor 1254, applied topically in 100 μg doses, on skin tumor initiation by DMBA. Again, inhibition was dependent on the time of pretreatment and maximum inhibition occurred with pretreatment at 18 hr prior to initiation.

Figure 1 shows HPLC profiles of metabolites formed upon incubation of [14C]DMBA with epidermal homogenates from Aroclor 1254 and TCDD-pretreated CD-1 mice. The doses utilized and the pretreatment times were identical to the conditions employed in the tumor experiments in which maximal inhibition was observed. These HPLC profiles demonstrate that chlorinated hydrocarbons such as Aroclor 1254 and TCDD are capable of inducing monooxygenases of the skin which are responsible for converting DMBA to a variety of hydroxylated

TABLE 8. *Effects of TCDD on skin tumor-initiation by BP*[a]

Pretreatment (μg/mouse)	Pretreatment time	Initiator	Number of mice[b]	Papillomas per mouse[c]	Percent of control[d]
None	—	None[e]	30	0.06	1.5
None	—	BP[f]	30	0.00	0
None	—	TCDD[g]	21	0.10	2.6
Acetone	5 min	BP	29	2.30	100
TCDD (1)	1 day	BP	28	1.90	83
TCDD (1)	3 days	BP	29	1.00	43
TCDD (1)	5 days	BP	30	0.80	35

[a] Pretreated mice were initiated with 100 nmol BP and promoted with twice weekly applications of 10 μg TPA.

[b] Number of mice surviving after 20 weeks of promotion; 30 mice were used per experimental group.

[c] Average number of papillomas per mouse after 20 weeks of promotion.

[d] Expressed as a percentage of the papillomas per mouse in the BP-initiated, TPA-promoted group.

[e] Mice in this group received only twice weekly applications of 10 μg TPA.

[f] Mice in this group were only initiated with 100 nmol BP; no promoter was given.

[g] Mice in this group were initiated with 2 μg TCDD and promoted twice weekly with 10 μg TPA for 32 weeks.

TABLE 9. *Effects of Aroclor 1254 on skin-tumor initiation by DMBA*[a]

Pretreatment (μg/mouse)	Pretreatment time	Initiator	Number of mice[b]	Papillomas per mouse[c]	Percent of control[d]
None	—	None[e]	30	0.06	1.5
None	—	DMBA[f]	30	0.00	0
None	—	Aroclor 1254	29	0.20	2.6
Acetone	5 min	DMBA	29	3.80	100
Aroclor 1254 (100)	5 min	DMBA	28	3.60	95
Aroclor 1254 (100)	18 hr	DMBA	30	2.1	55
Aroclor 1254 (100)	3 days	DMBA	30	3.3	88

[a] Pretreated mice were initiated with 10 nmol DMBA and promoted twice weekly with 10 μg of TPA.

[b] Number of mice surviving after 20 weeks of promotion; 30 mice were used for each experimental group.

[c] Average number of papillomas per mouse after 20 weeks of promotion.

[d] Expressed as a percentage of the papillomas per mouse in the DMBA-initiated, TPA-promoted group.

[e] Mice were only treated twice weekly with 10 μg TPA.

[f] Mice were only initiated with 10 nmol DMBA; no promoter was given.

[g] Mice were initiated with 100 μg Aroclor 1254 and promoted twice weekly with 10 μg TPA for 32 weeks.

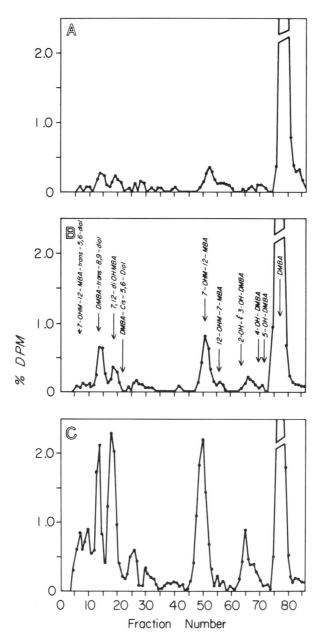

FIG. 1. HPLC profiles of [¹⁴C]DMBA metabolites generated *in vitro* using mouse epidermal homogenates from variously pretreated female CD-1 mice. Profile **A**: mice were pretreated topically with 0.2 ml acetone 18 hr prior to sacrifice. Because of extremely low activity in homogenates from uninduced mice, disintegrations per min values for each fraction collected before fraction 75 are multiplied by a factor of 3 to permit display of the data as % DPM. Profile **B**; mice were pretreated topically with 100 μg Aroclor 1254 in 0.2 ml acetone 18 hr prior to sacrifice. Profile **C**; mice were pretreated topically with 1 μg TCDD 72 hr prior to sacrifice. The retention times of various synthetic standard compounds (either known or suspected metabolites of DMBA) are depicted as arrows above peak fractions in which they elute in this system. Further details of the methodology can be found in ref. 24.

products. Furthermore, a good correlation between the increased rates of oxidative metabolism induced by Aroclor 1254 and TCDD and the inhibition of DMBA tumor initiation was observed.

To further understand the inhibitory effects of pretreatment with Aroclor 1254 and TCDD on skin tumor initiation by PAH, the effects of TCDD on covalent binding of [³H]DMBA to mouse epidermal DNA, RNA and protein were investigated. These experiments are summarized in Table 10. TCDD was applied topically to CD-1 mice (1 μg per mouse) 3 days prior to application of [³H]DMBA. After topical application of [³H]DMBA, mice were sacrificed 3 and 24 hr later. Under these conditions (which mimicked the tumor experiments described above), TCDD pretreatment was found to significantly reduce the covalent binding of DMBA to epidermal DNA (60 to 70%) and RNA (45 to 55%) but not to protein. All these experiments, when taken together, suggest that pretreatment with Aroclor 1254 and TCDD results in an increased rate of inactivation of the DMBA molecule relative to the activation rate in mouse skin. It should be noted that Kouri et al. (51) reported that TCDD enhanced the formation of MCA-induced sarcomas at the site of injection when the two compounds were administered concurrently to "nonresponsive" D2 mice. This effect was attributed to the ability of TCDD to enhance MCA metabolism in this system but seems somewhat unlikely in view of the timing. Further work is required to clarify the discrepancies between the results obtained with these two test systems (initiation-promotion on mouse skin vs. subcutaneous sarcoma formation) as well as metabolic differences between the two strains of mice.

In summary, the anticarcinogenic effects of Aroclor 1254 and TCDD were correlated with their ability to induce the monooxygenases of the skin as assessed by HPLC. Furthermore, the quantity of [³H]DMBA bound to DNA and RNA

TABLE 10. *Effect of pretreatment with TCDD on covalent binding of [³H]DMBA to mouse epidermal DNA, RNA, and protein[a]*

Treatment	Time (hr)[b]	Hydrocarbon bound to macromolecule (pmol/mg × 10²)[c]		
		DNA	RNA	Protein
DMBA	3	4.79	2.88	69.5
DMBA	24	12.63	7.16	38.8
DMBA + TCDD[d]	3	1.78 (37)	1.56 (54)	63.8
DMBA + TCDD[d]	24	3.52 (28)	3.16 (44)	39.4

[a]Mice were treated topically with 10 nmol [³H]DMBA (10 μCi) and sacrificed 3 and 24 hr later.

[b]Time of sacrifice after application of [³H]DMBA; 40 mice were used for each experimental group.

[c]Numbers in parentheses are percentages of values found in the group not receiving TCDD pretreatment.

[d]Mice in this group received 1 μg TCDD, applied topically, 72 hr prior to application of [³H]DMBA.

(but not protein) in the presence and absence of TCDD pretreatment correlated well with the tumor response under similar conditions. Although these data point to induction of oxidative biotransformation as a possible mechanism for the inhibitory effects exhibited by chlorinated hydrocarbons, it is important to emphasize that other mechanisms could be operating as well. Possibilities include induction in epidermal tissues of nonoxidative metabolic pathways such as epoxide hydratase, glutathione-*S*-transferase, UDP-glucuronosyltransferase, and others. Other possibilities include effects on DNA-repair systems and on the distribution of the carcinogen to the critical target site(s).

An intriguing aspect of these studies is the notion that compounds with little or no toxicity could be developed that still retain the capacity to inhibit carcinogenesis by virtue of enzyme-inducing properties. Furthermore, derivatives with differential-inducing properties may be a possibility; for example, compounds that induce specific detoxifying pathways, compounds that are specific inducers for a particular target tissue, and/or combinations thereof.

SUMMARY

Inhibition of chemical carcinogenesis has been studied in several tissues including liver, mammary gland, subcutaneous tissues, and skin. A wide variety of chemicals are known or suspected carcinogens and many different types of chemicals have been shown to modify tumorigenesis. This chapter has concentrated on chemicals that modify carcinogenesis by PAH with particular emphasis on the skin as a model system for studying this interaction. The two-stage, initiation-promotion system of carcinogenesis in mouse skin allows a more critical evaluation of the inhibitory mechanism. Effects on initiation and/or promotion can be studied individually.

The mechanisms of inhibition of carcinogenesis by flavonoids, antioxidants, PAH, and chlorinated hydrocarbons are still not fully understood. However, information presented in this chapter suggests that three potentially important mechanisms may be operating: (a) inhibition of enzymes responsible for formation of electrophilic intermediates, (b) induction of enzymes involved in detoxifying pathways, and (c) competitive interaction between structurally similar compounds for bioactivating metabolism or for critical intracellular targets. Other possibilities also have been discussed. A primary event occurring as a result of the inhibitory interaction appears, in the case of PAH, to be a decrease in the covalent binding of the hydrocarbon to DNA. This is most clearly demonstrated for the flavones and chlorinated hydrocarbons although also indirectly for the antioxidants and PAH.

The experimental studies presented in this chapter as well as other chapters of this book suggest that many factors can play a role in the inhibition of chemical carcinogenesis. The response to a particular inhibitor depends on the animal test system utilized, dose of modifier, dose of carcinogen, time and sequence of exposure, and route of administration as well as other parameters.

The final goal is an understanding of the chemical nature, mechanisms, and specificity of inhibitors in addition to the parameters mentioned above. With this type of information, steps can be made toward a rational approach to chemoprevention of chemical carcinogenesis in man. Some of the chemicals discussed in this chapter would obviously not be practical for use in humans. However, the hope is that further research and development will present us with derivatives that lack the undesirable characteristics although still retaining the capacity to inhibit carcinogenesis.

ACKNOWLEDGMENTS

Original research was supported by grants HD-04839 from the National Institute of Child Health and Human Development, National Institutes of Health, U.S.P.H.S. Training Grant GM-00109, by grant CA-20076 from the National Cancer Institute, U.S.P.H.S., and by the U.S. Department of Energy under contract with Union Carbide Corporation.

REFERENCES

1. Alfred, L. J., and DiPaolo, J. A. (1968): Reversible inhibition of DNA synthesis in hamster embryo cells in culture: Action of 1,2,-benzanthracene and 7,12-dimethylbenz(a)anthracene. *Cancer Res.*, 28:60–65.
2. Alfred, L. J., Donovan, P. J., Baker, M. S., and DiPaolo, J. A. (1969): Protection of cultured hamster embryo cells from 7,12-dimethylbenz(a)anthracene cytotoxicity and the induced synthesis of aryl hydrocarbon hydroxylase. *Cancer Res.*, 29:1805–1809.
3. Arcos, J. C., Conney, A. H., and Buu-Hoi, N. P. (1961): Induction of microsomal enzyme synthesis by polycyclic aromatic hydrocarbons of different molecular sizes. *J. Biol. Chem.*, 236:1291–1296.
4. Baird, W. M., and Dipple, A. (1977): Photosensitivity of DNA-bound 7,12-dimethylbenz(a)anthracene. *Int. J. Cancer*, 20:427–431.
5. Baker, J. E., and Mabie, J. M. (1973): Tribolium confusum: Food additives as ovicides. *J. Econ. Entomol.*, 66:765–767.
6. Berry, D. L., Bracken, W. R., Slaga, T. J., Wilson, N. M., Buty, S. G., and Juchau, M. R. (1977): Benzo(a)pyrene metabolism in mouse epidermis. Analysis by high pressure liquid chromatography and DNA binding. *Chem. Biol. Interact.*, 18:129–142.
7. Berry, D. L., DiGiovanni, J., Juchau, M. R., Bracken, W. M., Gleason, G. L., and Slaga, T. J. (1978): Lack of tumor-promoting ability of certain environmental chemicals in a two-stage mouse skin tumorigenesis assay. *Res. Commun. Chem. Pathol. Pharmacol.*, 20:101–107.
8. Berry, D. L., Slaga, T. J., Wilson, N. M., Zachariah, P. K., Namkung, M. J., Bracken, W. M., and Juchau, M. R. (1977): Transplacental induction of mixed-function oxygenases in extrahepatic tissues by 2,3,7,8-tetrachlorodibenzo-p-dioxin. *Biochem. Pharmacol.*, 26:1383–1388.
9. Berry, D. L., Zachariah, P. K., Namkung, M. J., and Juchau, M. R. (1976): Transplacental induction of carcinogen-hydroxylating systems with 2,3,7,8-tetrachlorodibenzo-p-dioxin. *Toxicol. Appl. Pharmacol.*, 36:569–584.
10. Bickers, D. R., Harber, L. C., Kappas, A., and Alvares, A. P. (1972): Polychlorinated biphenyls: Comparative effects of high and low chlorine containing Aroclors® on hepatic mixed function oxidase. *Res. Commun. Chem. Pathol. Pharmacol.*, 3:505–512.
11. Bickers, D. R., Kappas, A., and Alvares, A. P. (1974): Differences in inducibility of cutaneous and hepatic drug metabolizing enzymes and cytochrome P-450 by polychlorinated biphenyl and 1,1,1-trichloro-2,2-bis(p-chlorophenyl) ethane (DDT). *J. Pharmacol. Exp. Ther.*, 188:300–309.

12. Boutwell, R. K. (1964): Some biological aspects of skin carcinogenesis. *Prog. Exp. Tumor Res.,* 4:207–250.
13. Boutwell, R. K. (1976): The biochemistry of preneoplasia in mouse skin. *Cancer Res.,* 36:2631–2635.
14. Bowden, G. T., Slaga, T. J., Shapas, B. G., and Boutwell, R. K. (1974): The role of aryl hydrocarbon hydroxylase in skin tumor-initiation by 7,12-dimethylbenz(a)anthracene and 1,2, 5,6-dibenzanthracene using DNA binding and thymidine-^{3}H incorporation into DNA as criteria. *Cancer Res.,* 34:2634–2642.
15. Boyland, E. (1950): The biological significance of metabolism of polycyclic compounds. *Biochem. Soc. Symp.,* 5:40–54.
16. Brookes, P., and Lawley, P. D. (1964): Evidence for the binding of polynuclear aromatic hydrocarbons to the nucleic acids of mouse skin: Relation between carcinogenic power of hydrocarbons and their binding to deoxyribonucleic acid. *Nature,* 202:781–784.
17. Burki, K., Liebelt, A. G., and Bresnick, E. (1973): Induction of aryl hydrocarbon hydroxylase in mouse tissues from a high and low cancer strain and their F_1 hybrids. *J. Natl. Cancer Inst.,* 50:369–380.
18. Buty, S. G., Thompson, S., and Slaga, T. J. (1976): The role of epidermal aryl hydrocarbon hydroxylase in the covalent binding of polycyclic hydrocarbons to DNA and its relationship to tumor-initiation. *Biochem. Biophys. Res. Commun.,* 70:1102–1108.
19. Cawthorne, M. A., Bunyan, J., Sennitt, M. V., and Green, J. (1970): Vitamin E and hepatotoxic agents. 3. Vitamin E, synthetic antioxidants and carbon tetrachloride toxicity in the rat. *Br. J. Nutr.,* 24:357–384.
20. Collings, A. J. and Sharratt, M. (1970): The BHT content of human adipose tissue. *Food. Cosmet. Toxicol.,* 8:409–412.
21. Conney, A. H., Miller, E. C., and Miller, J. A. (1957): Substrate-induced synthesis and other properties of benzpyrene hydroxylase in rat liver. *J. Biol. Chem.,* 228:753–766.
22. Daudel, P., Duquesne, M., Vigny, P., Grover, P. L., and Sims, P. (1975): Fluorescence spectral evidence that benzo(a)pyrene-DNA products in mouse skin arise from diol-epoxides. *FEBS Lett.,* 57:250–253.
23. Diamond, L., and Gelboin, H. V. (1969): Alpha-napthoflavone: An inhibitor of hydrocarbon cytotoxicity and microsomal hydroxylase. *Science,* 166:1023–1025.
24. DiGiovanni, J., Slaga, T. J., Berry, D. L., and Juchau, M. R. (1977): Metabolism of 7,12-dimethylbenz(a)anthracene in mouse skin homogenates analyzed with high pressure liquid chromatography. *Drug Metab. Dispos.,* 5:295–301.
25. DiGiovanni, J., Slaga, T. J., Berry, D. L., and Juchau, M. R. (1978): The effects of 2,3,7,8-tetrachlorodibenzo-*p*-dioxin (TCDD) and Aroclor 1254 on 7,12-dimethylbenz(a)anthracene metabolism and tumor initiating activity in mouse skin. *Abst. Am. Assoc. Cancer Res.,* 19:110.
26. DiGiovanni, J., Slaga, T. J., Viaje, A., Berry, D. L., Harvey, R. G., and Juchau, M. R. (1978): The effects of 7,8-benzoflavone on skin tumor initiating activities of various 7- and 12-substituted derivatives of 7,12-dimethylbenz(a)anthracene. *J. Natl. Cancer Inst.,* 61:135–140.
27. DiGiovanni, J., Viaje, A., Berry, D. L., Slaga, T. J., and Juchau, M. R. (1977): Tumor-initiating ability of 2,3,7,8-tetrachlorodibenzo-p-dioxin (TCDD) and Aroclor 1254 in the two-stage system of mouse skin carcinogenesis. *Bull. Environ. Contam. Toxicol.,* 18:552–557.
28. Falk, H. L., Kotin, P., and Thompson, S. (1964): Inhibition of carcinogenesis. *Arch. Eviron. Health,* 9:169–179.
29. Feuer, G., and Kellen, J. A. (1974): Inhibition and enhancement of mammary tumorigenesis by 7,12-dimethylbenz(a)anthracene in the female Sprague-Dawley rat. *Int. J. Clin. Pharmacol.,* 9:62–69.
30. Fowler, B. A., Hook, G. E. R., and Lucier, G. W. (1977): Tetrachlorodibenzo-p-dioxin induction of renal microsomal enzyme systems: Ultrastructural effects of pars recta (S_3) proximal tubule cells of the rat kidney. *J. Pharmacol. Exp. Ther.,* 203:712–721.
31. Gelboin, H. V., Wiebel, F., and Diamond, L. (1970): Dimethylbenz(a)anthracene tumorigenesis and aryl hydrocarbon hydroxylase in mouse skin: Inhibition by 7,8-benzoflavone. *Science,* 170:169–171.
32. Gelboin, H. V., Wiebel, F. J., and Kinoshita, N. (1972): Microsomal aryl hydrocarbon hydroxylases: On their role in polycyclic hydrocarbon carcinogenesis and toxicity and the mechanism of enzyme induction. *Biochem. Soc. Symp.,* 34:103–133.
33. Goldstein, J. A., Hickman, P., Bergman, H., McKinney, J. D., and Walker, M. P. (1977):

Separation of pure polychlorinated biphenyl isomers into two types of inducers on the basis of induction of cytochrome P-450 or P-448. *Chem. Biol. Interact.,* 17:69–87.

34. Harman, D. (1968): Free radical theory of aging: Effect of free radical reaction inhibitors on the mortality rate of male LAF$_1$ mice. *J. Gerontol.,* 23:476–482.

35. Heidelberger, C., and Moldenhauer, M. G. (1950): The interaction of carcinogenic hydrocarbons with tissue constituents: IV. A quantitative study of the binding to skin proteins of several [^{14}C]-labeled hydrocarbons. *Cancer Res.,* 16:442–449.

36. Heidelberger, C. (1975): Chemical carcinogenesis. *Annu. Rev. Biochem.,* 44:79–121.

37. Hendricks, J. D., Putnam, T. P., Bills, D. D., and Sinnhuber, R. O. (1977): Inhibitory effect of a polychlorinated biphenyl (Aroclor 1254) on aflatoxin B$_1$ carcinogenesis in rainbow trout *(Salmo gairdneri). J. Natl. Cancer Inst.,* 59:1545–1551.

38. Hill, W. T., Stanger, D. W., Pizzo, A., Riegel, B., Shubik, P., and Wartman, W. B. (1951): Inhibition of 9,10-dimethyl-1,2-benzanthracene skin carcinogenesis in mice by polycyclic hydrocarbons. *Cancer Res.,* 11:892–897.

39. Hill, W. T., Stanger, D. W., Pizzo, A., Reigel, B., and Wartman, W. B. (1952): Inhibition of skin carcinogenesis in mice by mixtures of strong carcinogens. *Cancer Res.* 12:270–271.

40. Hook, G. E. R., Haseman, J. K., and Lucier, G. W. (1975): Induction and suppression of hepatic and extra-hepatic microsomal foreign-compound-metabolizing enzyme systems by 2,3,7,8-tetrachlorodibenzo-p-dioxin. *Chem. Biol. Interact.,* 10:199–214.

41. Huberman, E., and Sachs, L. (1977): DNA binding and its relationship to carcinogenesis by different polycyclic hydrocarbons. *Int. J. Cancer,* 19:122–127.

42. Huh, T. Y., and McCarter, J. A. (1960): Phenanthrene as an anti-initiating agent. *Br. J. Cancer,* 14:591–595.

43. Huggins, C., Grand, L., and Fukunishi, R. (1964): Aromatic influences on the yields of mammary cancers following administration of 7,12-dimethylbenz(a)anthracene. *Proc. Natl. Acad. Sci. USA,* 51:737–742.

44. Ito, N., Nagasaki, H., Arai, M., Makiura, S., Sugihara, S., and Hirao, K. (1973): Histopathologic studies on liver tumorigenesis induced in mice by technical polychlorinated biphenyls and its promoting effect on liver tumors induced by benzene hexachloride. *J. Natl. Cancer Inst.,* 51:1637–1646.

45. Jaffe, W. G. (1946): The influence of wheat germ oil on the production of tumors in rats by methylcholanthrene. *Exp. Med. Surg.,* 4:278–282.

46. Jerina, D. M., Daly, J. W., Witkop, B., Zaltzman-Nirenberg, P., and Udenfriend, S. (1970): 1,2-Napthalene oxide as an intermediate in the microsomal hydroxylation of napthalene. *Biochemistry,* 9:147–155.

47. Kimura, N. T., Kanematsu, T., and Baba, T. (1976): Polychlorinated biphenyl(s) as a promoter in experimental hepatocarcinogenesis in rats. *Z. Krebsforsch,* 87:257–266.

48. Kinoshita, N., and Gelboin, H. V. (1972): Aryl hydrocarbon hydroxylase and polycyclic hydrocarbon tumorigenesis: Effect of the enzyme inhibitor 7,8-benzoflavone on tumorigenesis and macromolecular binding. *Proc. Natl. Acad. Sci. USA,* 69:824–828.

49. Kinoshita, N., and Gelboin, H. V. (1972): The role of aryl hydrocarbon hydroxylase in 7,12-dimethylbenz(a)anthracene skin tumorigenesis: On the mechanism of 7,8-benzoflavone inhibition of tumorigenesis. *Cancer Res.,* 32:1329–1339.

50. Kotin, P., Falk, H. L., Lijinsky, W., and Zechmeister, L. (1956): Inhibition of the effect of some carcinogens by their partially hydrogenated derivatives. *Science,* 123:102.

51. Kouri, R. E. (1976): Relationship between levels of aryl hydrocarbon hydroxylase activity and susceptibility to 3-methylcholanthrene and benzo(a)pyrene-induced cancers in inbred strains of mice. In: *Polynuclear Aromatic Hydrocarbons,* edited by R. Freudenthal and P. Jones, pp. 139–151. Raven Press, New York.

52. Lijinsky, W., Cefis, F., Garcia, H., and Saffiotti, U. (1965): Skin tumorigenesis by dibenz(a,h)anthracene modified by its hydrogenated derivatives. *J. Natl. Cancer Inst.,* 34:7–12.

53. Lucier, G. W., McDaniel, O. S., and Hook, G. E. R. (1975): Nature of the enhancement of hepatic uridine diphosphate glucuronyltransferase activity by 2,3,7,8-tetrachlorodibenzo-p-dioxin in rats. *Biochem. Pharmacol.,* 24:325–334.

54. Makiura, S., Aoe, H., Sugihara, S., Hirao, K., Arai, M., and Ito, N. (1974): Inhibitory effect of polychlorinated biphenyl on liver tumorigenesis in rats treated with 3′-methyl-4-dimethylaminoazobenzene, N-2-fluorenylacetamide and diethylnitrosamine. *J. Natl. Cancer Inst.,* 53:1253–1257.

55. Marniemi, J., Nokkala, M., Vainio, H., and Hartiala, K. J. W. (1977): Stimulation of hepatic drug hydroxylation and conjugation by a cutaneously applied PCB-mixture (Clophen A 50). *Chem. Biol. Interact.,* 18:247–251.

56. Mclean, A. E. M., and Marshall, A. (1971): Reduced carcinogenic effects of aflatoxin in rats given phenobarbitone. *Br. J. Exp. Pathol.,* 52:322–329.

57. Meechan, R. J., McCafferty, D. E., and Jones, R. S., (1953): 3-Methylcholanthrene as an inhibitor of hepatic cancer induced by 3'-methyl-4-dimethylaminobenzene in the diet of the rat: A determination of the time relationships. *Cancer Res.,* 13:802–806.

58. Metcalfe, S. M. (1971): Cell culture as a test system for toxicity. *J. Pharm. Pharmacol.,* 23:817–823.

59. Miller, E. C., and Miller, J. A. (1966): Mechanisms of chemical carcinogenesis: Nature of proximate carcinogens and interactions with macromolecules. *Pharmacol. Rev.,* 18:805–838.

60. Miller, E. C., Miller, J. A., Brown, R. R., and McDonald, J. C. (1958): On the protective action of certain polycyclic aromatic hydrocarbons against carcinogenesis by aminoazo dyes and 2-aceytlaminofluorene. *Cancer Res.,* 18:469–477.

61. National Academy of Sciences (1972): Committee on Biologic Effects of Atmospheric Pollutants. Washington, D.C.

62. Nebert, D. W., Benedict, N. F., and Gielen, J. E. (1972): Aryl hydrocarbon hydroxylase, epoxide hydrase, and 7,12-dimethylbenz(a)anthracene-produced skin tumorigenesis in the mouse. *Mol. Pharmacol.,* 8:374–379.

63. Nebert, D. W., Robinson, J. R., Niwa, A., Kumaki, K., and Poland, A. (1975): Genetic expression of aryl hydrocarbon hydroxylase activity in the mouse. *J. Cell. Physiol.,* 85:393–414.

64. Nishizumi, M. (1976): Enhancement of diethylnitrosamine hepatocarcinogenesis in rats by exposure to polychlorinated biphenyls or phenobarbital. *Cancer Lett.,* 2:11–16.

65. Okey, A. B. (1972): Dimethylbenzanthracene-induced mammary tumors in rats: Inhibition by DDT. *Life Sci.,* 11:833–843.

66. Peraino, C., Fry, R. J. M., and Staffeldt, E. (1971): Reduction and enhancement by phenobarbital of hepatocarcinogenesis induced in the rat by 2-acetylaminofluorene. *Cancer Res.,* 31:1506–1512.

67. Poland, A., and Glover, E. (1974): Comparison of 2,3,7,8-tetrachlorodibenzo-p-dioxin, a potent inducer of aryl hydrocarbon hydroxylase, with 3-methylcholanthrene. *Mol. Pharmacol.,* 10:349–359.

68. Richardson, H. L., Stier, A. R., and Borsos-Nachtnebel, E. (1952): Liver tumor inhibition and adrenal histologic responses in rats to which 3'-methyl-4-dimethylaminoazobenzene and 20-methylcholanthrene were simultaneously administered. *Cancer Res.,* 12:356–361.

69. Riegel, B., Wartman, W. B., Hill, W. T., Reeb, B. B., Shubik, P., and Stanger, D. W. (1951): Delay of methylcholanthrene skin carcinogenesis in mice by 1,2,5,6-dibenzofluorene. *Cancer Res.,* 11:301–303.

70. Selkirk, J. K., Huberman, E., and Heidelberger, C. (1971): An epoxide is an intermediate in the microsomal metabolism of the carcinogen, dibenz(a,h)anthracene. *Biochem. Biophys. Res. Commun.,* 43:1010–1016.

71. Selkirk, J. K., Croy, R. G., Roller, P. P., and Gelboin, H. V. (1974): High pressure liquid chromatographic analysis of benzo(a)pyrene metabolism and covalent binding and the mechanism of action of 7,8-benzoflavone and 1,2,-epoxy-3,3,3-trichloropropane. *Cancer Res.,* 34:3474–3480.

72. Shamberger, R. J. (1970): Relationship of selenium to cancer. 1. Inhibitory effect of selenium on carcinogenesis. *J. Natl. Cancer Inst.,* 44:931–936.

73. Shamberger, R. J. (1972): Increase of peroxidation in carcinogenesis. *J. Natl. Cancer Inst.,* 48:1491–1497.

74. Shamberger, R. J., and Rudolph, G. (1966): Protection against cocarcinogenesis by antioxidants. *Experientia,* 22:116.

75. Shamberger, R. J., Baughman, F. F., Kalchert, S. L., Willis, C. E., and Hoffman, G. C. (1973): Carcinogen-induced chromosomal breakage decreased by antioxidants. *Proc. Natl. Acad. Sci. USA,* 70:1461–1463.

76. Sims, P., Grover, P. L., Kuroki, T., Huberman, E., Marquardt, H., Selkirk, J. K., and Heidelberger, C. (1973): The metabolism of benz(a)anthracene and dibenz(a,h)anthracene and their related "K-region" epoxides, cis-dihydrodiols and phenols by hamster embryo cells. *Biochem. Pharmacol.,* 22:1–8.

77. Sims, P., Grover, P. L., Swaisland, A., Pal, K., and Hewer, A. (1974): Metabolic activation of benzo(a)pyrene proceeds by a diol-epoxide. *Nature,* 252:326–327.
78. Slaga, T. J., and Boutwell, R. K. (1977): Inhibition of the tumor-initiating ability of the potent carcinogen 7,12-dimethylbenz(a)anthracene by the weak tumor initiator 1,2,3,4-dibenzanthracene. *Cancer Res.,* 37:128–133.
79. Slaga, T. J., and Bracken, W. M. (1977): The effects of antioxidants on skin tumor-initiation and aryl hydrocarbon hydroxylase. *Cancer Res.,* 37:1631–1635.
80. Slaga, T. J., Thompson, S., Berry, D. L., DiGiovanni, J., Juchau, M. R., and Viaje, A. (1977): The effects of benzoflavones on polycyclic hydrocarbon metabolism and skin tumor-initiation. *Chem. Biol. Interact.,* 17:297–312.
81. Speier, J. L., and Wattenberg, L. W. (1975): Modifications in microsomal metabolism of benzo-(a)pyrene in mice fed butylated hydroxyanisole. *J. Natl. Cancer Inst.,* 55:469–472.
82. Steiner, P. E. (1955): Carcinogenicity of multiple chemicals simultaneously administered. *Cancer Res.,* 15:632–635.
83. Steiner, P. E., and Falk, H. L. (1950): Summation and inhibition effects of weak and strong carcinogenic hydrocarbons: 1,2-Benzanthracene, chrysene, 1:2:5:6-dibenzanthracene, and 20-methylcholanthrene. *Cancer Res.,* 11:56–63.
84. Thompson, S., and Slaga, T. J. (1976): Mouse epidermal aryl hydrocarbon hydroxylase. *J. Invest. Dermatol.,* 66:108–111.
85. Turusov, V. S., and Chemeris, G. Y. (1976): Modification of toxic effects of DMBA by DDT and DDE. *Chem. Biol. Interact.,* 15:295–298.
86. Vainio, H. (1974): Enhancement of microsomal drug oxidation and glucuronidation in rat liver by an environmental chemical, polychlorinated biphenyl. *Chem. Biol. Interact.,* 9:379–387.
87. Wattenberg, L. W. (1972): Inhibition of carcinogenic and toxic effects of polycyclic hydrocarbons by phenolic antioxidants and ethoxyquin. *J. Natl. Cancer Inst.,* 48:1425–1430.
88. Wattenberg, L. W. (1971): Inhibition of carcinogenic effects of diethylnitrosamine (DEN) and 4-nitroquinoline-N-oxide (NQO) by antioxidants. *Fed. Proc.,* 31:633.
89. Wattenberg, L. W. (1973): Inhibition of chemical carcinogen-induced pulmonary neoplasia by butylated hydroxyanisole. *J. Natl. Cancer Inst.,* 50:1541–1544.
90. Wattenberg, L. W. (1974): Inhibition of carcinogenic and toxic effects of polycyclic hydrocarbons by several sulfur-containing compounds. *J. Natl. Cancer Inst.,* 52:1583–1587.
91. Wattenberg, L. W., and Leong, J. L. (1967): Inhibition of 9,10-dimethylbenzanthracene (DMBA) induced mammary tumorigenesis. *Fed. Proc.,* 26:692.
92. Wattenberg, L. W., and Leong, J. L. (1968): Inhibition of the carcinogenic action of 7,12-dimethylbenz(a)anthracene by beta-napthoflavone. *Proc. Soc. Exp. Biol. Med.,* 128:940–943.
93. Wattenberg, L. W., and Leong, J. L. (1970): Inhibition of the carcinogenic action of benzo(a)pyrene by flavones. *Cancer Res.,* 30:1922–1925.
94. Wattenberg, L. W., Page, M. A., and Leong, J. L. (1968): Induction of increased benzpyrene hydroxylase activity by flavones and related compounds. *Cancer Res.,* 28:934–937.
95. Weinstein, I. B., Jeffrey, A. M., Jennette, K. W., Blobstein, S. H., Harvey, R. G., Harris, C., and Autrup, H. (1976): Benzo(a)pyrene diol epoxides as intermediates in nucleic acid binding *in vitro* and *in vivo. Science,* 193:592–595.
96. Wiebel, F. J., Leutz, J. C., and Gelboin , H. V. (1975): Aryl hydrocarbon (benzo(a)pyrene) hydroxylase: A mixed function oxygenase in mouse skin. *J. Invest. Dermatol.,* 64:184–189.

Carcinogenesis, Vol. 5: Modifiers of Chemical Carcinogenesis, edited by T. J. Slaga. Raven Press, New York, 1980.

9

Interactions of Radiation and Chemical Carcinogens

Robert L. Ullrich

Biology Division, Oak Ridge National Laboratory, Oak Ridge, Tennessee 37830

Throughout their lifetimes, human beings are generally exposed in their environment to repeated low doses of many potential and known carcinogenic agents. Although the effects of many individual chemical, physical, or biological agents with carcinogenic potential have been studied extensively, the potential interactions of these agents have received relatively little attention. This is probably not because the significance of such potential interactions has not been appreciated but rather because the task of designing and interpreting such experiments is formidable. There are almost infinite combinations of agents, dose, and treatment regimens that could be selected, and it is quite likely that the results could differ, depending upon the regimen selected. Furthermore, interpretation of such results is impossible without an adequate understanding of the effects of the individual agents. Because of these difficulties, the experiments which have been performed have been limited in scope, and the interpretations placed on the data have, for the most part, been restricted to deciding whether or not any type of interaction occurred. As a result, few general principles that might be applied to the human situation or contribute to an understanding of carcinogenic mechanisms have emerged. This chapter will examine the current state of understanding regarding interactions that can occur after combined exposure to radiation and chemical carcinogens.

The first report of a suspected interaction between radiation and chemical carcinogens in humans has been attributed to Bruusgaard in 1922, who suggested that the high incidence of skin cancer among sailors was due to a combination of the high doses of sunlight and coal tar to which sailors were exposed (11). More recently, epidemiological studies of uranium miners have indicated an interaction between ionizing radiation exposures and cigarette smoke (2). In these studies, a significant excess of lung cancer has been found primarily among those miners who were cigarette smokers, with the incidence for smoking miners being greater than that expected for simple additivity of the effects of the two agents.

Although these reports support the belief that interactions are possible at high occupational exposure levels, such studies are not likely to provide information concerning the possibility of interactions at the much lower levels to which the general population is exposed, nor are epidemiological studies likely to provide sufficient information to elucidate the mechanisms of the interactions. Information on the probability of interaction, the kinds of interactions which might occur, and their mechanistic basis is more likely to emerge from experimental studies. A number of such investigations have been performed utilizing a variety of chemical agents and either ultraviolet (UV) or ionizing radiation. The present discussion of these investigations will be divided into those studies dealing with interactions between chemicals and UV radiation and those studies dealing with chemicals and ionizing radiation. Only *in vivo* tumor induction studies will be included, since *in vitro* transformation systems are not sufficiently well defined at the present time to allow proper interpretation of interactions which might occur.

RADIATION CARCINOGENESIS

Before studies on interactions are discussed, it might be helpful to briefly discuss some aspects of tumor induction with UV or ionizing radiation alone. This presentation will be quite brief and limited to only a few of the more general aspects of radiation carcinogenesis. For more comprehensive reviews see Urbach et al. (66) and Black and Chan (5) for information on carcinogenesis with UV light, and Upton (65) and Storer (63) for information on carcinogenesis with ionizing radiation.

UV Radiation

Radiation can be divided into two types, nonionizing and ionizing. Of the nonionizing radiations, only UV is known to have carcinogenic properties. Absorption of UV radiation by a molecule results in electron excitation. It is reasonable to conclude that it is the absorption of UV radiation and the resultant excitation in the macromolecular constituents of the cell that eventually results in its carcinogenic effects.

The first suggestion of an association between UV light and skin cancer came from clinical observation. This association appears to have been first described in 1896 almost simultaneously by Unna and by Dubreuilh (21,64). Subsequent clinical reports in the period 1900 to 1928 expanded on this association (66). It was not until 1928 that an experimental study reported by Findlay provided the first direct demonstration of the carcinogenic potential of UV light (30). In his studies, Findlay found that daily irradiation of mice with UV light could induce skin tumors. Subsequent studies have confirmed and expanded these results.

Roffo (53) contributed the first information about the relationship between wavelength and tumor induction when he found that skin tumors in mice exposed to UV light could be blocked by an ordinary window-glass filter, indicating that the major carcinogenic effect is with wavelengths shorter than 320 nm. In more recent studies, wavelengths between 280 and 320 nm have generally been the most efficient for tumor induction in a variety of animals (8,32,54).

Some of the most comprehensive experiments were performed by Blum, Grady, and Kirby-Smith at the National Cancer Institute during the period 1941 to 1944 (6,7). In these studies, Blum found that by designating the time between the first dose and the appearance of a tumor of a certain volume as his experimental end point, he could quantitatively assess a number of factors which might influence UV carcinogenesis. In these studies, it was seen that a single dose of UV light was not sufficient to induce tumors during the lifetime of the experimental animals. A second observation was that differences in dose, intensity, or interval between doses did not alter the shape or slope of the dose-response relationship, but rather shifted their relative position along the abscissa. A decrease in dose or intensity or an increase in the interval between doses resulted in a shift of the dose-response relationships to the left, as illustrated in Fig. 1. Blum suggested from these data that much of the effect of the multiple doses, particularly the later exposures, was to enhance or promote tumor expression after the initial induction process. This concept will be discussed further in the section on Interactions.

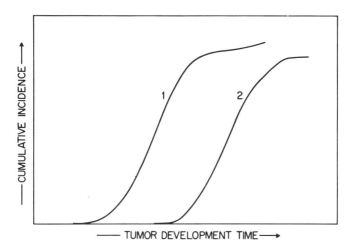

FIG. 1. Cumulative incidence of skin tumors in mouse skin exposed to multiple doses of UV radiation. Curve 2 represents the result of lower dose, lower intensity, or an increase in the interval between doses.

In 1975 Hsu et al. reported that skin tumors could be produced within 16 weeks after exposure of hairless mice to single large doses of UV light (38). However, tumors appeared only in the mice that had considerable evidence of tissue damage and arose only around the edge of the severely damaged tissues. Because of the severe destruction required, the relationship between the events involved in this type of tumor induction and those involved after multiple UV light exposures is unclear.

The mechanism of action of UV light in inducing tumors, as for all carcinogenic agents, is largely unknown. It is reasonable to conclude, as stated earlier, that the absorption of UV light and the resultant electron excitation in the macromolecular constituents of the cell eventually result in the carcinogenic effect, but the events between absorption and tumor formation or even the target macromolecules whose excitation and damage eventually result in tumor formation are unknown. By far, the most extensively studied effect of UV light on DNA is the formation of pyrimidine dimers, which appear to be one of the principle photoproducts in UV-irradiated DNA (67). Cells are apparently capable of repairing this damage through a number of repair processes (5), and dimers have been implicated in the lethal (57) and mutagenic effects (68) of UV light. More recently it has been suggested that pyrimidine dimer formation is likely to lead to skin tumor formation if the dimers are not excised or if they lead to defective repair or replication (27,42,69). However, at present the evidence for a relationship between DNA damage, repair, and carcinogenesis is largely inferential.

One study which appears to support this suggestion was reported by Zajdela and Latajet (69). These investigators painted a solution of caffeine, an inhibitor of postreplication repair, on the skin of mice during UV irradiation and found that caffeine-treated skin developed fewer tumors than unpainted control skin on the same animals. From these data the authors have hypothesized that skin tumor formation is initiated by DNA repair which allows cell survival but which leads to error in DNA replication and ultimately to an increased probability of malignant change. However, it is probable that other factors such as increased cell killing (51) or effects on DNA synthesis (14) produced by treatment with UV light plus caffeine could also account for the reduced tumor induction.

Ionizing Radiation

Unlike UV light, whose effects are mediated via electron excitations, ionizing radiation effects are primarily a result of ion-pair production and subsequent free radical formation which leads to molecular change, although excitation also occurs. The effects may be direct on the molecule or may be indirectly produced. The indirect route is mediated by direct radiation effects on water (radiolysis of water) and interactions of the products of radiolysis with other molecules. Ionizing radiation may be either electromagnetic (e.g., γ rays and X-rays) or particulate (e.g., α particles, β particles, protons, or neutrons). Besides being categorized as electromagnetic or particulate, ionizing radiations may be characterized by the nature of the energy loss along their track length. The energy release per unit track length is commonly known as the linear energy transfer (LET). Because ionizations are responsible for the ultimate effect, the nature of the energy deposition (i.e., the LET) of a particular radiation can make a quantitative difference in the biological response, since the patterns of energy deposition affect the density of the ionizations along the track. Radiation such as X-rays and γ rays have a low LET, and therefore the density of ionization is low. High-LET radiation such as α particles and neutrons have densely clustered ionizations along their track.

As for UV light, the first record of a radiation-induced cancer came from human experience (33). Subsequently many other cases manifested themselves, at first primarily as skin cancer on the hands of radiologists, who exposed their hands repeatedly while focusing their equipment (35). Radiation-induced leukemogenesis was also noted quite early (18). Soon after the first observations in humans, studies on the experimental induction of tumors in animals began. These studies have indicated that under the appropriate conditions of animal model, radiation dose, and exposure schedule radiation can induce tumors in nearly every tissue. Because of the variety of tumors induced, these studies have also indicated that the particular mechanism through which radiation can influence neoplastic development varies with the target tissue and tumor type (13). In many tissues, such as the skin, lungs, liver, and brain, the induction process seems to be a result of direct local radiation effects in the target tissues. In other tissues, carcinogenesis not only depends on local changes but may also be greatly influenced by systemic effects. For example, many endocrine tissue tumors not only depend on irradiation of the target tissue, but also seem to require an additional disturbance of the hormonal balance (13). In fact, in the case of ovarian tumor induction, direct irradiation of the ovary does not seem to be essential, suggesting that the most important element for tumor induction in this case is the systemic radiation effect (20). Thymic lymphoma is also a neoplasm that requires a complex interaction of local and systemic effects for induction. In this case, the mechanism may be even more complex than that for ovarian tumor induction, since in addition to direct and systemic effects, a virus has also been implicated in its pathogenesis (39,40). In spite of the diverse and complex processes involved in radiation carcinogenesis, the dose-response relationship has a somewhat similar form for most experimentally induced tumors. For low-LET radiation this relationship is generally curvilinear, with a rapidly rising component in the intermediate dose range followed by a plateau or decline in incidence in the high-dose region (63,65), as illustrated in Fig. 2. This decrease has been generally attributed to excessive injury and cell killing. In fact, the shape of the entire dose-response relationship is a result of a combination of both transformation and cell-killing effects (36). In the low-dose range, as also shown in Fig. 2, the dose response is more shallow than in the intermediate region and can usually be adequately described by a

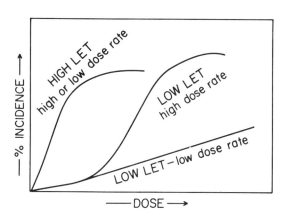

FIG. 2. Generalized dose-response curves for tumor induction after exposure to ionizing radiation.

linear relationship, whereas the response in the intermediate region is more closely approximated by a dose-squared relationship. With decreasing dose rate or with dose fractionation, the dose response is less with a similar acute exposure, particularly in the intermediate dose range; therefore, the overall relationship takes on a more linear form. High-LET radiation is generally more effective than low-LET radiation, and the dose response for tumor induction is generally more linear and somewhat less dependent on dose rate in many cases (65,63).

As for other carcinogens, the basis for the induction of tumors is unknown. It is known that as a result of the chemical changes which may be produced by ionizations in a biological system, the large biologically important macromolecules undergo a variety of structural alterations that can ultimately affect their function. The effects of radiation on the cellular DNA are probably the most important and are most likely responsible for the primary cellular effects and eventually for carcinogenesis.

For low-LET radiation, most effects at the cellular and molecular level display two-hit induction kinetics and are dose-rate dependent, whereas for high-LET radiation the induction kinetics are generally single hit in nature and, as would be expected because of the single-hit kinetics, are less dependent on dose rate (9,10,23,52). One current hypothesis that attempts to explain these results suggests that the effects are the result of interaction of two sublesions in the nucleus (41). This can be illustrated by use of double-stranded DNA damage as a specific example. Double-strand damage may occur when there is independent damage to both strands in close proximity or when a single particle with a high LET produces damage to both strands simultaneously as a result of its dense ionization track. The probability of producing independent damage to both strands in close proximity with low-LET radiation is lower when the total dose is low than when it is high, simply because of the random nature of ionization events. With low dose rates this probability is also low, even at moderate to high total doses, since in most cells there are enzyme systems capable of repairing much of the single-strand DNA damage (22), resulting in the number of possible interacting lesions. Because effects are produced in both strands by a single event with high-LET radiation, dose rate and dose make little difference with high-LET radiation in terms of the probability of producing double-strand damage rather than single-strand damage.

INTERACTIONS

Interactions with UV Light

Studies examining the interactions of UV radiation and chemicals date back to the first experimental UV light carcinogenesis studies of Findlay referred to earlier (30). In these studies it was observed that when mice were treated with tar before exposure to UV light, there was a reduction in the latent period and an increased probability for induction of skin tumors by UV light. The subsequent literature has presented conflicting results, with UV light showing both enhancing and inhibitory effects on chemical carcinogenesis, depending upon the particular study. These conflicting results appear to be primarily due to the photodynamic activity of most chemical carcinogens (19,25,66). This activity was first reported in 1935 by Lewis, who noted that when 20-methylcholanthrene, 7,12-dimethylbenz*(a)*anthracene (DMBA), or benzo*(a)*pyrene (BP) were added to tissue cultures, the cells developed photosensitivity to long-wavelength UV light (340 to 390 nm) (43). It has since been demonstrated that most skin carcinogens are photodynamically active (29,48,56). In addition to the demonstrated photosensitization, exposure to UV light can reduce the carcinogenicity of these compounds by photochemical degradation, again as a result of their photodynamic activity (19,66). It therefore appears that UV light can act in two diametrically opposite ways, namely, by degradation of the carcinogen to a less carcinogenic compound or through photosensitization which can enhance the carcinogenic response. Because of these effects experiments on interactions have been complicated. Experiments designed to examine true carcinogenic interactions must be designed to ensure that neither photodegradation of the carcinogen nor photosensitization to UV light by the carcinogen are involved. The subsequent discussion will be limited to those experiments that have properly separated the application of chemical carcinogen from the direct influence of the UV light exposure.

Experiments by Epstein and Epstein in 1962 (26) demonstrated that multiple doses of UV light which were not carcinogenic by themselves could increase the incidence of skin tumors produced by a single dose of a 0.5% solution of DMBA from 18% (4/22) to 63% (12/19). In these studies, the DMBA and UV light treatments were separated by 14 days. In subsequent experiments (24) with hairless mice it was found that a single application of DMBA 6 weeks prior to the beginning of a carcinogenic UV light exposure could accelerate the rate of appearance of tumors; however, the final incidence was not affected, since virtually all mice irradiated developed tumors regardless of whether or not they received prior DMBA treatment. Although the interpretation of this second experiment is less clear, the first experiment of Epstein and Epstein suggests that a portion of the activity of multiple exposures to UV radiation is related to a tumor-enhancing or -promoting activity. The general applicability of the enhancement phenomenon, when multiple doses of UV light follow an initiating dose of chemical carcinogens, is at present not known; however, these data are consistent with the original hypothesis of Blum (6) regarding the enhancing activity of multiple UV light doses. The validity of this concept has been demonstrated recently by Fry and his colleagues using UV light plus 8-methoxypsoralen (8-MOP) as a photosensitizer and 12-*O*-tetradecanoylphorbol-13-acetate (TPA) as a promoting agent (34). In these experiments the skin tumor incidence with UV light plus 8-MOP treatments three times per week for 12 weeks was markedly less than with five exposures per week for 24 weeks. However, when promotion with TPA began after 12 weeks of UV light plus 8-MOP three times per week, the incidence was similar to that found with the 24-week exposure. These data indicate quite convincingly that the role of later exposures is associated with tumor expression. Interestingly, in these same studies, when comparing two strains which had markedly different sensitivity to tumor induction by UV light plus 8-MOP, the strain-dependent difference was much less marked when UV light plus 8-MOP treatment was followed by TPA treatment.

Stenback et al. reported data suggesting that prior exposure to UV light can enhance the effectiveness of certain chemical carcinogens. The first series of experiments examined the effect of UV light on initiation by DMBA in two-stage carcinogenesis when croton oil was used as the promoting agent (62). In these studies a single dose of UV light prior to initiation with DMBA enhanced the two-stage skin carcinogenesis, whereas multiple doses did not cause an enhancement. A single or multiple UV light dose *after initiation* decreased the effectiveness of the two-stage carcinogenesis scheme. The decreased effectiveness when UV light was given 1 hr after initiation was likely due to photochemical degradation of the carcinogen. The enhancement found in these experiments with a single prior exposure to UV light suggests an interaction between UV light and chemical carcinogens that is greater than additive, since the single UV light exposure was not in itself carcinogenic. When UV light treatment was given 10 times prior to initiation and promotion, ulceration and scarring of the skin was observed. This increased tissue injury may explain the lack of enhancement by pretreatment with multiple UV radiation doses. In later studies (61), Stenbeck showed a similar enhancement with pretreatment with single doses of UV light when DMBA was used as a complete carcinogen or when BP was used as the initiator in two-stage carcinogenesis. The basis for this interaction between UV radiation and chemical carcinogen, when UV light is given as a single dose before the course of chemical carcinogen treatment, has not been investigated. Increased DNA damage or susceptibility to damage as a result of UV-light-induced lesions might explain this enhancement, but changes in the metabolism of DMBA could also play a role. An alternative explanation may be that these single doses of UV radiation initiate additional tumors, which are then promoted during the course of chemical treatment along with the chemically initiated tumors. Such a summation effect would be similar to those described by Saffiotti and Shubik (55) and by Poel (49) after sequential treatment with chemical carcinogens.

Studies have also demonstrated that UV light can act as an initiator in two-stage carcinogenesis when croton oil or TPA is used as a promoting agent. The first such study was reported by Epstein and Roth (28), who subjected hairless mice to a single exposure of UV light followed by biweekly application of croton oil beginning 2 weeks after UV light exposure. No tumors were seen at 18 months in UV-irradiated or croton-oil-treated mice, but 23% of the mice receiving both treatments showed malignant skin tumors. These results have been confirmed by Pound (50). The recent studies of Fry et al. using TPA, referred to earlier, also indicate that tumors initiated by UV light plus 8-MOP can be promoted with chemical promoting agents (34).

Interactions with Ionizing Radiation

The first attempt to study possible interactions between ionizing radiation and chemical carcinogens was reported in 1932 by Cramer (17). In these experiments he found that when radium exposures followed twice-weekly tarring, fewer tumors developed and those that developed appeared at a later time than after tarring alone. Although the doses of radium were not known, they were estimated to be between 4,000 and 8,000 rads, which is quite a high dose. Whatever the actual dose may have been, it was apparent that a great deal of tissue destruction occurred at the exposure levels used, suggesting that much of the reduction in incidence was a result of extensive cell killing and tissue destruction. That this might have been the case in Cramer's work was pointed out by Mottram in 1937 (47). His studies employed much lower radiation doses (approximately 0, 160, 480, and 1440 rads) 60 days after twice-weekly treatment with a 0.5% solution of BP; tumor incidences of 25,30,65, and 75%, respectively, were found. These data indicate that radiation could interact with a chemical carcinogen to increase the tumor response if the radiation dose were not high enough to cause tissue destruction. Unfortunately the nature or degree of the interaction (i.e., additive, synergistic, etc.) could not be ascertained, since no group with irradiation only was included.

More recent studies examining carcinogenic interactions have also used the skin as a model system. Cloudman et al. apparently found additive effects on murine skin tumor induction when carcinogenic levels of both methylcholanthrene (MCA) and β-irradiation were combined (15). In these studies, treatment with MCA always followed the radiation exposure. Argus et al., on the other hand, reported that X-irradiation of mouse skin, whether preceding or following

DMBA treatment, decreased the tumor yield from that induced by DMBA alone (1). More recent data reported by Burns indicated an additive effect for X-irradiation combined with DMBA in the rat skin tumor system (12). The inhibitory effects seen by Argus et al. are puzzling, since the radiation doses used were not sufficient to cause severe tissue destruction and were in fact comparable to those used by other investigators who have reported positive interactions in the skin.

As early as 1953, studies by Shubik et al. (60) indicated that small doses of β-rays, which by themselves were not tumorigenic, could produce tumors when followed by twice-weekly painting with croton oil, just as Berenblum had earlier demonstrated for subcarcinogenic doses of chemical carcinogens (3). Subsequently, Berenblum reported that nonleukemogenic single doses of X-rays, when followed by a urethan treatment which was only slightly leukemogenic, could markedly enhance the incidence of leukemia (4). Treatment with urethan prior to irradiation did not produce such effects. These data suggest that for this system radiation can serve as an initiator and urethan as a promoter. Recent studies by McGregor have shown that cigarette tar can also have promoting or enhancing effects on skin tumor induction by β-ray exposure in rats (46).

All of these data on initiation and promotion indicate that even subcarcinogenic doses of radiation can have latent carcinogenic effects. Studies reported by Hoshino and Tanooka in 1964 suggest that these latent effects may remain for long periods (37). The experiments of Hoshino and Tanooka examined the interaction of β-rays and 4-nitroquinoline 1-oxide after various intervals between exposure to the two agents, ranging from 11 to 408 days. As shown in Table 1, neither treatment by itself produced any tumors, but combined treatment

TABLE 1. *Tumor incidence in mouse skin exposed to* β *irradiation*[a] *and subsequent 4-nitroquinoline 1-oxide painting*[b] *for various intervals*

Interval (days)	No. of mice		No. of papillomas	No. of malignant tumors	Tumor incidence[c] (%)
	At the start	At 1st tumor appearance			
11	100	95	7	12 (11, 1)[d]	12.6
30	100	56	8	8 (7, 1)	14.3
63	100	91	5	10 (8, 2)	11.0
124	100	90	10	12 (11, 1)	13.3
234	100	47	4	8 (8, 0)	17.0
408	100	25	5	2 (2, 0)	8.0[e]

[a] β-ray dose at the skin surface, 2.7 krads.
[b] 4-Nitroquinoline 1-oxide dose, 2 mg in 20 fractions.
[c] (No. of malignant tumors per no. of mice at 1st tumor appearance) $\times$ 100.
[d] Numbers in parentheses: 1st number, squamous cell carcinoma; 2nd number, fibrosarcoma of the skin.
[e] 95% confidence limit: upper, 26%; lower, 1%. The χ^2 test of this value versus other whole-tumor incidence gives $p > 0.10$, indicating that the difference is not statistically significant.
From Hoshino and Tanooka (37).

resulted in an average incidence of malignant skin tumors of 12.4%. More importantly, the tumor incidence level was essentially the same for all intervals. The results of these experiments indicate that latent carcinogenic effects of β-irradiation can persist for long periods after radiation exposure. This demonstration of persistent lesions suggests that exposures to multiple carcinogens at low levels which themselves may not induce a tumor could eventually combine to be tumorigenic. The demonstration of a persistent late effect has important implications not only when interactions are being considered, but also for radiation carcinogenesis. As discussed earlier, fractionation or protraction of a radiation dose generally produces fewer tumors than a similar single dose. In view of the above, this dose-rate effect may be related to factors influencing tumor expression rather than being a reflection of the tumor-initiating effects of the radiation.

Although many of the experiments on interactions have used the skin, interactions have been studied using other systems as well. Shellabarger (58) and later Shellabarger and Straub (59) examined the interactions of radiation with MCA in the Sprague-Dawley rat mammary tumor system. In their experiments the carcinogenic effects of MCA and X-irradiation or neutron irradiation were essentially additive, whether the radiation exposure preceded or followed treatment with MCA.

Cole and Foley found that urethan and X-rays were additive for lung tumorigenesis in mice if each was used at a relatively low dose level, but when higher radiation doses were used, the incidence of lung adenomas was lower than in those animals treated with urethan alone (16,31). They attributed the latter results to an increased cytotoxicity at higher radiation doses. In addition to these studies using external irradiation of the lung, interactions in the lung have also been observed using internally deposited radioisotopes. McGandy et al. (45) reported that multiple intratracheal instillations of ^{210}Po, an α-emitter, and BP given simultaneously on a ferric oxide carrier induced an incidence of lung tumors twice that expected from the additive effect of either carcinogen alone. In another experiment, a single instillation of ^{210}Po followed 18 weeks later by seven weekly instillations of BP also produced a greater than additive or synergistic response.

As discussed earlier in the section on ionizing radiation, it has been observed that for low-LET radiation, protracted or fractionated irradiation is generally less effective than an acute exposure of a similar dose. However, no studies have been done comparing the influence of protracted and acute radiation exposures on interactions. Because the basis for the reduced dose-rate effect with protraction is not completely understood (i.e., whether the effect is due to a reduced carcinogenic effect or merely to reduced tumor expression), and because exposures are more likely to occur under conditions of chronic exposure, studies examining the influence of the radiation dose rate are likely to provide useful information relevant to mechanism as well as to risk. Although no studies have compared single and protracted exposures, the studies of McGandy et al. (45),

TABLE 2. *Incidence of cheek-pouch tumors*

Treatment	No. of animals	Tumor incidence (%)
None	5	0
Mineral oil	10	0
DMBA[a]	35	45.7
Radiation[b]	23	0
Radiation + DMBA[c]	40	72.5

[a]0.05 ml 0.1% DMBA in mineral oil three times per week for 11 weeks with no treatment during the 6th week.
[b]Acute 20-rad dose once a week for 17 weeks.
[c]Treatments [a] and [b] starting together and running concurrently.
Adapted from Lurie (44).

referred to above, suggest a marked interaction after multiple doses of ^{210}Po. More recently, Lurie has reported a study which examined the potential interaction of multiple low doses of radiation combined with DMBA; the hamster cheek pouch epithelium was the target tissue (44). The results of these studies, summarized in Table 2, suggest that multiple doses of low-level X-irradiation, which are themselves not carcinogenic, can act as a cocarcinogen when combined with a chemical carcinogen.

SUMMARY

It is apparent from the above discussion that, under the appropriate circumstances, when either UV or ionizing radiation is combined with chemical carcinogens, the times of tumor appearance are accelerated and/or the tumor incidences are increased. For UV irradiation this is generally true when care is taken to prevent photodecomposition of the chemical. In the studies outlined, UV radiation has been shown to be a promoting or enhancing agent for chemically initiated tumors and an initiating agent for chemically promoted tumors. When the levels of exposure of the two agents were carcinogenic by themselves, an accelerated response was observed, suggesting a summation effect.

Although decomposition of the chemical is not a factor when ionizing radiation is used, doses must be sufficiently low so as to not cause substantial tissue destruction and cell killing. Under these circumstances, ionizing radiation has been shown to be an initiating agent when followed by chemical promotion, and this latent effect may persist for long periods of time. The enhancing or promoting effects of multiple doses have not been studied per se. The only data which might suggest an enhancing or promoting effect are those of Lurie and McGandy for multiple doses of radiation and chemical. Unfortunately, in these studies the two agents were delivered simultaneously so that cocarcinogenesis and enhancing effects cannot be separated. When carcinogenic levels of ionizing radiation and chemical carcinogens have been given together, the effects have generally been additive. However, most of these data were obtained at relatively high carcinogenic doses of the two agents, and the importance of dose level has not been examined in any detail.

It is apparent from the foregoing discussion that, although a number of studies have been carried out, interactions between chemicals and radiation have not been examined in any systematic way. As a result, many of the basic questions about interactions are unanswered. Studies on the importance of timing, sequence, dose level, and for ionizing radiation, the influence of dose rate in a number of well-defined tumor systems are still needed. It is likely that these types of studies may provide not only information on interactions but also an insight into the basic mechanism of carcinogenesis. In fact, even though interaction studies have been limited, two points relevant to mechanisms have already emerged: The first, from studies with UV light and chemicals, suggests that much of the importance of multiple UV light exposures is related to tumor expression activities rather than initiation. The second, from studies with UV light and ionizing radiation in combination with chemicals, suggests that latent carcinogenic effects can occur even after apparently nontumorigenic low doses of these radiations and that these effects can persist for long periods.

ACKNOWLEDGMENT

This research was sponsored by the Department of Energy under contract with Union Carbide Corporation.

REFERENCES

1. Argus, M. F., Kane, J. F., Sakuntala, M., and Ray, F. E. (1962): Effect of ionizing radiation on 9,10-dimethyl-1,2-benzanthracene tumorigenesis. *Radiat. Res.*, 16:37–43.
2. Bair, W. J. (1970): Inhalation of radionuclides and carcinogenesis. In: *Inhalation Carcinogenesis*, edited by P. Nettesheim, M. G. Hanna, Jr., and J. R. Gilbert, pp. 77–97. USAEC Division of Technical Information, Symposium Series 18, National Technical Information Service, Springfield, Virginia, CONF-691001.
3. Berenblum, I. (1941): The mechanism of carcinogenesis. A study of the significance of carcinogenic action and related phenomena. *Cancer Res.*, 1:807–814.
4. Berenblum, I., and Trainin, N. (1960): Possible two-stage mechanism in experimental leukemogenesis. *Science,* 132:40–41.
5. Black, H. S., and Chan, J. T. (1977): Experimental ultraviolet light carcinogenesis. *Photochem. Photobiol.,* 26:183–199.
6. Blum, H. F. (1959): *Carcinogenesis by Ultraviolet Light.* Princeton University Press, Princeton, New Jersey.
7. Blum, H. F., Kirby-Smith, S., and Grady, H. G. (1941): Quantitative induction of tumors in mice with ultraviolet radiation. *J. Natl. Cancer Inst.,* 2:259–268.
8. Blum, H. F., and Lipincott, S. W. (1942): Carcinogenic effectiveness of ultraviolet radiation of wavelength 2537A. *J. Natl. Cancer Inst.,* 3:211–216.
9. Brewen, J. G., and Luippold, H. E. (1971): Radiation induced human chromosome aberrations: *In vitro* dose rate studies. *Mutat. Res.,* 12:305–341.

10. Brooks, A. L. (1975): Chromosome damage in liver cells from low dose rate alpha, beta and gamma irradiation: Derivation of RBE. *Science,* 190:1090–1092.
11. Bruusgaard, cited in Rasch, C. (1926): Some historical and clinical remarks on the effect of light on the skin and skin diseases. *Proc. R. Soc. Med.,* 20:11–20.
12. Burns, F. J., Strickland, P., and Albert, R. E. (1977): The combined carcinogenic action of ionizing radiation and DMBA on rat skin. *Radiat. Res.,* 70:607 (Abstr).
13. Casarett, G. W. (1965): Experimental radiation carcinogenesis. *Prog. Exp. Tumor Res.* 7:49–82.
14. Cleaver, J. R., and Thomas, G. H. (1969): Single strand interruptions in DNA and the effects of caffeine in Chinese hamster cells irradiated with ultraviolet light. *Biochem. Biophys. Res. Commun.,* 36:203–208.
15. Cloudman, A. M., Hamilton, K. A., Clayton, R. S., and Brues, A. M. (1955): Effects of combined local treatment with radioactive and chemical carcinogens. *J. Natl. Cancer Inst.,* 15:1077–1083.
16. Cole, L. J., and Foley, W. A. (1969): Modification of urethan-lung tumor incidence by low x-radiation doses, cortisone, and transfusion of isogenic lymphocytes. *Radiat. Res.,* 39:391–399.
17. Cramer, W. (1932): Experimental observations on the effect of radium on a precancerous skin area. *Br. J. Radiol.,* 5:618–630.
18. Cronkite, E. P., Maloney, W., and Bond, V. P. (1960): Radiation leukemogenesis: An analysis of the problem. *Am. J. Med.,* 5:673–682.
19. Davies, R. E., and Dodge, H. A. (1972): Modification of chemical carcinogenesis by phototoxicity and photochemical decomposition of carcinogen. *Proc. 1st. Annu. Meet., Am. Soc. Photobiol.,* June 1973, p. 138.
20. Deringer, M. K., Lorenz, E., and Uphoff, D. E. (1955): Fertility and tumor development in (C57LXA) F_1 hybrid mice receiving x-radiation to ovaries, to whole body and to whole body with ovaries shielded. *J. Natl. Cancer Inst.,* 15:931–941.
21. Dubreuilh, W. (1896): Des hyperkeratoses circongerites. *Ann. Dermatol. Syphiligr. (Ser. 3),* 7:1158–1204.
22. Dugle, D. L., Gillespie, C. J., and Chapman, J. D. (1976): DNA strand breaks, repair and survival in x-irradiated mammalian cells. *Proc. Natl. Acad. Sci. USA,* 73:809–812.
23. Elkind, M. M., and Whitmore, G. G. (1967): *The Radiobiology of Cultured Mammalian Cells.* Gordon and Breach, London.
24. Epstein, J. H. (1965): Comparison of the carcinogenic and co-carcinogenic effects of ultraviolet light on hairless mice. *J. Natl. Cancer Inst.,* 34:741–745.
25. Epstein, J. H. (1966): Ultraviolet light carcinogenesis. In: *Advances in Biology of Skin,* Vol. 7, edited by W. Montagna and R. Dobson, pp. 215–236. Pergamon, New York.
26. Epstein, J. H., and Epstein, W. L. (1962): Co-carcinogenic effect of ultraviolet light on DMBA tumor initiation in albino mice. *J. Invest. Dermatol.,* 39:455–460.
27. Epstein, W. L., Fukuyama, K., and Epstein, J. H. (1971): Ultraviolet light, DNA repair and skin carcinogenesis in man. *Fed. Proc.,* 30:1766–1771.
28. Epstein, J. H., and Roth, H. L. (1968): Experimental ultraviolet light carcinogenesis. *J. Invest. Dermatol.,* 50:387–389.
29. Epstein, S., Small, M., Falk, H. L., and Monk, N. (1964): On the association between photodynamic and carcinogenic activities in polycyclic compounds. *Cancer Res.,* 24:855–862.
30. Findlay, G. M. (1928): Ultraviolet light and skin cancer. *Lancet,* 2:1070–1073.
31. Foley, W. A., and Cole, L. J. (1966): Urethan-induced lung tumors in mice: X-radiation dose dependent inhibition. *Radiat. Res.,* 27:87–91.
32. Freeman, R. G., Hudson, H. T., and Carnes, R. (1970): Ultraviolet wavelength factors in solar radiation and skin cancer. *Int. J. Dermatol.,* 9:232–235.
33. Frieben, A. (1902): Demonstration lines canceroids des rechten Handrückens, das sich nach langdauernder Einwirkung von Röntgenstrahlen entwickelt hatte. *Fortschr. Geb. Röntgenstr.,* 6:106.
34. Fry, R. J. M., Ley, R. D., and Grube, D. D. (1978): Photosensitized reactions and carcinogenesis. In: *Ultraviolet Radiation Carcinogenesis.* Natl. Cancer Inst. Monogr. *(in press).*
35. Furth, J., and Lorenz, E. (1954): Carcinogenesis by ionizing radiations. In: *Radiation Biology,* Vol. 1, edited by A. Hollaender, pp. 1145–1201. McGraw-Hill, New York.
36. Gray, L. H. (1965): Radiation biology and cancer. In: *Cellular Radiation Biology,* pp. 7–25. Williams and Wilkins Co., Baltimore, Maryland.

37. Hoshino, H., and Tanooka, H. (1975): Internal effect of β-irradiation and subsequent 4-nitroquinoline 1-oxide painting on skin tumor induction in mice. *Cancer Res.,* 35:3663–3666.
38. Hsu, T., Forbes, P. D., Harber, L. C., and Lakow, E. (1975): Induction of skin tumors in hairless mice by a single exposure to ultraviolet radiation. *Photochem. Photobiol.,* 21:185–188.
39. Kaplan, H. S. (1959): Some implications of indirect induction mechanisms in carcinogenesis: A review. *Cancer Res.,* 19:791–803.
40. Kaplan, H. S. (1961): Systemic interactions in radiation leukemogenesis. *Acta Unio. Int. Contra Cancrum,* 17:143–147.
41. Kellerer, A. M., and Rossi, H. H. (1972): The theory of dual radiation action. *Curr. Top. Radiat. Res. Q.,* 8:85–158.
42. Lehman, A. R. (1974): Postreplication repair of DNA in mammalian cells. *Life Sci.,* 15:2005–2016.
43. Lewis, M. R. (1935): The photosensitivity of chick embryo cells growing in media containing certain carcinogenic substances. *Am. J. Cancer,* 25:305–309.
44. Lurie, A. G. (1977): Enhancement of DMBA tumorigenesis in hamster cheek pouch epithelium by repeated exposures to low level x-radiation. *Radiat. Res.,* 72:499–511.
45. McGandy, R. B., Kennedy, A. R., Terzaghi, M., and Little, J. B. (1974): Experimental respiratory carcinogenesis: Interaction between alpha radiation and benzo(a)pyrene in the hamster. In: *Experimental Lung Cancer: Carcinogenesis and Bioassays,* edited by E. Karbe and J. F. Park, pp. 485–491. Springer-Verlag, New York.
46. McGregor, J. F. (1976): Tumor-promoting activity of cigarette tar in rat skin exposed to irradiation. *J. Natl. Cancer Inst.,* 56:429–430.
47. Mottram, J. C. (1937): Production of epithelial tumors by irradiation of a precancerous skin lesion. *Am. J. Cancer,* 30:746–748.
48. Mottram, J. C., and Doniach, I. (1938): The photodynamic action of light upon the incidence of tumors in painted mice. *Lancet,* 1:1156–1159.
49. Poel, W. W. (1963): Skin as a test site for bioassay of carcinogens and carcinogen precursors. *Natl. Cancer Inst. Monogr.,* 10:611–625.
50. Pound, A. W. (1970): Induced cell proliferation and the initiation of skin tumor formation in mice by ultraviolet light. *Pathology,* 2:269–273.
51. Rauth, A. M. (1967): Evidence for dark-reactivation of ultraviolet light damage in mouse L cells. *Radiat. Res.,* 31:121–138.
52. Ritter, M. A., Cleaver, J. E., and Tobias, C. A. (1977): High LET radiations induce a large proportion of non-rejoining DNA breaks. *Nature,* 266:653–655.
53. Roffo, A. H. (1939): Uber die physikalische Actiologie der Krebskrankheit mit besonderer Betonung des Zusammenhangs mit Sonnenbestrahlungen Strahlen Therapien. *Strahlentherap.,* 66:328–333.
54. Rusch, H. P., Kline, B. E., and Bauniann, C. A. (1941): Carcinogenesis by ultraviolet rays with reference to wavelength and energy. *Arch. Pathol.,* 31:135–146.
55. Saffiotti, U., and Shubik, P. (1956): The effects of low concentrations of carcinogen in epidermal carcinogenesis. A comparison with promoting agents. *J. Natl. Cancer Inst.,* 16:961–969.
56. Santamaria, L. (1960): Photodynamic action and carcinogenicity. In: *Recent Contributions to Cancer Research In Italy,* Vol. I, edited by P. Bucalossi and U. Veronesi, pp. 167–288. Rome.
57. Setlow, R. B., and Carrier, W. L. (1964): The disappearance of thymic dimers from DNA: An error-correcting mechanism. *Proc. Natl. Acad. Sci. USA,* 51:226–231.
58. Shellabarger, C. J. (1967): Effect of 3-methylcholanthrene and x-irradiation, given singly or combined, on rat mammary carcinogenesis. *J. Natl. Cancer Inst.,* 38:73–77.
59. Shellabarger, C. J., and Straub, R. F. (1972): Effect of 3-methylcholanthrene and fission neutron irradiation, given singly or combined, on rat mammary carcinogenesis. *J. Natl. Cancer Inst.,* 48:185–187.
60. Shubik, P., Goldfarb, A. R., Ritchie, A. C., and Lisco, H. (1953): Latent carcinogenic action of beta-irradiation on mouse epidermis. *Nature,* 171:934–935.
61. Stenback, F. (1975): Studies on the modifying effect of ultraviolet radiation on chemical skin carcinogenesis. *J. Invest. Dermatol.,* 64:253–257.
62. Stenback, F., Garcia, H., and Shubik, P. (1973): Studies on the influence of ultraviolet light on initiation in skin tumorigenesis. *J. Invest. Dermatol.,* 61:101–104.
63. Storer, J. B. (1975): Radiation carcinogenesis. In: *Cancer,* Vol. 1, edited by F. F. Becker. Plenum, New York.

64. Unna, P. G. (1896): *Histopathology of the Diseases of the Skin.* pp. 719–730, Edinburgh.
65. Upton, A. C. (1968): Radiation carcinogenesis. In: *Methods in Cancer Research,* Vol. 4, edited by H. Busch. Academic Press, New York.
66. Urbach, F., Forbes, P. D., Davies, R. E., and Berger, D. (1976): Cutaneous photobiology: Past, present and future. *J. Invest. Dermatol.,* 67:209–224.
67. Wacker, A., Dellweg, H., and Weinblum, D. (1961): Uber die strahlensensibilisierende Wirkung des 5-Bromuracils. *J. Mol. Biol.,* 3:787–789.
68. Witkin, E. M. N., Sicurella, N. A., and Bennett, G. M. (1963): Photoreversibility of induced mutations in a non-photoreactivable strain of *Escherichia coli. Proc. Natl. Acad. Sci. USA,* 50:1055–1059.
69. Zajdela, F., and Latarjet, R. (1973): Effect inhibiteur de la cafeine sur l'induction de cancers cutanes par les rayens ultraviolets chez la souris. *C. R. Acad. Sci. [D] (Paris),* 277:1073–1076.

Carcinogenesis, Vol. 5: Modifiers of Chemical
Carcinogenesis, edited by T. J. Slaga.
Raven Press, New York, 1980.

10

Mechanisms of Cocarcinogenesis Involving Endogenous Retroviruses

Raymond W. Tennant and Ralph J. Rascati

Biology Division, Oak Ridge National Laboratory, Oak Ridge, Tennessee 37830

Interactions between viruses and chemical carcinogens were recognized soon after the first tumor viruses were isolated [see Casto and DiPaolo (11) for review]. Such interactions generally result in a higher incidence of tumors in animals exposed to both agents than in animals exposed to either agent alone. At the systemic level, probably more than one mechanism is involved, leading to an increased frequency of transformed cells and to their enhanced proliferation. It has not been possible to define specific mechanisms because the virus–chemical interaction is influenced by many variables, including the order in which the animal is exposed to the agents, the age at exposure, the type of virus or chemical, and the relative size or proliferative state of the target cell population (57).

A number of studies have been done with various DNA tumor viruses and chemical carcinogens in cell cultures in order to define molecular mechanisms. Such studies have implicated an increased number of sites of integration of viral DNA into the host genome, cellular DNA damage caused by viruses and chemicals, and resultant repair synthesis as potential mechanisms of cocarcinogenesis (11). RNA tumor viruses (retroviruses), unlike the DNA viruses, exist as integrated genes in the genome of normal individuals in many mammalian species, and it is possible that similar viruses may be endogenous in most or all primate species [see Aaronson and Stephenson (2) for a review]. This basic difference in the biology of the RNA viruses implicates additional mechanisms of cocarcinogenesis.

The biology of endogenous RNA viruses has been characterized best in mice, because the use of inbred strains has permitted both genetic and molecular studies of these viruses. In mice of the AKR strain, one of at least two loci, designated as *Akv-1,* has been genetically mapped (96). BALB/c mice contain complete and/or partial gene sequences for at least three biologically distinct endogenous viruses (7,61,100,102,103), but the biological role of the viruses, including their role in neoplasia, remains undetermined. Although a few viruses have demonstrated oncogenicity after direct recovery from tumor tissue (33,75) or from chemically induced cells (101), most fail to demonstrate tumorigenicity, particularly after passage in cell culture. In addition, the determination of the oncogenic potential of the viruses is usually assessed in culture, where the appropriate target cells may not be present for transformation by these viruses. Nevertheless, the wide distribution of multiple copies of endogenous retroviruses suggests that virus–carcinogen interactions may be important in the etiology of certain types of cancer.

Many factors can influence virus–carcinogen interactions both *in vivo* and in cell culture systems (104); a major determinant is the host range of the virus. Three primary classes have been defined: *Ecotropic* viruses can reinfect the same species of cells from which they are induced or recovered. The ability of mouse ecotropic viruses to infect mouse cells is also regulated by the *Fv-1* gene locus, which consists of at least two alleles (n and b). This locus specifies dominant resistance of $Fv-1^n$ cells to B-tropic virus and $Fv-1^b$ cells to N-tropic virus. *Xenotropic* viruses (61) can be induced or recovered from cells but cannot exogenously reinfect the species of cells from which they are derived. *Amphotropic* viruses (43) have host range properties of both ecotropic and xenotropic viruses; therefore mouse amphotropic viruses can infect both murine and nonmurine cells and are subject to *Fv-1* gene restriction. Evidence also exists for a variety of recombinants of these host range types (25,44,45) and for phenotypically mixed viruses (52,53,86) that can result from exogenous virus infection coupled with induction of endogenous virus. In addition, evidence indicates that some retroviruses have sequences for a specific cell-transforming gene designated as *src,* (111) which codes for a transformation specific protein (82), so that only limited transcription of the viral genome in the appropriate target cell could be required to initiate transformation. This review summarizes recent experimental results related to cocarcinogenesis and some potential mechanisms of virus–carcinogen interactions.

RADIATION–VIRUS TUMORIGENESIS

Studies beginning in the 1950s on the pathogenesis of leukemias and lymphomas arising in mice after exposure to whole-body X-irradiation (32,33,59) and chemicals, including hydrocarbon carcinogens, urethan, and 4-nitroquinoline 1-oxide (4-NQO) [reviewed by Kaplan (56–58)], provided the conceptual basis for endogenous viruses. Initial studies demonstrated that radiogenic lymphomas developed by an indirect induction mechanism and not by somatic mutation in the cells of the target organ, the thymus. The search for a postulated latent leukemogenic agent that was activated in the host by X-irradiation led to the discovery that cell-free extracts possessed a low but significant and reproducible leukemogenic activity when inoculated into nonirradiated newborn mice of the strain of origin. These results in C57BL strain mice (58) were reproduced in the C3H and RF strains (32,110). The leukemogenic activity of the extracts could be amplified by serial passage *in vivo* (63,68), and the agent was identified as a C-type virus (10) which was designated radiation leukemia virus (RadLV). Haran-Ghera (38) demonstrated that RadLV could be also recovered from nonlymphomatous tissues such as bone marrow as early as 7 days after the last X-ray exposure of C57BL/6 mice. In addition, the development of osteogenic sarcomas in mice exposed to bone-seeking radionuclides has been shown to be virus associated (24).

Although virus induction appears to be necessary for the development of radiogenic lymphoma, extensive studies by Kaplan, Haran-Ghera, and their associates (39–41,56–58,60) have defined several parameters essential to lymphoma induction: (a) virus host range, (b) target cells susceptible to transformation, (c) the thymic microenvironment, (d) a genetically susceptible host, (e) impairment of immune responsiveness, and (f) a number of constitutional factors including strain, sex, age, nutrition, and hormonal balance.

The first RadLV isolates could be propagated only *in vivo,* and the only available assay was lymphoma induction (64). The sensitivity of the bioassay was increased at least 1,000-fold when the virus was inoculated directly into the thymus (42,56), and leukemogenicity was increased by serial intrathymic passage of RadLV. Subsequently RadLV-induced lymphomas established in culture have been a source of virus with biological characteristics of the parent RadLV (34). Recent advances using intrathymic injection and immunofluorescence assay of thymic frozen sections (15) and the establishment of thymic epithelial reticular cell cultures that can release virus which may transform thymocytes in culture (36,37,39,112) have led to an increased understanding of the nature of these viruses. RadLV which is highly leukemogenic and selectively replicates in the thymus is designated as *thymotropic* (T^+) (16). RadLV proliferation was detected specifically in the "blastoid population" of the thymic outer cortex, the area in which neoplastic cells are first detected (18). The thymotropic RadLV preferentially infected mice of the $Fv-1^{bb}$ genotype and is thus a B-tropic isolate (17,21), but it poorly infected C57BL mouse embryo fibroblast cells in culture (nonfibrotropic, F^-). Cultivation in fibroblasts resulted in the loss of leukemogenic potential (66). Infection of C57BL fibroblasts by high multiplicities of RadLV yielded a virus preparation designated BL/Ka (6) which is fibrotropic (F^+), thymotropic (T^+), and leukemogenic (L^+) (23). However, this preparation was subsequently determined to be a mixture of thymotropic–leukemogenic (T^+L^+) RadLV-like virus and fibrotropic–nonleukemogenic (F^+L^-) virus, together with virions that are phenotypic mixtures of the two types (A. Decleve, *personal communication*). Several other viruses also have been isolated from lymphoid tissues of normal or X-irradiated C57BL/Ka strain mice (68) and from C57BL embryo fibroblast cultures that had been treated with 5-iodo-2′-deoxyuridine (IdUrd) (29) or X-rays (20). Unlike RadLV, these isolates, a B-tropic [BL/Ka (B)], an N-tropic [BL/Ka (N)], and a xenotropic [BL/Ka (X)] agent, are nonthymotropic (T^-) and nonleukemogenic (L^-) when injected into weanling C57BL mice. It is significant that no T^+L^+ virus has been reported isolated from cultured fibroblasts. In addition, both of the ecotropic isolates (B- and N-tropic) originally contained xenotropic virus that was eliminated by limit dilution passage in C57BL/Ka and SC-1 cells. The BL/Ka (B) isolate is the only one of the T^-L^- C57BL agents that can replicate *in vivo* in bone marrow cells when injected into newborn rather than weanling mice (Decleve, personal communication). The BL/Ka (X) and BL/Ka (N) isolates are the most readily recoverable virus from C57BL mice; this is paradoxical, because the spread of these viruses is specifically restricted at the cell membrane or by the $Fv-1^b$ locus. Another virus similar to the mink cell focus-inducing (MCF) isolate reported by Hartley et al. (44) in the AKR strain was also derived from C57BL/6 thymus reticular epithelial cells (35). A summary of the properties of C57BL isolates is given in Table 1.

Comparison of the biological and immunological properties of the wild-type RadLV derived from C57BL/Ka lymphomas *in vivo* and of the RadLV-LTC obtained from cell cultures of RadLV-induced lymphomas indicates that both T^+L^+ viruses are distinct from the T^-L^- fibrotropic BL/Ka (B), BL/Ka (N), and BL/Ka (X) isolates (19,22). Differences were detected between the envelope glycoprotein gp70 of the T^+L^+ viruses and those of the T^-L^- fibrotropic viruses. However, the "gag" gene proteins (virion proteins p12, p15, p30, and p10) of T^+L^+ viruses appear to be identical to the T^-L^- BL/Ka (B) virus. In addition, characterization of isolates derived from IdUrd-treated C57BL/Ka fibroblasts indicates that recombinant viruses can emerge in the process of isolation and propagation of induced viruses. Modulation of host range, plaque-forming ability, and electrophoretic mobility of some low-molecular-weight virion proteins can also occur (29). Thus, the emergence of a particular variant is dependent on the cell of origin, the method of isolation (infection by cell-free extracts or by cocultivation), and the cell types in which the induced viruses are propagated.

In the isolation of most endogenous agents it is not possible to determine whether the emergence of the predominant fibrotropic virus represents *de novo* induction and selection, adaptation, or host-induced modification of an endogenous thymotropic agent. Adaptation to growth in cells restrictive at the $Fv-1$ locus has been reported (69) and appears to represent the loss of, or alteration of, the virion target(s) of the $Fv-1$ gene product. The apparent loss of thymotropism and thymic cell oncogenicity by adaptation to growth in fibroblastic cells could represent both the loss of or alteration in gp70 molecules which mediate cell-specific attachment (111) and/or in potential oncogenic gene sequences which may be preferentially expressed in cells in specific differentiated states (106). The evidence favors a loss of such functions, since in the $Fv-1$ system the change in tropism is irreversible, and in the case of RadLV adapted to fibroblasts, no thymotropic reversion has been reported.

It is paradoxical that most radiation-induced C57BL/Ka thymic lymphomas do not express viral antigens (63,67) detectable by immunofluorescence or radioimmune competition assays (51,52). This is in direct contrast to the results of leukemia induction by the laboratory-adapted tumor virus strains (Friend,

TABLE 1. *Properties of viral isolates from C57BL mouse tissues and cell cultures*

| Isolate | Source | Host range (tropism) | | | | Serologic specificity |
		Ecotropic	Xenotropic	Fibrotropic	Thymotropic	
RadLV[b]	Thymoma extract	B	+	–	+	Specific for RadLV
RadLV-LTC (RadLV/VL3)	Cell culture of RadLV-induced lymphoma	B	+	+	+	Specific for RadLV
BL/Ka (B)	Cell line (RadLV) infected	B	+	+	+	Ecotropic + xenotropic
BL/Ka (B)[a]	Antixenotropic serum + RadLV	B	–	+	–	Ecotropic
BL/Ka (N)[a]	NIH Swiss mouse embryo fibroblasts + lymphoma extract	N	–	+	–	Ecotropic
BL/Ka (X)	Mink lung cells cocultivated with C57BL thymus	–	+	+	–	Xenotropic
BL/Ka (6)	C57BL cell line + RadLV	B	+	+		
RadLV*	C57BL cell line + RadLV	Similar to BL/Ka (B)		+	+	Ecotropic + xenotropic

[a]Cloned.
[b]Radiation leukemia virus, the generic term for all viruses isolated from radiation-induced thymomas and other cells.

Rauscher, Moloney, etc.) or spontaneously in the AKR strain, where high levels of virus are generally expressed in all tumor cells (33). One hypothesis presented to explain this apparent paradox (22) is that RadLV is activated in a replication-defective form (RadLV-O) in which only the oncogenic segment of the RadLV genome is expressed initially. This hypothesis is based upon experiments in which RadLV was injected into thymectomized weanling mice. Although the bone marrow cells remained totally negative by indirect immunofluorescence, it was possible by grafting a thymus or by transfer of the cells to a secondary syngeneic host to demonstrate high levels of virus in the secondary thymus (65). In these experiments, virus could be found in a cryptic state in the bone marrow cells for up to 2 months. In addition, it was found *in vitro* that cultured lymphoma cells derived from nonvirus-producing radiation-induced tumors could remain virus negative in culture for many months, or could release T^+L^+ particles. Virus release occurred spontaneously after subculture of the nonproducer cells or after infection by BL/Ka (B).

Finally, host susceptibility patterns are determined by the *Fv-1* locus and by the *SRV* gene [the dominant allele of which occurs in C57BL mice (21)]. In addition to the effects of *Fv-1*, *SRV*, and possibly other loci, the target cell specificity of T^+L^+ viruses may reside in a differentiation-specific restriction system which determines the cytotropic patterns of the viruses (14). Among other speculations advanced are: (a) that the product(s) of a putative leukemia *(leuk)* gene interact with only specific sequences of the cellular genome and

TABLE 2. *Agents that have been shown to induce endogenous virus in mouse cells*

Agent	Dose (μg/ml)	Reference
IdUrd	20–100	71,105
BrUrd	20–100	71,105
5-Iododeoxycytidine	100	105
Mitomycin C	1,3	105
MCA	50	105
DMBA	10	105
Puromycin	10	1
Cycloheximide	10	1
Anisomycin	100	1
Sparsomycin	100	1
HU	0.4–4 mM	85,85a,109
Carbamoyloxyurea	0.1–2 mM	85
Formamidoxine	1–10 mM	85
γ-Radiation	20 rads/hr	74,108,109
X-Radiation	1,000 rads/7 min	108,109
L-Canavanine	300	4,5
O-Methylthreonine	1,000	5
Hydroxynorvaline	300	5
7,8-Dihydroxybenzo(*a*)pyrene	1	R. J. Rascati and R. W. Tennant *(unpublished)*
7,8-Diol-9,10-epoxybenzo(*a*)pyrene	0.15	R. J. Rascati and R. W. Tennant *(unpublished)*

that such an interaction is effective only if these sequences are transcriptionally active, i.e., as in certain classes of lymphocytes. Thus, cells differentiated along other pathways could not be affected because such regions would never be expressed; and (b) that integration sites for endogenous virus that spreads to adjacent cells could be altered by cellular transcriptional patterns, or that some integration sites are preferentially used which predispose to neoplastic transformation. Thus, the radiation tumorigenesis system demonstrates the complexity of the endogenous retrovirus problem, including the wide variety of virus host-range types and target cell differences that exist. Complexity may also arise in the induction process itself, and the method of induction can, in at least some circumstances, determine the nature of the induced virus. It is important, therefore, to understand the mechanism(s) by which the various inducing agents produce their effect. A wide variety of agents have been shown to induce virus expression and a partial summary of them is given in Table 2.

VIRUS INDUCTION BY HALOGENATED PYRIMIDINES AND INHIBITORS OF PROTEIN SYNTHESIS

The most potent virus-inducing agents are the halogenated pyrimidines; it has been shown that IdUrd or 5-bromo-2'-deoxyuridine (BrdUrd) must be incorporated into DNA for virus induction, since thymidine and drugs that inhibit DNA synthesis also inhibit induction (71,105). The period of inducibility corresponds to the S-phase of the cell cycle (8,31,97), and there is evidence that two discrete cycles of DNA replication are required (49). When IdUrd was incorporated into cells capable of two or more cycles of DNA synthesis, induction was observed; however, if only a single cycle occurred, then no induction was observed until the cells again divided. Inhibition of either cycle of DNA synthesis with cytosine arabinoside prevented induction. However, IdUrd needed to be present in the medium only during the first replication cycle, since only during this first cycle could induction be inhibited by excess thymidine. In the second replication cycle the presence of IdUrd was no longer required, and excess thymidine had no effect. Therefore, it appears that the first round of DNA synthesis allows the incorporation of IdUrd into the DNA. If no further DNA synthesis occurs, then no induction is observed, but a stable intermediate state has been formed; when DNA synthesis resumes, even up to 4 days later, virus can be expressed. Therefore, the second round of DNA synthesis is required for expression of the virus and does not require the continuing presence of IdUrd. This requirement for DNA synthesis has also been observed for exogenous infection of chicken cells with Rous sarcoma virus (48). Furthermore, cell division itself is not required, since cells pretreated with mitomycin C to prevent division are still capable of virus induction (31).

The mechanism of virus induction by halogenated pyrimidines is as yet unknown. It has been demonstrated that IdUrd produces mutations (28), but the high frequency of induction (1 to 15%) as compared with the frequency of mutation (0.001%) and the observation that other mutagens (Table 3) do not induce virus expression argue against mutation as the immediate and sole cause of induction. Since exposure of halogenated pyrimidine substituted DNA to high-intensity light causes single-strand breaks and increases the level of induction (105), it is possible that they act through this mechanism. However, physical agents, such as X-, and γ-irradiation which also cause strand breaks, have very low frequencies of induction (0.01 to 0.03%) (74,105,108,109).

The IdUrd induction process does not require reverse transcription, since polynucleotide inhibitors of the reverse transcriptase enzyme do not prevent induction even though they effectively inhibit exogenous infection (76,107). Therefore, induction proceeds from the already reversely transcribed and presumably already integrated endogenous viral genome, which is under some form of transcriptional control. One hypothesis is that halogenated pyrimidine incorporation into DNA alters the binding of a repressor-like protein to DNA. This has been observed in bacterial systems (70) and is further supported by the

TABLE 3. *Agents that have not been shown to induce endogenous virus in mouse cells*

Agent	Dose (μg/ml)	Reference
5-Fluorodeoxyuridine	0.002–20	55,105
Cytosine arabinoside	0.1–20	105
8-Azaguanine	20	105
Cyclic dibutyryl adenosine monophosphate	12	105
Cyclophosphamide	5–50	105
Uracil mustard	0.1–10	105
6-Mercaptopurine	0.12–12 (mg/ml)	105
Ethyl methansulfonate	4–200	105
Methyl methanesulfonate	4–200	105
Isopropyl methanesulfonate	4–200	R. J. Rascati and R. W. Tennant *(unpublished)*
6-Azathymine	0.25–25 (mg/ml)	105
6-Azauridine	0.17–17 (mg/ml)	105
Hydrocortisone	10^{-5} M	50
Dexamethasone	10^{-5} M	50
Nitrosocarbaryl	10	83
Carbaryl	10	R. J. Rascati and R. W. Tennant *(unpublished)*
Nitrosoethylurea	10	R. J. Rascati and R. W. Tennant *(unpublished)*
N-Methyl-N′-nitro-N-nitrosoguanidine	10	84, R. J. Rascati and R. W. Tennant *(unpublished)*
Dibenz(*a*)anthracene	—	84
BP derivatives other than 7,8-dihydroxy	10	84, R. J. Rascati and R. W. Tennant *(unpublished)*
L-homoarginine and other amino acid analogs	1–4 mM	4,5
Amino acid deprivation	—	5

ability of protein synthesis inhibitors such as cycloheximide and puromycin (1,31) and certain amino acid analogs such as L-canavanine, hydroxynorvaline, and O-methylthreonine (4,5) to induce virus expression at high frequencies. When protein synthesis is inhibited or analogs are used to produce altered, defective proteins, the normal turnover of such proteins is interrupted so that degradation without replacement of the putative repressor takes place. The virogenes would thus become available for transcription and expression. Since no alteration is made in the DNA, induction by these methods is more transient (1,3,8). When protein synthesis resumes or analogs are removed, functional repressor is again synthesized and virus expression is terminated.

INDUCTION BY OTHER AGENTS

Different classes of viruses respond differently to the various treatments. For example, in cells from BALB/c mice a class of ecotropic viruses is induced by halogenated pyrimidines but not by protein synthesis inhibitors, whereas a class of xenotropic virus is induced by both. Yet another xenotropic class is not induced by either treatment (2). Therefore, as has been demonstrated with the RadLV of C57BL mice, the endogenous viruses can be differentially regulated, and their detection can be affected by the method of induction.

We have shown that hydroxyurea (HU) will induce virus from AKR cells, that induction is proportional to dose over a limited range of concentrations (85,85a,109), and that it correlates with the cytotoxicity of the HU treatment (85). Other laboratories have reported that HU damages the DNA of both prokaryotic (93–95) and eukaryotic (9,13) cells and also that HU can degrade DNA *in vitro* (54). Although we have not been able to detect degradation of AKR DNA *in vivo* directly, we have demonstrated that treatment with HU results in unscheduled DNA synthesis (i.e., repair); this indicates that some alteration in the DNA has occurred (85a). It is paradoxical that HU, which inhibits DNA synthesis, can cause induction since induction appears to require DNA synthesis. However, when HU is removed, DNA synthesis must occur for virus expression. If cells are maintained in serum-free media after removal of HU, no virus expression is observed.

We have previously reported that low-dose-rate γ-irradiation and acute X-irradiation, which also damage DNA, can induce virus expression, and that cells exposed to γ-irradiation must be actively dividing in order to be induced (74,108,109). Irradiation of serum-starved cells does not lead to virus induction (74), indicating a requirement for cellular DNA synthesis. This requirement was further substantiated by work with acute X-irradiation. X-ray treatment was given in short pulses (1,000 rads/7 min) at various times during the cell cycle of synchronized AKR cell cultures. If the X-rays were given during S-phase, significant levels of induction were observed (109). At other periods of the cell cycle induction was not observed or was drastically reduced. Again, as discussed previously, DNA synthesis or some cellular function, which only occurs during the period of DNA synthesis, is required for virus expression. Since lesions caused by the radiation are available for repair, the probability of replication occurring through the damaged region prior to repair of the lesion would be greater during S-phase than at other times. This hypothesis would explain the reduced level of induction when cells were irradiated during periods of the cell cycle other than S. It would also explain the requirement for serum during γ-irradiation mediated induction, since in the absence of serum, lesions would be available for repair for a large period of time prior to initiation of DNA synthesis. In the presence of serum the probability of DNA replication occurring prior to repair of any given lesion would be increased, and therefore the probability of induction would increase.

If lesions leading to induction could be stabilized in some manner, induction would be enhanced in mass cultures because lesions introduced into cells prior to S-phase would still be available for induction when those cells entered into S-phase. Two methods have been used to stabilize lesions to test this hypothesis. In the first approach repair synthesis inhibitors such as quinacrine (12) were used. In this case, induction by γ-irradiation was enhanced in actively dividing cells and could also be observed in cells irradiated in the absence of serum if serum was added immediately after irradiation (109). Under these conditions, lesions introduced into the DNA may not be repaired prior to the onset of DNA replication and could therefore induce virus expression. A similar observation using caffeine was reported during UV induction of SV40 virus from hamster cells and probably also represents inhibition of repair of damage (118). The second approach involved the incorporation of halogenated pyrimidines during repair of DNA in the absence of replicative DNA synthesis. A representative experiment using this approach is shown in Table 4. Cells were plated in serum-free, isoleucine-free medium, held for 4 days, and then X-irradiated (1,000 rads/7 min) with or without IdUrd (50 μg/ml). The results show that unirradiated cells were only minimally capable of DNA synthesis, as evidenced by the low

TABLE 4. *Stimulation of X-ray induction of endogenous retrovirus by IdUrd in nondividing AKR cells[a]*

Treatment	pfu/10^6 cells [b,c]
None	0
Iododeoxyuridine (50 μg/ml)	3
X-ray (1,000 rads)	28
X-ray (1,000 rads) plus IdUrd (50 μg/ml)	100

[a]Cells were seeded in serum-free, isoleucine-free medium and held for 4 days. They were then treated as indicated and given complete medium supplemented with 5% fetal calf serum. After 5 days induction was scored by the XC-syncytial plaque assay.

[b]Results are normalized for number of survivors.

[c]pfu: plaque-forming units.

induction frequency observed with IdUrd. Irradiated cells were induced to express virus if serum was added immediately after irradiation, but again only at a low level. However, induction was stimulated fourfold when cells were irradiated in the presence of IdUrd. The most likely explanation for this synergistic effect is that IdUrd was incorporated into lesions repaired prior to the onset of scheduled DNA replication. These "repaired" lesions, therefore, retained their ability to cause virus expression, as in the incorporation of IdUrd during DNA replication. Cells irradiated in the absence of IdUrd were repaired normally, and the radiation-induced lesions were, therefore, not available for induction when replication occurs. In these cells only unrepaired lesions can cause virus induction. When both irradiation and IdUrd were given, unrepaired and at least some of the repaired lesions were capable of induction, thus stimulation was observed.

A similar observation was made for HU-mediated induction. In this case, serum-starved cells were treated with HU (2 mM) and IdUrd (50 μg/ml) for 24 hr, then washed and refed with either serum-free or complete media. At 24-hr intervals cells fed with serum-free medium were refed with complete medium. Nine days after treatment all cultures were examined for virus induction. The results from a typical experiment are given in Table 5. Cells treated with IdUrd alone showed a low level of induction, indicating a residual level of replication. This induction was stable (i.e., a stable intermediate had been formed) throughout the starvation period. With HU alone, however, induction was observed only if serum was added immediately after treatment, indicating a requirement for DNA synthesis as discussed above. If as little as 24 hr elapsed between

TABLE 5. *Stimulation of HU-mediated induction by IdUrd and the formation of a stable intermediate*[a]

Period of starvation after treatment (days)	pfu/10^6 cells[b] after treatment with[c]		
	IdUrd (50 μg/ml)	HU (2 mM)	HU (2 mM) plus IdUrd (50 μg/ml)
0	12	9	180
1	11	0	192
2	13	0	178
3	12	0	156
4	12	0	132

[a] Cells were subcultured at a density of 5×10^5 cells/100-mm dish in serum-free, isoleucine-free medium containing either IdUrd, HU, or both as indicated. After 24 hr cells were washed, and one group was given complete medium supplemented with 5% fetal calf serum; the remaining groups were maintained in serum-free medium. At 24-hr intervals, groups of cultures were given complete medium containing 5% fetal calf serum. After 5 days each group was scored for induction by the XC-syncytial plaque assay.

[b] Results are normalized for number of surviving cells.

[c] pfu: plaque-forming units.

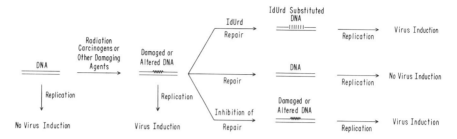

FIG. 1. Proposed model for induction by DNA-damaging agents.

HU treatment and serum addition, induction was completely eliminated. However, when both IdUrd and HU were present, induction was stimulated 9-fold over that with either treatment alone and was found to be stable even if 4 days were allowed to elapse between treatment and serum addition, indicating that a stable intermediate had been formed by the IdUrd incorporation. Two lines of evidence indicate that this observed stimulation is the result of incorporation of IdUrd during repair and not the result of residual replicative DNA synthesis. First, the combination of HU and IdUrd is synergistic. If the IdUrd-mediated induction were the result of residual DNA synthesis, the effects would be expected to be additive. Furthermore, since HU inhibits DNA synthesis, even less induction than that observed in cells treated with IdUrd alone would be expected. Second, experiments using BrdUrd indicate that the halogenated pyrimidines are incorporated in such a way that there is no significant shift in the density of substituted DNA (85a). This is indicative of repair synthesis, not replicative synthesis, and therefore provides indirect evidence that induction proceeds through an as yet undefined alteration in the DNA of the treated cells.

A model which accounts for the above observations is given in Fig. 1. DNA which is damaged by some treatment is capable of inducing virus expression only if replication occurs while the lesion is still present. If repair occurs prior to replication, induction is eliminated. Therefore, induction can be enhanced by one of three means: (a) introduction of the lesion during S-phase which would minimize the probability of repair prior to replication through the lesion, (b) inhibition of repair to retain the lesion in the DNA until S-phase, or (c) incorporation of IdUrd during repair to create a stable induction intermediate.

CHEMICAL CARCINOGENS

Work with chemical carcinogens indicates a similar interaction with viral genes. In the avian system, Weiss et al. (114), using several types of chicken cells, demonstrated the induction of infectious virus with methylcholanthrene

(MCA), 4-NQO, urethan, and X-irradiation. Altanerova (6), using hamster cells transformed with the Schmidt-Ruppin strain of Rous sarcoma virus but not producing infectious virus, demonstrated that treatment of the cells with MCA, benzo*(a)*pyrene (BP), 4-NQO, and azacytidine induced the release of virus particles, and that this virus was infectious and sarcomagenic in chickens. In AKR mouse embryo cells, virus has been induced by treatment with chemicals such as MCA (105,109) and dimethylbenz*(a)*anthracene (DMBA) (105). We have reported previously that MCA induces virus expression and that induction can be enhanced by the presence of IdUrd under conditions in which replicative DNA synthesis is limited. Furthermore, induction in the presence of IdUrd is proportional to the dose of MCA (109), indicating that IdUrd stimulates MCA-mediated induction, presumably by a repair substitution mechanism similar to that described above when IdUrd is used with either radiation or HU.

Since many potential carcinogens, particularly polycyclic hydrocarbons, must be metabolically converted to an active state in order to demonstrate carcinogenicity (72), demonstration of virus induction could also be dependent upon the ability of cultured cells to make such conversions. Huberman and Fogel (46), using cloned rat cells transformed by, but not producing, polyoma virus, showed that those subclones which could metabolize BP to water-soluble products were inducible for virus synthesis when treated with BP, MCA, or DMBA. However, subclones which have low hydrocarbon-metabolizing ability (only 0.1 μmol BP per 10^6 cells) were not inducible by those compounds. None of the subclones were inducible when treated with noncarcinogenic hydrocarbons; furthermore, 7,8-benzoflavone, which blocks BP metabolism, also inhibited virus induction. Using AKR cells (clone 2B), Spelsberg et al. (99) found evidence for metabolically dependent, high-affinity binding of [^{3}H]MCA and its metabolites to a specific, transcriptionally active subfraction of chromatin. The amount of covalent binding increased as a function of time, presumably allowing the compound to be metabolized, and was inhibited by 7,8-benzoflavone. These results also suggest that the metabolically dependent active intermediates, which may be responsible for cellular transformation, may also be the compounds that induce virus synthesis. However, this does not necessarily support a causal relationship, since different intermediates could be involved in each process or both processes could be independent events that are the result of the general affinity of the intermediates to bind to nucleic acid.

RETROVIRUS–CHEMICAL COCARCINOGENESIS

Freeman et al. (26,78) demonstrated that rat embryo cells infected with Rauscher murine leukemia virus could be transformed with diethylnitrosamine, and Price et al. (77) showed the same effect with MCA. In neither case were the cells transformed by chemical or virus alone but only when the two were used in combination. Similar results were obtained with rat embryo cells infected with xenotropic murine leukemia virus (81) and treated with MCA or 4-NQO.

In addition, the same results could be demonstrated in an NIH Swiss mouse cell line infected with the AKR strain of murine leukemia virus treated with either BP or smog extracts (89–91). The authors proposed that the postulated oncogenes of the RNA tumor virus genomes integrated into the cellular genome after infection (47) were derepressed by the action of these chemicals and that these derepressed oncogenes were the mediators of cellular transformation. When the transforming activities of a variety of carcinogens and noncarcinogens were tested in this system, they were found to conform to the transforming activities of these compounds measured *in vivo* (92).

Other information bears on the mechanism of the synergistic interaction between viruses and chemicals. First, it was noted in a cocarcinogenesis system that some carcinogens were more efficient in transformation at lower doses (88), suggesting that the decrease in toxicity at the lower doses might be important. Second, direct involvement of the retrovirus genome is supported by several lines of evidence: (a) Transformation occurs only when infected cells are treated with the chemical, that is, the virus fails to transform cells when added after chemical treatment (78); (b) Cordycepin and type-specific anti-Rauscher murine leukemia virus antisera, both of which inhibit virus infection, also inhibit cocarcinogenesis (79–81); and (c) Ethidium bromide, an inhibitor of provirus integration into the host genome, inhibits cocarcinogenic transformation if present at the time of virus inoculation, but is ineffective if added to preinfected cells (73).

CHEMICAL TRANSFORMATION OF CELLS WITHOUT EXOGENOUS VIRUS INFECTION

The foregoing results show that chemical carcinogens and retroviruses can act synergistically in certain cell systems to cause transformation under conditions at which neither treatment alone will cause transformation. However, in systems in which transformation occurs in the absence of infection by exogenously added retroviruses, the role played by the stably inherited endogenous viruses is uncertain. In studies of cell lines such as the mouse (C3H/10T$^{1/2}$ and BALB/c A31) lines and hamster embryo fibroblasts treated with such chemicals as MCA, DMBA, 5-fluorodeoxyuridine, the nitrosated derivative of the pesticide carbaryl, and BP, transformation has been found to occur without concomitant virus induction (55,83,84,87). The criteria used in each of the studies were the lack of infectious virus, extracellular reverse transcriptase activity, or expression of virus structural proteins. In hamster embryo fibroblasts, virus-specific RNA sequences were also not detected (87). In other experiments, however, Whitmire and Salerno (116) demonstrated that virus-group-specific antigen (P30 protein) was expressed in many of the tumor cells from animals treated with MCA, but the gs antigen was not observed in normal muscle tissues from the same animals. The percentage of cells expressing gs antigen appeared to be related to the mouse strain but not necessarily to the dose. Therefore, in strains that exhibit stringent genetic control over their endogenous viruses, fewer cells expressed viral antigens, whereas in strains that control their viruses less stringently, more cells expressed viral antigens. In other experiments, Freeman et al. (27), using rat embryo cells, demonstrated that low-passage cells could not be transformed by treatment with MCA unless the cells had been previously treated with BrdUrd. This double treatment also resulted in the induction of virus-group-specific antigen expression. In contrast, high-passage cells could be transformed by either MCA or DMBA alone without BrdUrd treatment. Virus-group-specific antigen expression was also induced in these cells. The authors concluded that low-passage cells exhibit tight control over their endogenous viruses and that these could not be induced to express viral antigens unless they were treated with BrdUrd, which was also required before transformation could be observed. In high-passage cells, however, the state of the genome had been altered so that the cells controlled virus expression less stringently and therefore both viral antigen expression and transformation could be induced with carcinogen alone. Mouse cells transformed spontaneously or by treatment with MCA or DMBA and which do not express virus as a result of carcinogen treatment were seven to ten times more inducible when subsequently treated with the halogenated pyrimidines BrdUrd or IdUrd (62,117). These observations suggest a role for endogenous virus expression in the transformation process; in support of this hypothesis it has been noted that streptonigrin and cordycepin prevented both virus induction and transformation in this system (79). More recently, it was observed that AKR/2B clones transformed with MCA produced 150 to 200 times as much virus-specific mRNA as nontransformed clones and that other cellular mRNAs were not similarly increased (30). One mechanism by which retroviruses could exert a cocarcinogenic effect is indicated by experiments involving rat cells chronically infected with exogenous Rauscher leukemia virus (113). In this system repair synthesis was observed as an increase in the molecular weight of DNA after treatment with the damaging agent (98), where size of the DNA was determined by velocity sedimentation in sucrose gradients. By use of 4-NQO or UV radiation, it was shown that a reduced rate of increase in the molecular weight of DNA synthesized after treatment occurred in the infected cells, which suggests some virus-mediated defect in post-replication, but not excision, repair. Therefore, in virus-infected cells the repair process appears to be partially defective, is reflected in a lower rate of increase in the molecular weight of DNA synthesized after chemical treatment, and does not appear to be due to a greater amount of DNA damage in the infected cells.

VIRUS IN CHEMICAL AND RADIATION CARCINOGENESIS— CAUSE AND EFFECT

The generality of these observations, particularly in the case of induced endogenous retrovirus, has not yet been determined. If retroviruses generally disrupt repair synthesis of DNA, then they could serve to indirectly increase the probability that exposure to a carcinogen could result in transformation. From the available results the determinant role of endogenous retroviruses or potential mutagens or carcinogens in the induction of specific types of tumors cannot be established. Many alternative mechanisms have been proposed to explain these interactions: (a) chemical or radiation induction of endogenous retrovirus that subsequently spreads to target cells, where a product of the putative tumorigenic, *onc* gene heritably alters cell transcriptional patterns; (b) retrovirus infection sensitizes cells to carcinogenic or mutagenic effects of chemicals or radiation; and (c) chemical or radiation damage to cellular DNA makes available new virus integration sites that alter cellular control processes.

It has been argued that although certain carcinogens have induced endogenous retrovirus expression, the viruses induced were not tumorigenic. The results on RadLV, however, indicate that the tumorigenicity of induced viruses can be affected by their passage history and that passage in nontarget cells may permanently impair or select against tumorigenic viruses which may have been induced initially. Therefore, target cell specificity must be accounted for, and the concepts of partial induction and noncoordinate expression of the various virogenes must also be considered in light of the frequent recombinational events involving retroviruses (25,44,45,115). Thus, although it may at first appear that viruses are not involved in certain transformation systems, it must be realized that this is based on our limited ability to identify endogenous viruses and virogene products. The actual situation may involve subtle regulation of only those virogenes responsible for oncogenesis in the absence of identifiable viral products. Since products of the putative viral *onc* gene have not yet been conclusively identified, their participation in chemical and physical carcinogenesis remains uncertain.

ACKNOWLEDGMENT

This work was supported jointly by the Virus Cancer Program of the National Cancer Institute and the Division of Biomedical and Environmental Research, U.S. Department of Energy, under contract W-7405-eng-26 with the Union Carbide Corporation.

REFERENCES

1. Aaronson, S. A., and Dunn, C. Y. (1974): High frequency C-type virus induction by inhibitors of protein synthesis. *Science,* 183:422–424.
2. Aaronson, S. A., and Stephenson, J. R. (1976): Endogenous type-C RNA viruses of mammalian cells. *Biochim. Biophys. Acta,* 458:323–354.
3. Aaronson, S. A., Anderson, G. R., Dunn, C. Y., and Robbins, K. C. (1974): Induction of type-C RNA virus by cycloheximide: Increased expression of virus-specific RNA. *Proc. Natl. Acad. Sci. USA,* 71:3941–3945.
4. Aksamit, R. R., and Long, C. W. (1977): Induction of endogenous murine type-C virus by an arginine analog: L-canavanine. *Virology,* 78:567–570.
5. Aksamit, R. R., Christensen, W. L., and Long, C. W. (1977): Characterization of type-C virus induction by aminoacid analogs. *Virology,* 83:138–149.
6. Altanerova, J. (1972): Virus production induced by various chemical carcinogens in a virogenic hamster cell line transformed by Rous sarcoma virus. *J. Natl. Cancer Inst.,* 49:1375–1380.

7. Benveniste, R. E., Callahan, R., Sherr, C. J., Chapman, V., and Todaro, G. J. (1977): Two distinct endogenous type-C viruses isolated from the Asian rodent *Mus cervicolor:* Conservation of virogene sequences in related rodent species. *J. Virol.,* 21:849–853.

8. Besmer, P., Smotkin, D., Haseltine, W., Fan, H., Wison, A. T., Pasking, M., Weinberg, R., and Baltimore, D. (1975): Mechanisms of induction of RNA tumor viruses by halogenated pyrimidines. *Cold Spring Harbor Symp. Quant. Biol.,* 39:1103–1107.

9. Cameron, J. L., and Jeter, J. R., Jr. (1973): Action of hydroxyurea and *N*-carbamoyloxyurea on the cell cycle of Tetrahymena. *Cell Tissue Kinet.,* 6:289–301.

10. Carnes, W. H., Lieberman, M., Marchildon, M., and Kaplan, H. S. (1968): Replication of type C virus particles in thymus grafts on C57BL mice inoculated with radiation leukemia virus. *Cancer Res.,* 28:98–103.

11. Casto, B. C., and DiPaolo, J. A. (1973): Virus, chemicals and cancer. *Prog. Med. Virol.,* 16:1–47.

12. Clarke, C. H., and Shankel D. M. (1974): Effects of ethidium, quinacrine and hycanthone on survival and mutagenesis of UV-irradiated *hcr⁺* and *hcr⁻* strains of E. coli B/r. *Mutat. Res.,* 26:473–481.

13. Coyle, M. D., and Strauss, B. (1970): Cell killing and the accumulation of breaks in the DNA of HEp-2 cells in the presence of hydroxyurea. *Cancer Res.,* 30:2314–2319.

14. Decleve, A., and Kaplan, H. S. (1977): Genetic control of naturally occurring murine ecotropic C-type virus replication *in vitro* and *in vivo:* A concise review. In: *Radiation-Induced Leukemogenesis and Related Viruses,* edited by J. F. Duplan, pp. 197–212. North-Holland Publishing Company, Amsterdam.

15. Decleve, A., Lieberman, M., Niwa, O., and Kaplan, H. S. (1974): Rapid in vivo assay for murine lymphatic leukemia viruses. *Nature,* 252:79–80.

16. Decleve, A., Sato, C., Lieberman, M., and Kaplan, H. S. (1974): Selective thymic localization of murine leukemia virus-related antigens in C57BL/Ka mice after inoculation with radiation leukemia virus. *Proc. Natl. Acad. Sci. USA,* 71:3124–3128.

17. Decleve, A., Niwa, O., Gelmann, E., and Kaplan, H. S. (1975): Replication kinetics of N- and B-tropic murine leukemia viruses on permissive and nonpermissive cells *in vitro. Virology,* 65:320–332.

18. Decleve, A., Travis, M., Weismann, I. L., Lieberman, M., and Kaplan, H. S. (1975). Focal infection *in situ* of thymus cell subclasses by a thymotropic murine leukemia virus. *Cancer Res.,* 35:3585–3595.

19. Decleve, A., Lieberman, M., Ihle, J. N., and Kaplan, H. S. (1976): Biological and serological characterization of radiation leukemia virus (RadLV). *Proc. Natl. Acad. Sci. USA,* 73:4675–4679.

20. Decleve, A., Niwa, O., Gelmann, E., and Kaplan, H. S. (1976): Radiation activation of endogenous leukemia viruses in cell culture: Acute X-ray irradiation. In: *Biology of Radiation Carcinogenesis,* edited by J. M. Yuhas, R. W. Tennant, and J. D. Regan, pp. 217–225. Raven Press, New York.

21. Decleve, A., Niwa, O., Kojola, J., and Kaplan, H. S. (1976): New gene locus modifying susceptibility to certain B-tropic murine leukemia viruses. *Proc. Natl. Acad. Sci. USA,* 73:585–590.

22. Decleve, A., Lieberman, M., Ihle, J. N., and Kaplan, H. S. (1977). Biological and serological characterization of the C-type RNA viruses isolated from the C57BL/Ka strain of mice: III. Characterization of the isolates and their interactions *in vitro* and *in vivo.* In: *Radiation-Induced Leukemogenesis and Related Viruses,* edited by J. F. Duplan, pp. 247–264. North-Holland Publishing Company, Amsterdam.

23. Decleve, A., Lieberman, M., and Kaplan, H. S. (1977): *In vivo* interaction between RNA viruses isolated from the C57BL/Ka strain of mice. *Virology,* 81:270–283.

24. Finkel, M. P., Reilly, C. A., and Biskis, B. O. (1976): Pathogenesis of radiation and virus-induced bone tumors. *Recent Results Cancer Res.,* 54:92–103.

25. Fischinger, P. J., Nomura, S., and Bolognesi, D. P. (1975): A novel murine oncornavirus with dual eco- and xenotropic properties. *Proc. Natl. Acad. Sci. USA,* 72:5150–5153.

26. Freeman, A. E., Price, P. J., Igel, H. I., Young, J. C., Maryak, J. M., and Huebner, R. J. (1970): Morphological transformation of rat embryo cells induced by diethylnitrosamine and murine leukemia viruses. *J. Natl. Cancer Inst.,* 44:65–78.

27. Freeman, A. E., Gilden, R. V., Vernon, M. L., Wolford, R. G., Hugunin, P. E., and Huebner, R. J. (1973): 5-Bromo-2′-deoxyuridine potentiation of transformation of rat-embryo cells in-

duced *in vitro* by 3-methylcholanthrene: Induction of rat leukemia virus gs antigen in transformed cells. *Proc. Natl. Acad. Sci. USA,* 70:2415–2419.

28. Freese, E. (1959): The specific mutagenic effect of base analogues on phage T4. *J. Mol. Biol.,* 1:87–105.
29. Gelmann, E. P., Decleve, A., and Kaplan, H. S. (1978): Biological and biochemical differences among ecotropic C-type RNA viral isolates chemically induced from C57BL/Ka mouse embryo cells *in vitro. Virology,* 85:198–210.
30. Getz, M. J., Reiman, H. M., Jr., Seigal, G. P., Quinlan, T. J., Proper, J., Elder, P. K., and Moses, H. L. (1977): Gene expression in chemically transformed mouse embryo cells: Selective enhancement of the expression of C-type RNA tumor virus genes. *Cell,* 11:909–921.
31. Greenberger, J. S., and Aaronson, S. A. (1975): Cycloheximide induction of xenotropic type-C virus from synchronized mouse cells: Metabolic requirements for virus activation. *J. Virol.,* 15:64–70.
32. Gross, L. (1959): Serial cell-free passage of a radiation activated mouse leukemia agent. *Proc. Soc. Exp. Biol. Med.,* 100:102–107.
33. Gross, L. (1970): *Oncogenic Viruses,* 2nd ed. Pergamon Press, London.
34. Haas, M. (1974): Continuous production of radiation leukemia virus in C57BL thymoma tissue culture lines: Purification of the leukemogenic virus. *Cell,* 1:79–83.
35. Haas, M. (1978): Leukemogenic activity of thymotropic, ecotropic and xenotropic radiation leukemia virus isolates. *J. Virol.,* 25:705–709.
36. Haas, M., and Hilgers, J. (1975): *In vitro* infection of lymphoid cells by thymotropic radiation leukemia virus grown *in vitro. Proc. Natl. Acad. Sci. USA,* 72:3546–3550.
37. Haas, M., Sher, T., and Smolinsky, S. (1977): Leukemogenesis *in vitro* induced by thymus epithelial reticulum cells transmitting murine leukemia viruses. *Cancer Res.,* 37:1800–1807.
38. Haran-Ghera, N. (1966): Leukemogenic activity of centrifugates from irradiated mouse thymus and bone marrow. *Int. J. Cancer,* 1:81–87.
39. Haran-Ghera, N. (1967): The mechanism of radiation action in leukemogenesis: I. The role of radiation in leukemia development. *Br. J. Cancer,* 21:739–749.
40. Haran-Ghera, N. (1977): Target Cells involved in radiation and radiation leukemia virus leukemogenesis. In: *Radiation-Induced Leukemogenesis and Related Viruses,* edited by J. F. Duplan, pp. 79–89. North-Holland Publishing Company, Amsterdam.
41. Haran-Ghera, N., and Peled, A. (1968): The mechanism of radiation action in leukemogenesis: IV. Immune impairment as a coleukemogenic factor. *Isr. J. Med. Sci.,* 4:1181–1187.
42. Haran-Ghera, N., Lieberman, M., and Kaplan, H. S. (1966): Direct action of a leukemogenic virus on the thymus. *Cancer Res.,* 26:438–442.
43. Hartley, J. W., and Rowe, W. P. (1976): Naturally occurring murine leukemia viruses in wild mice: Characterization of a new "amphotropic" class. *J. Virol.,* 19:19–25.
44. Hartley, J. W., Walford, N. K., Old, L. J., and Rowe, W. P. (1977): A new class of murine leukemia virus associated with development of spontaneous leukemia. *Proc. Natl. Acad. Sci. USA,* 74:789–792.
45. Hopkins, N., Schindler, J., and Gottlieb, P. K. (1977): Evidence for recombination between N- and B-tropic murine leukemia viruses. *J. Virol.,* 21:1074–1078.
46. Huberman, E., and Fogel, M. (1975): Activation of carcinogenic polycyclic hydrocarbons in polyoma virus-transformed cells as a prerequisite for polyoma virus induction. *Int. J. Cancer,* 15:91–98.
47. Huebner, R. J., and Todaro, G. J. (1969): Oncogenes of RNA tumor viruses as determinants of cancer. *Proc. Natl. Acad. Sci. USA,* 64:1087–1094.
48. Humphries, E. H., and Temin, H. M. (1974): Requirement for cell division for initiation of transcription of Rous sarcoma virus RNA. *J. Virol.,* 14:531–546.
49. Ihle, J. N., Kenney, F. T., and Tennant, R. W. (1974): Evidence for a stable intermediate in leukemia virus activation in AKR mouse embryo cells. *J. Virol.,* 14:451–456.
50. Ihle, J. N., Lane, S. E., Kenney, F. T., and Farrelly, J. G. (1975) Effects of glucocorticoids on activation of leukemia virus in AKR mouse embryo cells. *Cancer Res.,* 35:442–446.
51. Ihle, J. N., Joseph, D. R., and Pazmino, N. H. (1976): Radiation leukemia in C57BL/6 mice. II. Lack of ecotropic virus expression in the majority of lymphomas. *J. Exp. Med.,* 144:1406–1423.
52. Ihle, J. N., McEwan, R., and Bengali, K. (1976): Radiation leukemia in C57BL/6 mice. I. Lack of serological evidence for the role of endogenous ecotropic viruses in pathogenesis. *J. Exp. Med.,* 144:1391–1405.

53. Ishimoto, A., Hartley, J. W., and Rowe, W. P. (1977): Detection and quantitation of phenotypically mixed viruses: Mixing of ecotropic and xenotropic murine leukemia viruses. *Virology,* 81:263–269.
54. Jacobs, S. J., and Rosenkranz, H. W. (1970): Detection of a reactive intermediate in the reaction between DNA and hydroxyurea. *Cancer Res.,* 30:1084–1094.
55. Jones, P. A., Benedict, W. F., Baker, M. S., Mondal, S., Rapp, U., and Heidelberger, C. (1976): Oncogenic transformation of C3H/10T1/2 clone 8 mouse embryo cells by halogenated pyrimidine nucleosides. *Cancer Res.,* 36:101–107.
56. Kaplan, H. S. (1967): On the natural history of the murine leukemias: Presidential address. *Cancer Res.,* 27:1325–1340, 1967.
57. Kaplan, H. S. (1974): Leukemia and lymphoma in experimental and domestic animals. *Ser. Haematol.,* 7:94–163.
58. Kaplan, H. S. (1977): Interaction between radiation and viruses in the induction of murine thymic lymphomas and lymphatic leukemias. In: *Radiation-Induced Leukemogenesis and Related Viruses,* edited by J. F. Duplan, pp. 1–18. North-Holland Publishing Company, Amsterdam.
59. Kaplan, H. S., and Brown, M. B. (1952): A quantitative dose-response study of lymphoid tumor development in irradiated C57 black mice. *J. Natl. Cancer Inst.,* 13:185–191.
60. Kaplan, H. S., and Lieberman, M. (1976): The role of lymphoid and haematopoietic target cells in viral lymphomagenesis of C57BL/Ka mice. II. Neoplastic transformation of bone marrow-derived cells in the thymic microenvironment. *Blood Cells,* 2:301–317.
61. Levy, J. A. (1973): Xenotropic viruses associated with NIH Swiss, NZB, and other mouse strains. *Science,* 182:1151–1153.
62. Lieber, M. M., Livingston, D. M., and Todaro, G. J. (1973): Superinduction of endogenous type-C virus by 5-bromodeoxyuridine from transformed mouse clones. *Science,* 181:443–444.
63. Lieberman, M., and Kaplan, H. S. (1959): Leukemogenic activity of filtrates from radiation-induced lymphoid tumors of mice. *Science,* 130:387–388.
64. Lieberman, M., and Kaplan, H. S. (1966): Lymphoid tumor induction by mouse thymocytes infected *in vitro* with radiation leukemia virus. *Natl. Cancer Inst. Monogr.,* 22:549–554.
65. Lieberman, M., and Kaplan, H. S. (1976): The role of lymphoid and haematopoietic target cells in viral lymphomagenesis of C57BL/Ka mice. I. Susceptibility to viral replication. *Blood Cells,* 2:291–299.
66. Lieberman, M., Niwa, O., Decleve, A., and Kaplan, H. S. (1973): Continuous propagation of radiation leukemia virus on a C57BL mouse embryo fibroblast line, with attenuation of leukemogenic activity. *Proc. Natl. Acad. Sci. USA,* 70:1250–1253.
67. Lieberman, M., Kaplan, H. S., and Decleve, A. (1976): Anomalous viral expression in radiogenic lymphomas of C57BL/Ka mice. In: *Biology of Radiation Carcinogenesis,* edited by J. M. Yuhas, R. W. Tennant, and J. D. Regan, pp. 237–244. Raven Press, New York.
68. Lieberman, M., Decleve, A., Gelmann, E. P., and Kaplan, H. S. (1977): Biological characterization of the C-type viruses isolated from the C57BL/Ka strain of mice. II. Induction and propagation of the isolates. In: *Radiation-Induced Leukemogenesis and Related Viruses,* edited by J. F. Duplan, pp. 231–246. North-Holland Publishing Company, Amsterdam.
69. Lilly, F., and Pincus, T. (1973): Genetic control of murine viral leukemogenesis. *Adv. Cancer Res.,* 17:231–277.
70. Lin, S. Y., and Riggs, A. D. (1972): *Lac* operator analogues: Bromodeoxyuridine substitution in the *lac* operator affects the rate of dissociation of the *lac* repressor. *Proc. Natl. Acad. Sci. USA,* 69:2574–2576.
71. Lowy, D. R., Rowe, W. P., Teich, N., and Hartley, J. W. (1971): Murine leukemia virus: High frequency activation *in vitro* by 5-iododeoxyuridine and 5-bromodeoxyuridine. *Science,* 174:155–156.
72. Miller, J. A. (1970): Carcinogenesis by chemicals: An overview. *Cancer Res.,* 30:559–576.
73. Mishra, N. K., Pant, K. J., Thomas, F. O., and Price, P. J. (1976): Chemical-viral co-carcinogenesis: Requirement for leukemia virus expression in accelerated transformation. *Int. J. Cancer,* 18:852–858.
74. Otten, J. A., Quarles, J. M., and Tennant, R. W. (1976): Cell division requirement for activation of murine leukemia virus in cell cultures by irradiation. *Virology,* 70:80–87.
75. Peters, R. L., Spahn, G. J., Rabstein, L. S., Kelloff, G. J., and Huebner, R. J. (1973): Oncogenic potential of murine type-C RNA virus passaged directly from naturally occurring tumors of BALB/c CR mice. *J. Natl. Cancer Inst.,* 51:621–629.

76. Pitha, P. M., Pitha, J., and Rowe, W. P. (1975): Lack of requirement of reverse transcriptase function for the activation of murine leukemia virus by halogenated pyrimidines. *Virology,* 63:568–572.
77. Price, P. J., Freeman, A. E., Lane, W., and Huebner, R. J. (1971): Morphological transformation of rat embryo cells by the combined action of 3-methylcholanthrene and Rauscher leukemia virus. *Nature (New Biol.),* 230:144–146.
78. Price, P. J., Suk, W. A., and Freeman, A. E. (1973): Type-C RNA tumor viruses as determinants of chemical carcinogenesis: Effects of sequential treatment. *Science,* 117:1003–1004.
79. Price, P. J., Suk, W. A., Peters, R. L., Martin, C. E., Bellew, T. M., and Huebner, R. J. (1975): Cordycepin inhibition of 3-methylcholanthrene-induced transformation *in vitro. Proc. Soc. Exp. Biol. Med.,* 150:650–653.
80. Price, P. J., Beller, T. M., King, M. P., Foreman, A. E., Gilden, R. V., and Huebner, R. J. (1976): Prevention of viral-chemical co-carcinogenesis *in vitro* by type-specific anti-viral antibody. *Proc. Natl. Acad. Sci. USA,* 73:152–155.
81. Price, P. J., Suk, W. A., Peters, R. L., Gilden, R. V., and Huebner, R. J. (1977): Chemical transformation of rat cells infected with xenotropic type-C RNA virus and its suppression by virus specific antiserum. *Proc. Natl. Acad. Sci. USA,* 74:579–581.
82. Purchio, A. F., Erikson, E., and Erikson, R. L. (1977): Translation of 35S and of subgenomic regions of avian sarcoma virus RNA. *Proc. Natl. Acad. Sci. USA,* 74:4661–4665.
83. Quarles, J. M., and Tennant, R. W. (1975): Effects of nitrosocarbaryl on BALB/3T3 cells. *Cancer Res.,* 35:2637–2645.
84. Rapp, U. R., Nowinski, R. C., Renznikoff, C. A., and Heidelberger, C. (1975): Endogenous oncornaviruses in chemically induced transformation: I. Transformation independent of virus production. *Virology,* 65:392–409.
85. Rascati, R. J., and Tennant, R. W. (1978): Induction of endogenous murine retrovirus by hydroxyurea and related compounds. *Virology,* 87:208–211.
85a. Rascati, R. J., and Tennant, R. W. (1979): Involvement of DNA damage in hydroxyurea-mediated induction of endogenous murine retrovirus. *Virology,* 94:273–281.
86. Rein, A., Kashimiri, S. V. S., Bassin, R. H., Gerwin, B. I., and Duran-Trosie, G. (1976): Phenotypic mixing between N- and B-tropic murine leukemia viruses: I. Infectious particles with dual sensitivity to Fv-1 restriction. *Cell,* 7:373–379.
87. Reitz, M. S., Saxinger, W. C., Ting, R. C., Gallo, R. C., and DiPaolo, J. A. (1977): Lack of expression of type-C hamster virus after neoplastic transformation of hamster embryo fibroblasts by benzo(*a*)pyrene. *Cancer Res.,* 37:3585–3589.
88. Rhim, J. S. (1974): Combined chemical and RNA viral carcinogenesis. In: *Chemical and Viral Oncogenesis,* Proceedings of the XI International Cancer Congress, Florence 1974, pp. 128–134. Excerpta Medica, Amsterdam.
89. Rhim, J. S., Cho, H. Y., Joglekar, M. H., and Huebner, R. J. (1972): Comparison of the transforming effect of benzo(*a*)pyrene in mammalian cell lines *in vitro. J. Natl. Cancer Inst.,* 48:949–957.
90. Rhim, J. S., Cho, H. Y., Rabstein, L., Gordon, R. J., Beyan, R. J., Gardner, M. B., and Huebner, R. J. (1972): Transformation of mouse cells infected with AKR leukemia virus induced by smog extracts. *Nature,* 239:103–107.
91. Rhim, J. S., Gordon, R. J., Beyan, R. J., and Huebner, R. J. (1973): Transformation of mouse cells infected with AKR leukemia virus by benzene extract fractions of city air particles. *Int. J. Cancer,* 12:485–492.
92. Rhim, J. S., Park, D. K., Weisburger, E. K., and Weisburger, J. H. (1974): Evaluation of an *in vitro* assay system for carcinogens based on prior infection of rodent cells with non-transforming RNA tumor virus. *J. Natl. Cancer Inst.,* 52:1167–1173.
93. Rosenkranz, H. S. (1970): Some biological effects of carbamoyloxyurea—an oxidation product of hydroxyurea. *Biochim. Biophys. Acta,* 195:266–267.
94. Rosenkranz, H. S., Jacobs, S. J., and Carr, H. S. (1968): Studies with hydroxyurea: VIII. The deoxyribonucleic acid of hydroxyurea-treated cells. *Biochim. Biophys. Acta,* 161:428–441.
95. Rosenkranz, H. S., Hjurth, R., and Carr, H. S. (1971): Studies with hydroxyurea: The biological and metabolic properties of formamidoxine. *Biochim. Biophys. Acta,* 232:48–60.
96. Rowe, W. P. (1973): Genetic factors in the natural history of murine leukemia virus infection: G.H.A. Clowes Memorial Lecture. *Cancer Res.,* 33:3061–3068.
97. Schwartz, S. A., Panem, S., and Kirsten, W. H. (1975): Distribution and virogenic effects of

5-bromodeoxyuridine in synchronized rat embryo cells. *Proc. Natl. Acad. Sci. USA,* 72:1829–1833.

98. Setlow, R. B., and Setlow, J. K. (1972): Effects of radiation on polynucleotides. *Annu. Rev. Biophys. Bioeng.,* 1:293–345.

99. Spelsberg, T. C., Zytkovicz, T. H., and Moses, H. L. (1977): Effects of metabolism on the binding of polycyclic hydrocarbons to nuclear subfractions of cultured AKR mouse embryo cells. *Cancer Res.,* 37:1490–1496.

100. Stephenson, J. R., Crow, J. D., and Aaronson, S. A. (1974): Differential activation of biologically distinguishable endogenous mouse type-C RNA viruses: Interaction with host cell regulatory factors. *Virology,* 61:411–419.

101. Stephenson, J. R., Greenberger, J. S., and Aaronson, S. A. (1974): Oncogenicity of an endogenous C-type virus chemically activated from mouse cells in culture. *J. Virol.,* 13:237–240.

102. Stephenson, J. R., Tronick, S. R., and Aaronson, S. A. (1974): Isolation from BALB/c mouse cells of a structural polypeptide of a third endogenous type-C virus. *Cell,* 3:347–351.

103. Stephenson, J. R., Cabradilla, C. D., and Aaronson, S. A. (1976): Genetic factors influencing endogenous type-C RNA viruses of mouse cells: Control of viral polypeptide expression in the C57BL/10 strain. *Intervirology,* 6:258–269.

104. Steves, R., and Lilly, F. (1977): Interactions between host and viral genomes in mouse leukemia. *Annu. Rev. Genet.,* 11:277–296.

105. Teich, N., Lowy, D. R., Hartley, J. W., and Rowe, W. P. (1973): Studies of the mechanism of induction of infectious murine leukemia virus from AKR mouse embryo cell lines by 5-iododeoxyuridine and 5-bromodeoxyuridine. *Virology,* 51:163–173.

106. Teich, N. M., Weiss, R. A., Martin, G. R., and Lowy, D. R. (1977): Virus infection of murine teratocarinoma stem cell lines. *Cell,* 12:973–982.

107. Tennant, R. W., Farrelly, J. G., Ihle, J. N., Pal, B. C., Kenney, F. T., and Brown, A. (1973): Effects of polyadenylic acids on functions of murine RNA tumor viruses. *J. Virol.,* 12:1216–1225.

108. Tennant, R. W., Otten, J. A., Quarles, J. M., Yang, W. K., and Brown, A. (1976): Cellular factors that regulate radiation activation and restriction of mouse leukemia viruses. In: *Biology of Radiation Carcinogenesis,* edited by J. M. Yuhas, R. W. Tennant, and J. D. Regan, pp. 227–236. Raven Press, New York.

109. Tennant, R. W., Rascati, R. J., and Lavelle, G. C. (1977): Mechanisms in endogenous leukemia virus induction by radiation and chemicals. In: *Radiation-Induced Leukemogenesis and Related Viruses,* edited by J. F. Duplan, pp. 179–188. North-Holland Publishing Company, Amsterdam.

110. Upton, A. C., Wolff, F. F., Furth, J., and Kimball, A. W. (1958): A comparison of the induction of myeloid and lymphoid leukemias in x-irradiated RF mice. *Cancer Res.,* 18:842–848.

111. Vogt, P. (1977): Genetics of RNA tumor viruses. In: *Comprehensive Virology,* edited by H. Fraenkel-Conrat and R. R. Wagner, Vol. 10, pp. 341–455. Plenum Press, New York.

112. Waksal, S. D., Smolinsky, S., Cohen, I. R., and Feldman, M. (1976): Transformation of thymocytes by thymus epithelium derived from AKR mice. *Nature,* 263:512–514.

113. Waters, R., Mishra, N., Bouck, N., DiMayorca, G., and Regan, J. D. (1977): Partial inhibition of postreplication repair and enhanced frequency of chemical transformation in rat cells infected with leukemia virus. *Proc. Natl. Acad. Sci. USA,* 74:238–242.

114. Weiss, R. A., Friis, R. R., Katz, E., and Vogt, P. K. (1971): Induction of avian tumor viruses in normal cells by physical and chemical carcinogens. *Virology,* 46:920–938.

115. Weiss, R. A., Mason, W. S., and Vogt, P. K. (1973): Genetic recombinants and heterozygotes derived from endogenous and exogenous avian RNA tumor viruses. *Virology,* 52:535–552.

116. Whitmire, C. E., and Salerno, R. A. (1972): RNA tumor virus gs antigen and tumor induction by various doses of 3-methylcholanthrene in various strains of mice treated as weanlings. *Cancer Res.,* 32:1129–1132.

117. Yoshikura, H., Zajedla, F., Perin, F., Perin-Roussel, O., Jacquinon, P., and Latarjet, R. (1977): Enhancement of 5-iododeoxyuridine-induced endogenous C-type virus activation by polycyclic hydrocarbons: Apparent lack of parallelism between enhancement and carcinogenicity. *J. Natl. Cancer Inst.,* 58:1035–1040.

118. Zamansky, G. B., Kleinman, L. F., Little, J. B., Black, P. H., and Kaplan, J. C. (1976): The effect of caffeine on the ultraviolet light induction of SV-40 virus from transformed hamster cells. *Virology,* 73:468–475.

Carcinogenesis, Vol. 5: Modifiers of Chemical Carcinogenesis, edited by T. J. Slaga.
Raven Press, New York © 1980.

11

Nutrition as a Modifier of Chemical Carcinogenesis

Johnnie R. Hayes and T. Colin Campbell

Division of Nutritional Sciences and Fields of Biochemistry and Toxicology, Cornell University, Ithaca, New York 14853

OVERVIEW

Nutrition and Diet

At the initiation of a discussion concerning the nutritional modification of chemical carcinogenesis, it is important that a careful distinction be made between the terms "nutrition" and "diet." "Nutrition" refers to the utilization of chemical components of food which cannot be synthesized by the ingesting organism and which are required for the maintenance of structural and biochemical integrity of cells, resulting in viability and reproductive potential. On the other hand, "diet" refers to the total composition of the ingested food, including nutrients, naturally occurring contaminants, and adventitious chemicals.

Although this discussion will be restricted primarily to the nutritional effect, other dietary factors are important modifiers of chemical carcinogenesis. Epidemiological investigations have implicated several aspects of diet in the etiology of cancer. Contamination of the diet by either natural products or adventitious chemicals is thought to play a prominent role in the causation of cancer. For instance, Peers and Linsell (125,126) have shown a linear relationship between the dietary levels of the hepatocarcinogenic aflatoxins and primary liver cancer in certain areas of Africa. Nitrites (84), nitrosamines (84), and saccharin (143) are other chemical components which may be important contributors to chemical carcinogenesis. In contrast, some food additives utilized to increase shelf life, usually termed antioxidants, such as butylated hydroxyanisole (BHA), prevent the induction of experimental tumors in rodents (19,185,186,187,191). Other naturally occurring nonnutrient constituents of foods have been implicated in modifying carcinogenicity. Cruciferous vegetables such as Brussels sprouts, cabbage, and cauliflower contain indoles which have been shown to increase the metabolism of carcinogenic polycyclic aromatic hydrocarbons (PAH) (123,

186,188) and inhibit neoplasia induced by 7,12-dimethylbenz(*a*)anthracene (DMBA) and benzo(*a*)pyrene (BP) (188).

Nutrients may play a nonnutrient role in respect to the host by serving as substrates for the growth of intestinal microflora. They may modify chemical carcinogenesis, not by direct effects on the metabolism of the host, but rather by altering either the metabolic capability of intestinal microflora or by altering the composition of the species and strains present in the intestine. This could result in altered bacterial metabolism of chemicals found in the intestine, yielding an altered carcinogenic potential. Reddy et al. (130,138,139) have shown that a high-meat, high-fat diet increased bacterial β-glucuronidase activity and total intestine microflora when compared with a meatless, low-fat diet. Hill (80) has suggested that intestinal bacteria may metabolize bile acids to carcinogenic unsaturated metabolites.

Dietary fiber has been implicated in the etiology of cancer of the colon and rectum (24). However, several studies designed to ascertain its contribution have shown that any protective effect may depend on the type of fiber and the particular chemical carcinogen. Colon tumors induced by 1,2-dimethylhydrazine were decreased in rats fed 15% wheat bran as compared to controls receiving 5% cellulose fiber (197). Dietary levels of 15% wheat bran or pectin did not influence methylnitrosourea-induced colon carcinogenesis, but inhibited that induced by azoxymethane when compared to diets containing 15% alfalfa or 5% cellulose (182). Diets containing 15% undegraded carrageenan increased the susceptibility of rats to both methylnitrosourea and azoxymethane, compared to controls receiving no dietary carrageenan (183).

A comprehensive discussion of dietary modification of chemical carcinogenesis is beyond the scope of this presentation and many suggested effects have not been mentioned, such as the pyrolytic products produced by cooking (10,159). However, it should be obvious that diet must be considered an important modifier of chemical carcinogenesis. This confounds studies of the effect of nutrition since many times it is difficult to isolate the contribution of diet from that of nutrition.

Methodological Approaches

A direct interaction between nutritional stress and cancer etiology is implied by many epidemiological investigations (6). These studies possess the advantage that large numbers of humans may be examined, rather than relying on animal data extrapolation. However, there are many confounding variables in this type of investigation, to say nothing of the relative insensitivity for investigations of individual nutrients. Epidemiological studies can only demonstrate associations and not prove causation. They do suggest important interactions, however, for laboratory investigation. At this time, these types of basic experimental investigations are desperately needed to validate or reject the suggested epidemiological findings.

Laboratory investigations have the advantage of controlling: (a) nutrient intake, (b) adventitious dietary chemicals, (c) animal age and health, (d) homogeneity of population, (c) ambient environment, and (d) carcinogen dosage protocol. They also allow the monitoring of both biochemical and pathological events during tumor initiation, promotion, and growth. To date, however, many laboratory investigations have been limited in their delineation of specific interactive mechanisms for several reasons. Among these, dietary composition has not been well controlled. There have been almost as many diet compositions used as there have been investigators. The compositions of these diets range from those comprised of various commercial laboratory chows to those purified to the extent that mixtures of individual amino acids are fed in place of protein. Specific nutrients may range from marginal deficiency to highly questionable excesses. Thus, comparisons of the many reports in the literature are severely compromised. Recently, standard diets have been recommended, such as the AIN-76 diet (7) and these should help considerably. Another example of inadequate control of the experimental nutritional protocol is the failure to ensure isocaloric intakes between control and experimental groups. Tannenbaum (167,169,171) was among the first to show that caloric restriction inhibited carcinogenesis. Other studies have shown that not only caloric restriction, per se, but also restriction of total food intake reduces tumor yield (152,171,190). Such studies have led to the suggestion that decreased body weight may be a more important determinant than caloric intake (39,166). This emphasizes the necessity to control for decreased body weight, especially in studies involving nutrient deficiencies, by use of the pair-feeding technique.

Whereas much of the early nutritional research dealt with nutrient deficiencies, it may be the nutritional excesses and imbalances which produce the more significant modifications of chemical carcinogenesis. Thus in the diet of Western societies nutrient excesses are implied that tend to be associated with major cancers, such as those of the colon and the breast.

INTERACTION BETWEEN NUTRITION AND CARCINOGEN METABOLISM

Metabolism and Activation of Chemical Carcinogens

Nutrient imbalances may influence various metabolic events involved in the initiation, promotion, and growth of tumors. These influences may be at the level of metabolism and activation of the carcinogen, alterations of the quantities or types of carrier proteins mediating the reaction of the ultimate carcinogen with its target, cocarcinogen and promoter availabilities, cell-mediated immunological destruction of neoplastic cells, hormonal control of tumor growth, and nutrition of the tumor itself. The hypothesis primarily considered in this discussion is that nutritional status may exert an influence through modification of enzyme activities responsible for the metabolism and activation of chemical carcinogens.

This hypothesis receives ample support from investigations that indicate that most carcinogens require metabolic activation to an ultimate carcinogen which produces the biochemical lesion (78,115,116), and that the primary enzyme system responsible for this activation, i.e., the mixed-function oxidase (MFO), is significantly influenced by nutritional status (26,27,89). A comprehensive survey of the literature on the effects of nutrition on the MFO system with respect to chemical carcinogenesis will not be attempted here because of the large numbers of nutrients that would have to be discussed and the preliminary nature of many of these findings.

James and Elizabeth Miller of the McArdle Laboratory for Cancer Research at the University of Wisconsin have pioneered the recognition that most chemical carcinogenesis requires enzymatic activation (115,116). Their basic hypothesis is that chemical carcinogens lacking inherent activity must be enzymatically activated to chemically reactive electrophilic species which possess the potential to react covalently and nonenzymatically with nucleophilic macromolecular sites. Such attack is thought to be required for the initiation of neoplasia. That the MFO system possesses the major catalytic activity for the production of reactive electrophiles capable of forming covalent adducts with DNA was demonstrated by Grover and Sims (63) and Gelboin (57), utilizing carcinogenic PAH. Since then, numerous laboratories have confirmed that the majority of chemical carcinogens undergo activation via mixed-function oxidation. There may also be other enzymatic reactions participating in the formation of the electrophiles. One example is 2-acetylaminofluorene (AAF) which requires MFO-catalyzed N-hydroxylation and sulfotransferase-catalyzed ester formation to produce the reactive electrophile N-sulfonoxy-2-acetylaminofluorene (115). Irving et al. (83) have suggested that the glucuronide of N-hydroxy-2-acetylaminofluorene may also serve as an activated intermediate and form adducts with DNA. Another possibility for this compound is an activation route via peroxidase-catalyzed nitroxide radical production followed by dismutation to produce the electrophiles N-hydroxy-2-acetylaminofluorene and 2-nitrosofluorene (16).

A preceding chapter in this volume has dealt with the detoxification and activation of chemical carcinogens; therefore, this chapter will be confined to a consideration of the effects of nutrients on the carcinogen reaction pathways.

Chemical carcinogens are typically lipophilic and are initially metabolized by the MFO system to more hydrophilic products (along with the activated electrophiles) in the so-called phase I reactions. These more hydrophilic products can undergo a series of reactions termed phase II that tend to increase their hydrophilic nature, allowing them to enter into the aqueous physiological routes of disposition. In general, the enzymes catalyzing both phase I and II reactions are located in the endoplasmic reticulum of the cell, facilitating their interactive efficiency. There is an abundance of reports in the literature concerning the effects of nutrition on the MFO or phase I reactions (26), but few concerning the cascade of phase II reactions, making the possible interactions speculative. However, it is obvious that phase II reaction rate limitations imposed by nutritional stress have the potential in some cases to alter the equilibrium of these interrelated reactions so that the balance of detoxification products and ultimate carcinogens is modified. Bock (22) has demonstrated that uridine-5'-diphosphate(UDP)-glucuronyltransferase-catalyzed glucuronide formation from hydroxylated products of the MFO metabolism of BP increases the total metabolism of BP. Formation of the glucuronide could shift the metabolism toward detoxification and away from activation.

Relationship Between Phase I and II Reactions

The complex relationships between Phase-I and Phase-II reactions, with respect to the production of the ultimate carcinogenic lesion, are illustrated in Fig. 1. A certain proportion of the parent carcinogen may undergo activation to highly reactive electrophilic products, with the quantity dependent on the molecular structure of the parent carcinogen and its relative affinity for the species of cytochromes P-450 catalyzing the activation. The activated ultimate carcinogen is the molecular species reacting nonenzymatically with key macromolecules such as DNA, RNA, and protein. However, there are detoxification pathways that may interpose between the production of the ultimate carcinogen

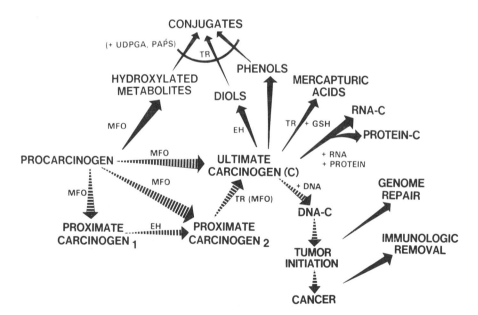

FIG. 1. Metabolism of chemical carcinogens. MFO, mixed-function oxidase; TR, transferase(s); EH, epoxide hydrase; GSH, glutathione; UDPGA, uridine diphosphoglucuronic acid; PAPS, (3'phosphoadenosine-5'-phosphosulfate); DNA-C, DNA-carcinogen adduct. Hatched arrows indicate reaction which may lead to neoplasia; the solid arrows indicate nonneoplastic events. DNA, as opposed to RNA and protein, has been somewhat arbitrarily chosen to illustrate specific as opposed to nonspecific covalent binding without adequate experimental proof.

and the formation of the macromolecular adduct. For instance, aryl epoxides may spontaneously rearrange to phenols, or microsomal epoxide hydrase may catalyze hydrolytic cleavage to form dihydrodiols, which in some cases, may be reoxidized to the bay region diol epoxides, yielding the ultimate carcinogen (86). Nutrient intake may alter the activity of epoxide hydrase (1), which could modify the steady-state levels of the ultimate carcinogen detoxified by this enzyme. Another possible mechanism for the detoxification of the ultimate carcinogen is via reaction with glutathione to yield an eventual mercapturic acid. The reaction with glutathione may occur spontaneously or be catalyzed by a group of soluble enzymes termed glutathione S-transferases. Production of glutathione conjugates may be modified by nutritional stress either through direct effects on the glutathione transferase activities and/or through alteration of the quantity or availability of glutathione. There have been little or no investigations of the former, even though they may represent as much as 10% of the extractable protein in the rat liver (85). These glutathione S-transferases may also act via an additional nonenzymatic mechanism by acting as noncritical nucleophilic scavengers. Glutathione S-transferase B of rat liver has been shown to be identical to ligandin (68), which derived its name from its ability to bind a large number of different ligands (90,98). The effects of nutritional stress on glutathione have been studied with respect to certain selected nutrients. For example, Allen-Hoffman and Campbell (4) have shown that low-protein diets supplemented with D,L-methionine increase glutathione levels while Chow (38) found decreased glutathione levels in vitamin E-deficient rats. Nutritional manipulations that tend to alter glutathione levels should result in levels of an ultimate carcinogen, that reacts with glutathione, inversely related to the direction of that alteration.

Additional quantities of activated carcinogen may be removed by forming covalent adducts with noncritical target sites on macromolecules. Protein, because of its high cellular concentration, may yield the largest number of noncritical sites, followed by RNA. Generally, DNA is considered the critical target for activated carcinogens, although the nonreplicating DNA in heterochromatin may act as a noncritical target site. Even critical sites on DNA may be rendered nonproductive through DNA repair processes, which can be considered detoxification mechanisms.

Another series of phase II reactions which may influence carcinogen metabolism and be modified by nutritional stress are the transferases. Both UDP-glucuronyltransferase and sulfotransferase can be involved in the conjugation of hydroxylated metabolites formed in Phase-I metabolism. These metabolites generally represent hydrophilic detoxified metabolites, with certain exceptions such as the reactive electrophile N-sulfonoxy-2-acetylaminofluorene. Nutritional stress may affect these transferases to alter the equilibrium between the detoxification and activation reactions. The effects of nutritional stress on these latter enzymes have received little attention. Riboflavin deficiency decreases (35), whereas dietary protein deficiency appears to increase UDP-glucuronyltransferase activity (198,199). If this is a general phenomenon and not substrate specific, then the metabolism of a carcinogen, which is not only activated but also hydroxylated to products forming glucuronides, may be shifted toward the detoxification pathway in protein-deficient animals.

Microsomal Mixed-Function Oxidase System

Phase I reactions illustrated in Fig. 1 must be considered key reactions in the activation of chemical carcinogens. That is *not* to say that the formation of adducts at critical nucleophilic macromolecular sites is dependent on the catalytic activity of the MFO system. Adduct formation will be a function of the critical rate limitation, whether spontaneous or catalytic activity, or a carrier-mediated event. This rate limitation will be dependent upon the specific carcinogen and its metabolic route and may be modified by a large number of environmentally controlled biochemical events, such as nutrition, enzyme induction, pathological conditions, etc.

The MFO system occurs in bacteria (76,142) and plants (13,112) as well as spanning the range of invertebrates (154) and vertebrates within the animal kingdom. Its occurrence throughout the phylogenetic tree indicates early evolutionary development, and its persistence emphasizes its importance in maintaining cellular homeostasis with respect to both endogenous and exogenous compounds. In vertebrates, its highest activity occurs in the liver but significant activities are also found in a variety of other tissues such as the skin, lung, kidney, and mucosal lining of the gastrointestinal tract. It is found as an integral component of the lipid-protein mosaic of the endoplasmic reticulum, and has been shown to be associated with the nuclear membrane (88,144).

A generally accepted hypothesis, proposed by Estabrook et al. (53), for the interaction of the components of the MFO system is shown in Fig. 2. The

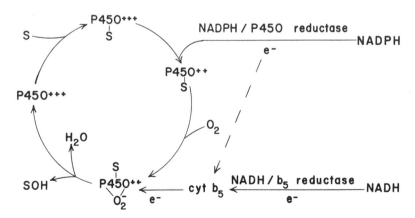

FIG. 2. Schematic representation of the interaction of components of the hepatic mixed-function oxidase system. NADPH, dihydronicotinamide adenine dinucleotide phosphate diaphorase; NADH, nicotinamide adenine dinucleotide, reduced form.

hemoprotein cytochrome P-450 serves as the terminal oxidase of the system and although determining its catalytic function, does not necessarily determine its reaction rate. Lipophilic substrates bind cytochrome P-450, possibly at more than one site, resulting in a substrate-cytochrome P-450 complex. This substrate P-450 complex is more readily reduced than cytochrome P-450 itself (46,58,62) and exhibits two or more substrate dependent difference spectra (141,151), reflecting shifts in its absolute spectra. Most substrates produce a difference spectra which has been termed Type I, characterized by a peak at 380 to 385 nm and a trough at 418 to 420 nm. Type II spectral changes are produced by heteroatoms, such as nitrogen, sulfur, selenium, or oxygen, characterized by a peak at 430 nm and a trough at 390 nm. Most compounds that produce the type II spectra change are not substrates but inhibitors of mixed function oxidation. Type I substrates appear to be binding to the apoprotein of P-450, whereas type II compounds bind the sixth coordination position of the iron, thereby inhibiting oxygen binding. A consequence of type I substrate binding is the increased reducibility of P-450, resulting either from a conformation change or an increase in the redox potential (46,58).

The substrate P-450 complex accepts an electron from NADPH-ferricytochrome P-450 reductase to yield the reduced ferriheme form, which is then capable of binding oxygen at the sixth coordination position of the iron. The ternary complex, substrate-P-450-oxygen undergoes a mechanistically undefined conversion to produce the "active-oxygen" complex which decomposes to yield the monooxygenated substrate, water, and ferrous cytochrome P-450. The nature of this mechanism is not understood and the identity of the active oxygen remains unknown (153,177). At the point of oxygen activation, the second electron transport chain involving NADH-cytochrome b_5 reductase and cytochrome b_5 may supply a second electron from NADH, or NADPH, by bypassing NADH-cytochrome b_5 reductase, although there is still some controversy about the source of the second electron (59,150).

An important determinant of mixed-function oxidation is the integration of the enzyme system within the architecture of the endoplasmic reticulum. Cytochrome P-450 appears to be buried deep within the membrane, but with at least some portion exposed at the membrane surface (176); on the other hand, the reductases and cytochrome b_5 appear to be bound to the membrane by hydrophobic tails, and are easily removed from the membrane by protease treatment (45,155). Franklin and Estabrook (54) have proposed that NADPH-ferricytochrome P-450 reductase is surrounded by several P-450 molecules and that cytochrome b_5 is in juxtaposition to this complex, forming a rigid assembly within the membrane. Recently, however, Yang (204) has proposed a nonrigid distribution requiring lateral diffusion of the reductase within the bulk lipid of the membrane.

Brown et al. (23), while studying dietary factors that influence microsomal enzyme activity, were the first to show that foreign compounds caused stimulation of the mixed-function oxidase system. Studies from many laboratories have shown that more than 200 drugs, insecticides, carcinogens, and other chemicals, most of which are MFO substrates, induce the MFO system. Among the bio-chemical alterations seen in response to these inducers are proliferation of the endoplasmic reticulum in many cases, increased activity of the NADPH ferricy-tochrome P-450 reductase and increased quantities of cytochrome P-450. Signifi-cantly not only does the quantity of cytochrome P-450 increase, but different forms of cytochrome P-450 are produced that appear to have altered substrate specificity (5).

It would appear that the increased MFO activity produced by induction would enhance carcinogenicity by increasing the yield of activated metabolites. How-ever, in most cases MFO inducers actually decrease carcinogenicity (188,189). This phenomena may, in part, be due to alterations of the species of P-450 activating the carcinogens and/or the effects of the inducer on the cascade of reactions involved in detoxification.

Systematic biochemical analysis of the properties and substrate specificity of the different forms of cytochrome P-450 had to await the development of methods for the isolation of the individual components of this complex enzyme system. Methods of fractionation, isolation, and reconstitution have now been developed, particularly in the laboratories of Coon and his associates (40,41, 101,158) and Lu and his colleagues (102,103). These studies have revealed that the activity of the system may be reconstituted with cytochrome P-450, NADPH-ferricytochrome P-450 reductase, and phosphatidylcholine. Of particular interest is the emerging evidence for the existence of multiple forms of cytochrome P-450 with distinct electrophoretic properties and substrate specificities, depend-ing on species and prior treatment with enzyme inducers (64,65,71).

It is obvious from the preceding description of the hepatic MFO system that there are many points within the system that may respond to nutritional stress. In a previous review of the interactions between nutrition and the MFO system (27), we found the intake of virtually every nutrient, when consumed at other than optimum levels, has been shown to affect the metabolism of xenobi-otics. Although much of these data have been generated utilizing drugs as sub-strates, it should be directly applicable to the metabolism of carcinogens. The MFO system does not mechanistically recognize carcinogens as being different from any other substrates. They differ from the drugs and other substrates in that certain of their metabolic products are capable of covalent interactions with critical cellular constituents leading to the production of a carcinogenic lesion. Even though the total quantity of ultimate carcinogen produced may be more important than its rate of production, it is still MFO mediated. Alterna-tively, the total quantity of carcinogen–macromolecular adduct formed may be more dependent on the rate of detoxification of the substrate or its activated product, as previously discussed, than on the rate of formation of the activated product.

It is obvious that there are several sites within the MFO system that would be sensitive to nutritional stress. For instance, nutritional alterations of either the quantity or quality of the proteins involved in the catalytic activity of the MFO system would be expected to alter its efficiency. Nutritional alteration of cofactor levels such as NADPH or NADH may impose restrictions on total enzyme activity. More subtle effects may be produced by nutritional modification of the enzyme system's environment. Alterations of either the lipid or protein elements of the endoplasmic reticulum could alter the fluidity of the membrane, changing the lateral mobility of the reductase, resulting in a new rate limitation. Alterations of MFO activity produced by dietary lipids have been studied by many workers. Alterations of dietary fat produced changes in the metabolism of several compounds with the direction of the alteration depending on the composition of the fat and particular substrate (2,33). Lang (93) found that rats treated with unsaturated fatty acids showed lower amounts of microsomal protein and phospholipid, with the phospholipids having altered fatty acid composition. Metabolism of BP was decreased, together with a reduction in the activity of UDP-glucuronyltransferase. He suggested that the effect on metabolism was in part due to modification of the microsomal membrane (93). Dietary cholesterol increases the activity of the MFO system, largely through alterations of microsomal membrane structure (92,94,95).

SPECIFIC NUTRIENT MODIFICATION OF CHEMICAL CARCINOGENICITY

Nutritional Modification of Chemical Carcinogenicity

All macronutrients, as well as many of the micronutrients, have been shown to modify chemical carcinogenicity; however, a detailed discussion of these interactions is beyond the scope of this discussion. Several reviews and symposia have recently addressed themselves to the role of nutrition in cancer cause and prevention, and the reader is directed to them for further discussions and different perspectives (6,8,29,39,48,179).

We have restricted our discussion to only two macronutrients, protein and fat, since they represent (a) nutrients which show varied world-wide and individual intakes with respect to both quantity and quality; (b) nutrients that have been implicated as modifying chemical carcinogenicity; (c) nutrients whose interactions with carcinogenicity have been investigated at the biochemical level, especially from the aspect of activation and detoxification of carcinogens; and (d) the authors' prejudice, because our laboratory has been engaged in elucidating the role of dietary protein in both activation and detoxification. The brevity of this discussion is not meant to deemphasize the significance of other nutrient interaction such as lipotropes (145,146), vitamin C (67,117) and the protective role of vitamin A and its analogs (18,119,156).

Effect of Dietary Protein

There are few epidemiological studies relating either the quantity or quality of dietary protein intake with cancer incidence. Few investigators have even questioned potential relationships; even those who did, have been unable to separate higher protein intakes from other dietary practices which tend to be associated with affluence. Epidemiological investigations have shown correlations between intake of animal fat and total fat and colon cancer (69). Since 42% of total fat calories come from meat, Wynder (200) has interpreted this and similar studies as implicating a role for animal fat. On the other hand, a high fat intake tends to occur with a high protein intake, because an excess of each is generally derived from animal products. Thus, the relative contribution of each to a carcinogenic effect is not clear.

Within the developed countries, there is little or no overt protein malnutrition; on the contrary there may be a tendency toward protein overnutrition. Moreover, within specific groups, there may be wide ranges of protein intake (60). Although there has been little change in the amount of protein consumed in the United States within the last 60 years, there has been a shift in the source of protein. There has been a decrease in the consumption of flour and cereal products which used to represent 50% of the protein, with a concomitant increase in the consumption of animal protein, which now represents 70% of the total protein intake (60). Thus, there has been an increase in the ingestion of utilizable protein. The situation is different within developing nations, where protein-calorie malnutrition is more prevalent.

Although the correlation coefficient between protein intake and certain major cancers such as those of the breast and large bowel is quite high, it must be remembered that many other factors must also be considered. Those countries which have had higher protein intakes also tend to be more industrialized and urbanized, thus giving rise to multiple environmental variables that may have to be considered. The relative extent to which a higher exposure to chemical carcinogens or an altered dietary pattern becomes involved in any excess cancer incidence is not at all clear. Moreover, the fact that only certain chemically induced tumors have been studied with respect to nutritional interaction must be kept in perspective when evaluating the more generalized role for any given nutrient.

A survey of the literature on the effects of protein nutrition on cancer development is confusing at best, and in several cases, contradictory. Much of the confusion is caused by inadequate experimental design, especially with respect to the nutritional design, as previously discussed (i.e., variable dietary composition, inadequate calorie and total food intake, etc.). Nevertheless, the emergence of general trends together with identification of relevant cellular mechanisms should allow the development of certain hypotheses.

In 1941, White and Mider (196) reported that a diet low in both protein and cystine decreased the incidence of leukemia in mice treated with 3-methyl-cholanthrene (MCA). White and Andervont (195) followed with a report indicating that diets low in cystine completely inhibited the development of spontaneous mammary gland tumors. Although food intake was similar between the low cystine diets and controls, the animals on the low cystine diets had 50% lower body weights, complicating the interpretation of the study. The animals fed the low cystine diets had irregular or no estrus cycles, leading these authors to question the role of hormones. To help delineate the effects of estrogen, White and White (194) fed the low-cystine diets and utilized diethylstilbestrol implants in both control and experimental groups. In these studies, instead of complete inhibition of spontaneous mammary gland tumors by the low-cystine diets, they found a 45% incidence as compared to a 92% incidence among the controls. This study indicates that the effects of the low-cystine diet may be mediated, in part, through an estrogenic effect. White and White (193) investigated protein quality further by feeding gliadin, a protein source low in lysine, and determined spontaneous mammary tumor development. They reported a 25% incidence rate in the low-lysine animals, as opposed to the 98% incidence found by Andervont (9) in mice on a chow diet.

Another example of an effect produced by protein quality is the study by Dunning et al. (49). They reported that the addition of 1.4% tryptophan to a diet containing a tryptophan-free casein hydrolysate produced a higher incidence of diethylstilbestrol-induced mammary tumors in rats. However, additions of 4.3% tryptophan yielded a lower incidence rate when compared to the casein controls, which may have been related to the decreased body weight of this group.

In a more recent study, Syrotuck and Worthington (165) reduced the dietary levels of three essential amino acids, isoleucine, leucine, and phenylalanine– tyrosine, and determined the effect on MCA carcinogenesis and resistance to a transplanted MCA tumor. They reported that the amino acid restrictions did not inhibit the carcinogenicity, but may have interfered with the potential immunity to the tumor. Although there are discrepancies between some of these reports, it nevertheless appears that low-quality protein may serve a protective role in chemical carcinogenesis.

Tannenbaum (172) was the first to suggest that, except for certain cases, the protective effect of protein deficiency was related to voluntary caloric restriction and decreased body weight. To further investigate this hypothesis, Tannenbaum and Silverstone (174) determined the effects of diets containing 9 to 45% casein so that no significant alterations in growth or body weight were evident. The influence of the diets was investigated with respect to four types of mouse tumors: (a) spontaneous mammary carcinomas, (b) BP-induced skin tumors, (c) BP-induced sarcomas, and (d) spontaneous hepatomas. They found no protein effect on the formation of spontaneous mammary carcinoma and BP-induced skin tumors or sarcoma formation. Spontaneous hepatoma formation was inhibited by the low-protein (9%) diet, leading the authors to speculate that the liver may be more sensitive to dietary protein levels. These studies reinforced Tannenbaum's hypothesis that many of the earlier studies, reviewed by Stern and Willheim (157), showed a protective effect of low protein because of voluntary decreases in total food consumption and decreased growth rate. However,

Tannenbaum's hypothesis has not received universal support. For instance, in these studies, the low levels of protein are only marginally deficient at best, and are probably adequate for maintenance. If the voluntary restriction of food intake seen in animals fed the low protein diets *ad libitum* is controlled by pair feeding the adequate protein diets, the effect on body weight is somewhat alleviated but not completely eliminated. Studies such as those by Tannenbaum and Silverstone (174) indicate that not all of the effect of protein deficiency is caused by restricted food intake and indicate the possibility for other mechanisms.

Studies investigating the role of dietary protein on the modification of chemical carcinogenicity have also been contradictory. Engel and Copeland (50) found tumor formation in response to 2-acetylaminofluorene to be inversely related to the percentage of dietary protein (9 to 60%). McLean and Magee (109) indicated that protein deficiency during the time of administration enhanced carcinogenesis of the kidney by decreasing the toxic effects on the liver. The numbers of 1,2-dimethylhydrazine-induced colon tumors were found to be decreased in rats receiving 7.5% as compared to those receiving 15 or 22% protein. Visek et al. (179) found that DMBA-induced mammary tumors developed more rapidly and in greater numbers as the percentage of dietary protein fed during the initiation period decreased from 45 to 7.5%. Low-protein diets have also been shown to increase the incidence of dimethylnitrosamine-induced kidney tumors (79).

Several laboratories have investigated the effect of low protein diets on hepatocarcinogenicity of the mycotoxin aflatoxin B_1 (AFB_1). Madhavan and Gopalan (105) were the first to show that low-protein (5% casein) diets protected against the hepatocarcinogenicity of aflatoxin (AF) but increased its toxicity (104). Wells et al. (192) found that an 8% casein diet protected rats from the hepatocarcinogenicity of AF whereas the severity of liver involvement increased as dietary casein was increased from 22 to 30%. Lee et al. (96), utilizing one of the most sensitive species, rainbow trout, found that diets containing 32 or 49.5% casein had no effect on hepatoma production by AF. On the other hand, when fish protein concentrate was fed at the same levels as the casein, the lower protein level had a protective effect. In contrast to these studies, Temcharoen et al. (175) found no significant difference in hepatoma rate between a 5 and 20% protein diet. They did find hyperplastic nodules in the 5% protein diet and none in the 20% protein diet. This study is in contrast with preliminary data from an investigation being carried out in our laboratory that agrees with the earlier studies (104).

Many of the apparent inconsistencies and ambiguities surrounding these studies are simply a result of a lack of knowledge of the carcinogenic process itself. Hence, more information on the interaction between nutrition and the biochemical mechanisms that lead to tumorigenesis are desperately needed. Protein nutrition may exert its effect at diverse levels and yield even multifaceted cascades of events. For example, dietary protein deficiency exerts an influence on initiation and possibly on promotion and tumor growth. Within these three major categories of events, it may be exerting its effect on several physiological and biochemical systems by alterations of specific enzymes, substrates, or cofactors.

Within the events comprising initiation, it is our hypothesis that protein nutrition may exert a major influence on the metabolic activation and detoxification of carcinogens and, thereby, alter the subsequent development of neoplasia. This is not to say that by knowing the effects of protein nutrition on a single metabolic event, predictions can be made about its effects on the carcinogenicity of a particular compound. As already indicated, the metabolic activation and detoxification of a carcinogen may involve a series of catalytic or spontaneous events and it is the net or coordinated effect of these events that leads to tumorigenesis. On the other hand, more complete knowledge of the effect of nutrition on these events, together with the knowledge of the metabolic route of a particular chemical, should lead to a better understanding of the more generalized relationship between nutrition and cancer.

The initial set of reactions in the cascade leading to the production of carcinogen–macromolecular adducts is mixed-function oxidation. Campbell (25) has recently reviewed the effect protein deficiency has on the MFO system. McLean and colleagues (106,110,111) were among the first to investigate the interaction between protein deficiency and the MFO system, and since then, several laboratories have extended these studies (25,27).

Figure 3 is a compilation of several studies (72,74,113) done in our laboratory

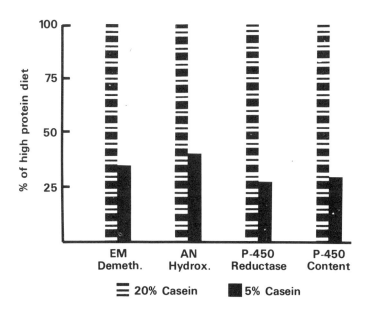

FIG. 3. Effect of dietary casein level on selected activities of the rat hepatic mixed-function oxidase system after 8 to 14 days of feeding.

and illustrates the effect of protein deficiency on the activity of the MFO system. There was a 60 to 70% decrease in the N-demethylation of ethylmorphine and aniline in the 5% casein group, compared to the 20% control groups. Both cytochrome P-450 reductase and cytochrome c reductase, measured by the ability of NADPH-ferricytochrome P-450 reductase to reduce exogenous cytochrome c, were decreased in the 5% protein group. When these decreases are coupled with the decrease in total microsomal protein content observed in the low-protein animals, the total MFO decrease per unit body weight may be as great as 75 to 80%, within the 14-day feeding period.

Protein deficiency decreased not only the basal MFO activities, but also the activities induced by both phenobarbital and MCA, compared to the animals fed 20% dietary casein (72,74,113). Although the percentage increases in activity produced by the inducers were similar for both the high- and low-protein diets, the induced activities were much lower for the latter.

The effects of protein deficiency on the MFO system are significant after feeding the diet for only 8 days (75), but may occur within 24 hr (107). These effects seem to be recoverable by refeeding the 20% casein diets with the recovery time dependent upon the extent of the deficiency (75).

Studies utilizing reconstituted enriched components of the MFO system from animals fed low- and high-protein diets have indicated that the mechanistic effects of protein deficiency may operate both on the specific enzyme activity and on the interactions between the components (120). Thus, the involvement of the endoplasmic reticulum membrane system in the enzyme activity is suggested, especially since protein malnutrition alters the functionality of membrane systems (11). This hypothesis has prompted further studies on the architecture of the membrane-bound enzyme system as related to protein deficiency. These studies (73) have indicated that the two diets produce differential energies of activation, thus indicating altered phase transitions of the membranes as well as altered hydrophobicities. Such changes could affect not only the lateral diffusion of the reductase within the membrane but also could modify substrate–membrane interactions.

From the preceding studies and those of others, it can be predicted that, in certain cases, metabolism of a carcinogen to its activated form by the MFO system should be restricted in animals fed low-protein diets. For instance, Czygan et al. (43) determined the capacity of isolated microsomes to alter the mutagenicity for bacteria of primary (proximate/ultimate) and secondary (procarcinogen) carcinogens as a function of dietary protein intake. They found the microsomal inactivation of N-methyl-N-nitro-N-nitrosoguanidine (primary) and the activation of dimethylnitrosamine (DMN) (secondary) were decreased by protein-deficient diets. Furthermore, the hepatic microsomal metabolism of AFB_1 is diminished by protein deficiency (1).

This is not to say that the activation of all carcinogens and subsequent lesion formation will be decreased with a protein-deficient diet. The final result will be dependent upon the site of carcinogen metabolism and activation and its particular metabolic route through the cascade of reactions initiated by the MFO system. The preponderance of data concerning the effects of protein deficiency on the metabolism of carcinogens has been generated employing liver preparations. Since the MFO system of other tissues such as the skin and intestinal mucosa may be differentially affected, carcinogens whose critical activation occurs in these nonhepatic tissues may not follow the predictions derived from the liver system. A possible example of this is seen in the work of McLean and his colleagues (160,161) studying the effects of protein deficiency on DMN, which requires metabolic activation to induce tumorigenesis. On a protein-free diet, a single dose of DMN produced a high incidence of kidney tumors in rats but on a commercial diet only 35% of the rats developed tumors (70). Swann and McLean (161) found liver metabolism of DMN to be depressed by 45% in the protein-free diet, whereas the decrease in kidney metabolism was only 23%. Moreover, they reported that the *in vivo* methylation of the *N*-7 position of guanine by DMN in kidney DNA was increased threefold, with only an insignificant increase in liver DNA alkylation, and deduced that the increase in renal tumors was caused by the relative increase in the amount of DMN metabolized by the kidney. On the basis of the relative effects of fasting, phenobarbital treatment, and ingestion of a low-protein diet on DMN metabolism both *in vitro* and *in vivo,* it was concluded that it is not the rate of DMN metabolism which is related to DMN toxicity but the amount of toxic metabolite formed (108). Paine and McLean (122) also have shown that lung MFO activity is decreased by feeding a low-protein diet but, similar to their earlier work, kidney MFO activity was not affected. However, they were able to show that the fat component of the diet could have accounted for the relatively higher kidney MFO activity and, perhaps, the renal carcinogenesis. Herein lies the most serious criticism of this series of studies in that the low-protein diets are semipurified but the high-protein (level not stated) diets are commercial preparations. It is not clear what role dietary lipid may have had, nor the effects of other nutrient components, which are presumably different in the stock diet. Moreover, *ad libitum* feeding is generally used and the relative effects of protein and caloric intake cannot be segregated.

Another, perhaps major determinant of the quantity of activated carcinogen-forming adducts with cellular macromolecules may be the cascade of reactions that influence detoxification of activated intermediates. Unfortunately, little data are available on these potentially critical reactions, making its discussion somewhat speculative. Epoxide hydrase may play an important role in detoxicating ultimate carcinogens which are epoxides. Adekunle et al. (1) have shown that protein deficiency depresses epoxide hydrase to an extent approximately equivalent to that of the MFO system. Therefore, the balance between activation of a carcinogen via epoxide formation and the catalytic destruction of the epoxide by epoxide hydrase may not be drastically altered by protein deficiency. The activity of UDP-glucuronyltransferase has been shown to be increased by protein deficiency although little effect on the sulfotransferases was noticed (198,199).

Any effect on these transferases, or their cosubstrates uridine diphosphogluc-uronic acid and 3'-phosphoadenosine-5'-phosphosulfate, could produce altera-tions in the balance between activation and detoxification as previously discussed. Decreases in cellular protein resulting from low-protein diets would lower the number of noncritical nucleophilic sites available for spontaneous adduct forma-tion resulting in larger quantities of the ultimate carcinogen being available for adduct formation with critical sites.

An example of the effect of protein nutrition on the metabolic disposition of a carcinogen and the eventual production of the tumor can be seen with AFB_1. The decreased hepatocarcinogenicity of AFB_1 in protein-deficient rats (104) may largely be dependent on alterations in its metabolism. AFB_1 is metabo-lized to a number of metabolites through a rather complex series of interrelating pathways (28) illustrated in Fig. 4. It is metabolized to a group of hydroxylated products, AFM_1, P_1, Q_1 and AFB_{2a}, by the MFO system and reduced to aflatoxi-col (AFOL) by soluble enzymes. These hydroxylated products can then be ex-creted or act as aglycones for the transferases to form more hydrophilic products. The critical reaction is the MFO-catalyzed activation of AFB_1 to the highly reactive electrophilic 2,3-epoxide (AFB-epoxide) illustrated in Fig. 5. This species

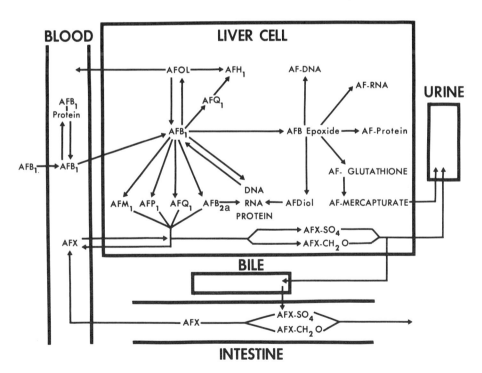

FIG. 4. Schematic representation of the biodisposition of AFB_1. AF, aflatoxin; AFOL, aflatoxiol; AFX, hydroxylatedmetabolite of AFB_1; AFDiol, dihydrodiol.

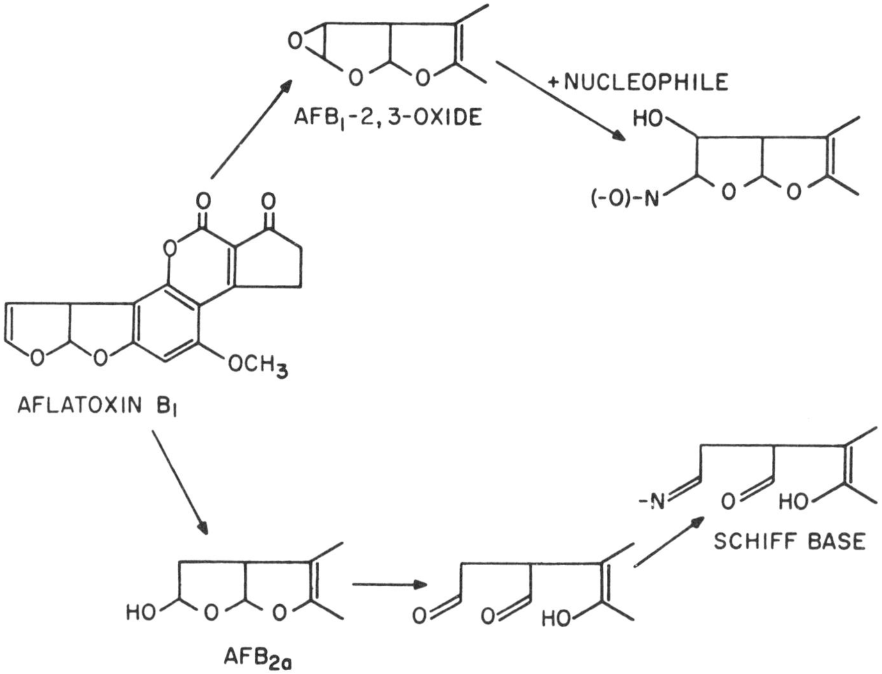

FIG. 5. Example of two metabolic routes giving rise to formation of AF adducts with macromolecules.

can then form covalent adducts at nucleophilic centers on either DNA, RNA, or protein, initiating the biochemical lesion and possibly leading to neoplasia. Metabolites such as AFB_{2a} and the AFB_1 dihydrodiol may also interact with cellular macromolecules. AFB_{2a} exists in resonance with its phenolate ion which contains a dialdehyde function capable of binding amino groups of protein through Schiff base formation (66,124) (Fig. 5). Adducts also form between AFB_{2a} and DNA and RNA but the nature of this binding has not been determined (73). It is possible, although no data are available, that the dihydrodiol produced from the spontaneous degradation of AFB-epoxide may also form adducts to macromolecules in a manner similar to AFB_{2a}.

Diets consisting of 5% casein have been shown to produce a 50% reduction in rat liver MFO-catalyzed metabolism of AFB_1 to its hydroxylated metabolites when compared to rats fed 20% casein (1). Since the toxicity and carcinogenicity of these metabolites are less than that of AFB_1, their production is normally considered a detoxification reaction. Decreased metabolism would then be expected to increase the toxicity and carcinogenicity of AFB_1. This is in agreement with the toxicity data but in contrast to that for carcinogenicity. Studies in the laboratory of the Millers (56,97,162,163,164) and that of Wogan (42,52) have indicated that AFB_1 is metabolized by the hepatic MFO system to AFB-epoxide which covalently binds nucleic acids. Therefore the decreased activity of the MFO system would be expected to reduce the quantity of AFB-epoxide formed and possibly the quantity of epoxide–macromolecular adducts. Preston et al. (128) were able to show that rats fed a 5% casein diet for 15 days showed a 70% reduction in the quantity of AF bound *in vivo* to rat liver chromatin. The low-protein diet causes significant reductions in AF adduct formation with total hepatic DNA, RNA, and protein as shown in Fig. 6. Although on the surface it might appear that the decreased binding to cellular macromolecules may be directly related to MFO activity, this conclusion would be too simplistic for reasons previously discussed. To determine which reaction becomes rate limiting in respect to adduct formation during protein deficiency, it is necessary to study the other routes involved in the biodisposition of AFB_1.

Although there is no convincing evidence that epoxide hydrase plays a role in the detoxification of AFB-epoxide, the possibility exists that it may. However, since the ratio of epoxide hydrase activity to MFO activity is not significantly changed in the protein-deficient rats, it is unlikely that it is a determinant in the decreased binding of AFB-epoxide to the macromolecules (1). A more important determinant is the detoxification of AFB-epoxide by conjugation with glutathione.

Several reports have indicated that a mercapturate of AF is formed (114,129) and a more recent report indicates that the glutathione conjugate may be the major metabolite of AFB_1 (44). Allen-Hoffmann (3) has studied the effects of

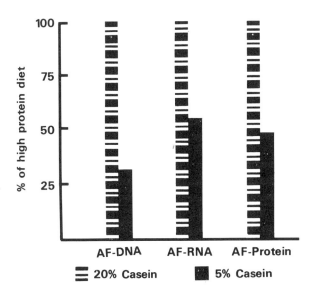

FIG. 6. Effect of dietary casein level on rat liver AF adduct formation with DNA, RNA, and protein. Rats were fed the diets for 15 days, injected i.p. (intraperitoneal) with 1 mg/kg AFB_1 and sacrificed 6 hr later.

dietary protein intake and glutathione levels on the formation of AF–macro-molecule adducts *in vivo.* They found that dietary protein depletion produced significantly elevated levels of hepatic glutathione. Hepatic glutathione was de-pleted by administration of AFB_1 to rats fed either high or low protein, indicating possible adduct formation. However, both experimental groups showed a similar degree of depletion. It would have been expected that if the depletion were caused by a glutathione conjugate with AFB-epoxide the low-protein animals would have shown a lower percent depletion because of less epoxide production. In addition, they found, as did Mitchell et al. (118) using bromobenzene, that the depletion was not stoichiometric with dosage level. This indicates that these responses are complex and need further clarification. Allen-Hoffman (3) was also able to show an inverse relationship between glutathione level and AF-nucleic acid adduct formation. Their data indicate that the higher hepatic gluta-thione levels in the protein-deficient rat may be a significant determinant of the low levels of nucleic acid adducts of AF found in these animals. Therefore, the lower quantity of AF-nucleic adducts found in the protein-deficient rat may depend not only on the lower levels of MFO activity, but also on the higher levels of glutathione. More studies are certainly required to determine the exact role of these reactions and other factors, such as carrier proteins, in the depression of the carcinogenicity of AFB_1 in protein-deficient rats.

Protein deficiency may affect the quantity of nucleic acid adducts via alteration of their degradation and persistence. A time course of the quantity of hepatic AF-DNA adducts formed after injection of AFB_1 by rats fed the adequate and low-protein diets for only 3.5 days is shown in Fig. 7. Maximal binding

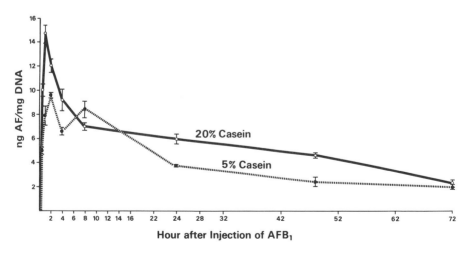

FIG. 7. Formation of covalent adducts between AF and DNA after a single i.p. injection of 1.0 mg/kg AFB_1 by rats fed either 5 or 20% casein for 3.5 days (0————20% casein, ●--------- 5% casein).

occurred at 1 hr after injection in the animals fed the adequate protein diets but was delayed until 2 hr in the low-protein group. During the first 4 hr, there was a 20 to 50% depression in total adducts formed by the low protein group. Maximal binding is followed by a degradation of the adducts until, at 72 hr after injection, there is no significant difference between the two dietary groups, indicating the degradation process may be somewhat retarded in the low-protein-fed rats. Adduct formation correlates with the carcinogenicity data only during the initial period and not with the more persistently bound material. This phenomena has also been seen employing other models in our laboratory (73). One problem encountered in interpreting data such as this is a lack of knowledge about the specific binding represented by these adducts.

Most studies (42,52,97) have indicated that the major site of adduct formation between DNA and AF is the N-7 position of guanine. Whether or not AF also forms the more persistent O-6 adduct of guanine (61) has not been ascertained, possibly because of the small numbers of adducts formed at this position.

Although these data have dealt with diets considered to be less than adequate in respect to dietary protein, diets that contain protein levels above optimum may also alter carcinogenicity. There have been no studies on the effects of high levels of dietary protein on AFB_1 carcinogenicity. However, Maso et al. (107) have titrated nucleic acid-AF adduct levels against dietary protein level as shown in Fig. 8. Adduct formation with DNA was found to be proportional to the level of dietary protein from 5 to 40% dietary casein. On the other hand, adduct formation with RNA was less at 40% casein than at 20% casein. If the carcinogenicity of AFB_1 correlates with AF-DNA adduct formation, as it appears to do, then these data would predict that rats with high protein intakes may show increased risks of hepatocarcinogenesis from AFB_1.

Although we have emphasized the metabolic events that may be affected by dietary protein during tumor initiation, it may also have ramifications during the promotion and growth phases. Generally, one of the aspects of promotion, whether it be by chemical promoters or other techniques such as partial hepatectomy, is an increase in cellular replication (36). Replication may be required to "set" or "freeze" the biochemical lesion in the genome, allowing eventual development of neoplasia. Since protein deficiency slows growth, and therefore cellular replication, decreased replication rates may act to inhibit neoplastic development in protein-deficient rats. This may, in part, contribute to the decreased spontaneous tumor development in protein-deprived rats reported by Ross and Bras (148) and Ross et al. (149). It is obvious that the effects of protein nutrition on promotion is an area much in need of further development.

The depression in growth seen in animals consuming low-protein diets may also result in depressed growth of tumor cells, increasing the likelihood of their destruction by processes such as cell-mediated immunity. In addition, altered amino acid requirements of a tumor cell may not be supplied in a low-protein diet, leading to inhibited growth or cellular death (91). Although difficult to ascertain because of various health-related complications, protein-calorie malnu-

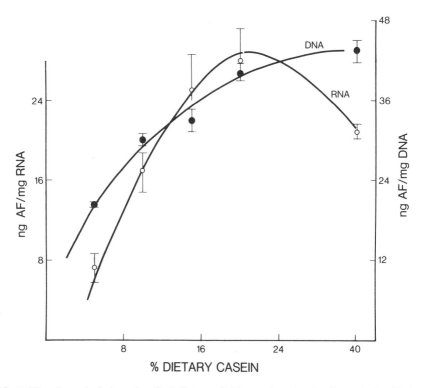

FIG. 8. Weanling rats fed semipurified diets containing various levels of casein for 15 days and then injected i.p. with [³H]-AFB₁ (1 mg/kg). Ten hours after injection, animals were sacrificed and DNA and RNA were isolated and counted to determine the covalently bound AFB₁ metabolite. Animals were fed *ad libitum;* intakes between 10 and 40% were not significantly different.

trition negatively affects the immune system in human populations (37,180). The role of immunological defects produced by protein deficiency on chemical carcinogenicity has not been determined. Jose and Good (87) have presented evidence that both protein and specific amino acid deficiency may actually enhance immunological-mediated destruction of tumor cells. Other factors, such as specific dietary protein effects on the target organ of a chemical carcinogen, may modify the susceptibility of an animal to tumorigenesis resulting from chemicals.

Protein deficiency, along with other nutrients, probably modifies chemical carcinogenicity in a multifaceted manner. Time and a more intense research effort will be required to isolate and evaluate these various factors. However, at this stage, it is evident that the effects of protein nutrition on metabolism of carcinogens must be considered a major determinant. To delineate the role of protein nutrition in the carcinogenicity of a particular carcinogen, it is necessary to have some knowledge of the metabolic pathway of the carcinogen and the effect of protein nutrition on that pathway. This knowledge will assist in explaining some of the contradictory data on the role of protein deficiency on chemical carcinogenicity. For example, Engel and Copeland (50) reported a higher incidence of mammary carcinoma induced by AAF in rats fed a low-protein diet. In retrospect, this may reflect the unusual activation of this carcinogen (briefly discussed earlier). The MFO system catalyzed conversion of AAF to the N-hydroxy-AAF may be assumed to be depressed, yielding decreased quantities of the proximate carcinogen. Nevertheless, the subsequent conversion to the various conjugates such as the sulfate ester (115), the glucuronide (83), and the N-acetoxy-AAF (116) may be increased by protein deficiency via its effects on certain of the transferases (198,199). Thus, more DNA adduct would be formed. Parenthetically, the AAF ultimate carcinogen also seems to be different from PAH in that it covalently binds to the C-8 position of guanine (144) rather than the N-7 position, the more common site of alkylation. To test this hypothesis further, studies on the effect of protein deficiency on the transferases, employing N-hydroxy-AAF as substrate are required.

Effect of Dietary Fat

The role of dietary fat in chemical carcinogenesis has recently received considerable attention, from both the aspect of epidemiological and laboratory animal investigations. Although a thorough review of this important dietary interrelation is beyond the scope of this discussion, we will briefly comment on its relationship to the metabolism of carcinogens.

The effect of dietary fat on carcinogenesis appears to be site specific and to date, most studies of this nutrient effect have been concerned with mammary gland and colon tumor formation. For mammary gland effects, a hormonal mechanism seems to be involved; for skin and colon carcinogenesis, dietary fat may act via carcinogen metabolism as one of the important mechanisms. Similar to dietary protein, fat may exert its influence both through quantity and composition.

Epidemiological investigations on dietary fat and certain cancers have demonstrated impressive correlations. However, these studies (21,80,200,202) lack the power to discriminate the effects from other nutrients such as fiber, protein, and soluble sugars. Cancers associated with higher dietary fat intake have been termed a disease of affluence because of their higher incidence in Western nations. Gortner (60) has stated that there has been an increase in the total fat consumed in the United States since 1909 and a shift in the type of fat consumed. Although saturated fat intake has increased since 1909, only a small change has occurred during the last several decades. Interestingly, there has been a larger increase in the intake of polyunsaturated fatty acids over the last several years because of an increase in the consumption of vegetable oils. A higher intake of animal fat, particularly that from beef, has been reported to be associated with a higher risk of colon cancer (69,200). On the other hand, Enig et al. (51) have stated that, since 1909, the increase in unsaturated fat has actually been four times that of saturated fat. These workers believe that better correlations between fat intake and cancer rates are obtained with total fat and vegetable fat rather than with animal fat. In particular, they have noted the increased consumption of trans fatty acids derived from processed vegetable oils. Unfortunately, many studies have not been particularly informative because of poor nutritional protocols such as lack of controlled calorie intake, inadequate attention being paid to the involvement of other nutrients, and the use of dietary fats of variable composition, both with respect to lipid components and with respect to nonlipid substances such as certain antioxidants, adventitious chemical residues, etc.

Tannenbaum (168) found that a high-fat diet failed to influence either spontaneous lung tumors or BP-induced sarcomas but did increase BP-induced skin tumors and spontaneous breast tumors. Several other studies have indicated that tumor production in laboratory animals is directly related to high-fat diets (20,31,55). Tannenbaum (170) and Carroll and Knor (30) have found that the effects of dietary fat levels were more significant via tumor promotion than through tumor initiation. Reddy et al. (131,137) have proposed that dietary fat-induced alterations in the composition of gastrointestinal flora are capable of influencing colon tumor formation. These effects may involve either the initiation and/or promotion phases. Although Tannenbaum (173) has concluded that the total quantity of dietary fat ingested may be more important than the type of fat, several studies have indicated that the degree of fatty acid saturation can also alter tumor yield (31,82,131).

Whereas dietary fat has been implicated in tumor promotion and growth, it may have a significant effect on the metabolic activation of chemical carcinogens (34). That is, dietary fat can produce alterations in the activity of the MFO system (26). For instance, diets deficient in essential fatty acids depress the activity of the hepatic microsomal MFO activity (32,121). Moreover, the microsomal MFO system exists in a lipid–protein membrane and its activity is influenced by the lipid-dependent interactions within the membrane. For instance, Lotlikar and colleagues (99,100) have demonstrated a phospholipid requirement for the ring and *N*-hydroxylation of AAF and demethylation of DMN by the hepatic MFO system. The tissue specificity of the dietary fat effects indicates that the MFO system of the skin and colon mucosa may be more responsive than that of the liver, although most studies investigating the effect of fat have utilized the hepatic MFO system.

There have been few studies designed to ascertain the role of dietary lipid on other reactions participating in the detoxification of carcinogens and non-MFO-mediated carcinogen activation. Like the MFO system, epoxide hydrase is found associated with the microsomal membrane, and may be similarly affected. Another microsomal enzyme that may be affected by microsomal lipids that are altered by dietary fat is UDP-glucuronyltransferase. Vessey and Zakim (178) have shown that the activity of UDP-glucuronyltransferase is regulated by microsomal phospholipids. Therefore, alterations of the fatty acid components of membrane phospholipids may have significant effects on this enzyme activity and should be investigated. As previously mentioned, modification of transferase activities may alter the balance between the detoxification and activation reactions of chemical carcinogens (22).

An example of the dietary-fat dependence of a nonmicrosomal enzyme participating in the activation of a chemical carcinogen is presented by Castro et al. (34). They tested the ability of 150,000 *g* supernatants from liver, lung, and kidney to convert *N*-hydroxy-2-fluorenylacetamide (N-OH-FAA) to a metabolite mutagenic to *Salmonella typhimurium*. Feeding either corn oil instead of beef tallow or 20% instead of 5% of either lipid source for 6 months increased the mutagenic activities for the hepatic supernatants. The kidney showed less response than did the liver, whereas lung activity was not sensitive to either fat quantity or composition.

The effect of dietary fat on colon carcinogenesis is illustrated by the work of Reddy et al. (132). Rats were fed either 5 or 20% corn oil or either 5 or 20% lard for two generations. Rats on the 20% fat diets had a higher incidence of dimethylhydrazine-induced colon tumors. Moreover, there was no significant difference in incidence rate between the corn oil and lard diets, indicating that quantity was a greater determinant than the type of fat. Bansal et al. (15) confirmed these studies and found that rats on high animal fat diets showed a higher degree of metastases.

One of the more interesting aspects of the interaction between dietary fat and chemical carcinogenesis is the interplay between carcinogen metabolism by the colon mucosa and intestinal microorganisms with respect to colon cancer. Reddy and colleagues (130,203) have suggested that fat may exert its effect through changes in the composition of intestinal microflora (81) that metabolize acid and neutral steroids found in the intestine (140). They have suggested (130) that colon microflora may affect carcinogenesis through metabolic conversion of bile acids and neutral steroids to products which then act as promoters, as well as through production of carcinogenic aglycones via β-glucuronidase activity. The microflora themselves may also activate chemical carcinogens which could then react with macromolecules of the colonic mucosa. For instance, Batzinger et al. (17) have demonstrated that 4-isothiocyano-4-nitrodiphenylamine is metabolized by intestinal microflora to a mutagenic product. Unlike conventional rats, germ-free animals do not excrete the mutagenic product into the urine. Studies utilizing germ-free rats and several carcinogens have yielded conflicting data on the role of microflora in chemical carcinogenesis. Colon tumors induced by 1,2-dimethylhydrazine (127,133) and 3,2'-dimethyl-4-amino-biphenyl (DMAB) (135) were decreased by germ-free conditions, whereas the incidence of colon tumors induced by DMAB (12), azoxymethane, and *N*-methyl-*N'*-nitro-*N*-nitrosoguanidine (MNNG) (14,133) were increased by germ-free conditions. These contradictory data will probably be better understood when additional information becomes available on the metabolic routes for these carcinogens with respect to the microflora-host interactions.

Reddy et al. (134) have shown that deoxycholic acid, a secondary bile acid found in high concentrations in stools of individuals consuming high-meat, high-fat Western diets, promotes MNNG-induced colon tumors in germ-free rats. They (136) have also shown that the primary bile acids, sodium cholate and sodium chenodeoxycholate, acted as promoters for MNNG-induced colon adenocarcinomas and adenomas in germ-free rats, although only increased numbers of adenomas were found in conventional rats. The bile acids themselves were not carcinogenic in either the germ-free or conventional rats. Alterations in quantities of either primary or secondary bile acids induced by the ingestion of various dietary fats would be expected to modify promotional activities.

The role of dietary fat in the activation and detoxification of carcinogens by the colon mucosa has received little attention. Intestinal mucosa contains an MFO system, similar to that of the liver, which can metabolize drugs and carcinogens (123,184). The role of this enzyme system in colon cancer as opposed to the microflora has not been ascertained. It would be assumed that the colon mucosal MFO system would be sensitive to dietary lipids as is the liver system, and alterations in its ability to activate carcinogens may affect colon cancer. Investigations are needed to determine the interplay between the mucosal enzyme system and the microflora to determine the contribution of each.

SUMMARY

Very recently, there has been an upsurge of interest in the potential relationships of diet and nutrition with cancer etiology. This interest has probably stemmed from two sources. First, much concern has been expressed by certain public and scientific sectors that there are significant food-borne chemical carcinogens. Second, epidemiological studies have revealed impressive correlations between dietary practices and certain major cancers, such as with those of the stomach, breast, and colon. Moreover, some of these studies have led to speculation that noncarcinogenic substances including certain nutrients, when ingested at inappropriate levels, may modify the course of neoplastic events. Thus, hypotheses on the influence of dietary lipid components, such as animal fat and trans fatty acids, dietary fiber, vitamin C, and vitamin A have emerged.

Following these earlier reports on various dietary associations, newer investigations are now being directed toward an understanding of fundamental mechanisms accounting for these important interactions. The possibilities range from an early effect on carcinogen metabolism through promotion of tumor growth to the eventual nourishment of the neoplastic tissue.

This brief commentary does not review the entire field; instead it has primarily focused on one potentially important mechanism, that is, the effect of nutrient intake on carcinogen metabolism. Thus, literature was reviewed to show that the total quantity of ultimate carcinogen produced can be readily influenced by the intakes of various nutrients. Such a modification of carcinogen metabolism involves a very complex series of reactions, where activation and detoxification may be closely interrelated and perhaps coordinated. For example, *in vitro* enzyme assays may indicate isolated activities which give clues to the role of carcinogen metabolism in the initiating event, but *in vivo* tumor studies often yield contrasting results. Thus, specific knowledge of carcinogen metabolism pathways, together with an understanding of relative enzyme rate limitations, must be at hand before a full understanding of nutrient effects can be appreciated.

This review has concentrated on a consideration of the effects of dietary lipid and protein as these may be related to carcinogen metabolism, in order to illustrate how this mechanism may become important to the eventual development of the neoplastic lesion. It is hoped that more fundamental studies will be forthcoming so that the various epidemiological associations recently publicized may be better understood.

Considering both the epidemiological and laboratory investigations, it is somewhat premature to recommend specific diets which may aid in the prevention of cancer. Nevertheless, we agree with the suggestions of Hegsted (77) and Wynder (201) that adoption of "prudent diets" (47) would be an initial step in the right direction.

REFERENCES

1. Adekunle, A. A., Hayes, J. R., and Campbell, T. C. (1977): Interrelationships of dietary protein level, aflatoxin B_1 metabolism, and hepatic microsomal epoxide hydrase activity. *Life Sci.,* 21:1785–1792.
2. Agradi, E., Spanuolo, C., and Galli, C. (1975): Dietary lipid and aniline and benzpyrene hydroxylations in liver microsomes. *Pharmacol. Res. Commun.,* 7:469–480.
3. Allen-Hoffmann, B. L. (1978): The relationship between hepatic glutathione levels and the formation of aflatoxin-macromolecule adducts *in vivo* as influenced by dietary protein intake. M. S. Thesis, Cornell University, Ithaca, N. Y.
4. Allen-Hoffmann, B. L., and Campbell, T. C. (1977): The relationship between hepatic glutathione levels and the formation of aflatoxin B_1-DNA adducts as influenced by dietary protein intake. *Fed. Proc.,* 36:1116.
5. Alvares, A. P., Schilling, G., Levin, W., and Kuntzman, R. (1967): Studies in the induction of CO-binding pigments in liver microsomes by phenobarbital and 3-methylcholanthrene. *Biochem. Biophys. Res. Commun.,* 29:521–526.
6. American Cancer Society and National Cancer Institute. (1975): Symposium on nutrition in the causation of cancer. *Cancer Res.,* 35:3231–3550.
7. American Institute of Nutrition. (1977): Report of the American Institute of Nutrition, Ad Hoc Committee on Standards for Nutritional Studies. *J. Nutr.,* 107:1340–1348.
8. American Institute of Nutrition Symposium. (1976): Nutrition and Cancer. *Fed. Proc.,* 35:1307–1338.
9. Andervont, H. B. (1941): Spontaneous tumors in a subline of strain C3H mice. *J. Natl. Cancer Inst.,* 1:737–744.
10. Andia, A. M. G., and Street, J. C. (1975): Dietary induction of hepatic microsomal enzymes by thermally oxidized fats. *J. Agric. Food Chem.,* 23:173–177.
11. Anonymous. (1978): Membrane changes and pathogenesis of protein-energy malnutrition. *Nutr. Rev.,* 36:297–299.
12. Asano, T., Pollard, M., and Madsen, D. C. (1975): Effects of cholestyramine on 1,2-dimethylhydrazine induced enteric carcinoma in germ-free rats. *Proc. Soc. Exp. Biol. Med.,* 150:780–785.
13. Baldwin, B. C. (1977): Xenobiotic metabolism in plants. In: *Drug Metabolism from Microbe to Man,* edited by D. V. Parke and R. L. Smith, pp. 191–217. Taylor & Francis Ltd., London.
14. Balish, E., Shin, C. N., and Croft, W. A. (1977): Effect of age, sex, and intestinal flora on the induction of colon tumors in rats. *J. Natl. Cancer Inst.,* 58:1103–1106.

15. Bansal, B., Rhoads, J. E., and Bansal, S. C. (1978): Effects of diet on colon carcinogenesis and the immune system in rats treated with 1,2-dimethylhydrazine. *Cancer Res.*, 38:3293–3303.
16. Bartsch, H. and Hecker, E. (1971): On the metabolic activation of the carcinogen N-hydroxy-N-2-acetylaminofluorene. III. Oxidation with horseradish peroxidase to yield 2-nitrosofluorene and N-acetoxy-N-2-acetylaminofluorene. *Biochim. Biophys. Acta*, 237:567–578.
17. Batzinger, R. P., Bueding, E., Reddy, B. S., and Weisburger, J. H. (1978): Formation of a mutagenic drug metabolite by intestinal microorganisms. *Cancer Res.*, 38:608–612.
18. Becci, P. J., Thompson, H. J., Grubbs, C. J., Squire, R. A., Brown, C. C., Sporn, M. B., and Moon, R. C. (1978): Inhibitory effect of 13-cis-retinoic acid on urinary bladder carcinogenesis induced in C57BL/6 mice by N-butyl-N-(4-hydroxybutyl)-nitrosamine. *Cancer Res.*, 38:4463–4466.
19. Benson, A. M., Batzinger, R. P., Ou, S-Y. L., Bueding, E., Cha, Y.-N, and Talalay, P. (1978): Elevation of hepatic glutathione-S-transferase activities and protection against mutagenic metabolites of benzo(a)pyrene by dietary antioxidants. *Cancer Res.*, 38:4486–4495.
20. Benson, J., Lev, M., and Girand, C. G. (1956): Enhancement of mammary fibroadenomas in the male rat by a high fat diet. *Cancer Res.*, 16:135–137.
21. Berg, J. W. (1975): Can nutrition explain the pattern of international epidemiology of hormone-dependent cancers? *Cancer Res.*, 35:3345–3350.
22. Bock, K. W. (1978): Increase of liver microsomal benzo(a)pyrene monooxygenase activity by subsequent glucuronidation. *Naunyn-Schmiedebergs Arch. Pharmacol.*, 304:77–79.
23. Brown, R. R., Miller, J. A., and Miller, E. C. (1954): The metabolism of methylated aminoazo dyes. IV. Dietary factors enhancing demethylation *in vitro*. *J. Biol. Chem.*, 209:211–217.
24. Burkitt, D. P. (1971): Epidemiology of cancer of the colon and rectum. *Cancer*, 23:3–13.
25. Campbell, T. C. (1978): Effects of dietary protein on drug metabolism. In: *Nutrition and Drug Interrelations*, edited by J. N. Hathcock and J. Coon, pp. 409–422. Academic Press, New York.
26. Campbell, T. C., and Hayes, J. R. (1974): Role of nutrition in the drug metabolizing enzyme system. *Pharmacol. Rev.*, 26:171–197.
27. Campbell, T. C., and Hayes, J. R. (1976): The effect of quantity and quality of dietary protein on drug metabolism. *Fed. Proc.*, 35:2470–2474.
28. Campbell, T. C., and Hayes, J. R. (1976): The role of aflatoxin metabolism in its toxic lesion. *Toxicol. Appl. Pharmacol.*, 35:199–222.
29. Carroll, K. K. (1975): Experimental evidence of dietary factors and hormone-dependent cancers. *Cancer Res.*, 35:3374–3383.
30. Carroll, K. K., and Khor, H. T. (1970): Effects of dietary fat and dose level of 7,12-dimethylbenz(a)anthracene on mammary tumor incidence in rats. *Cancer Res.*, 30:2260–2264.
31. Carroll, K. K., and Khor, H. T. (1971): Effects of level and type of dietary fat on incidence of mammary tumors induced in female Sprague-Dawley rats by 7,12-dimethylbenz(a)anthracene. *Lipids*, 6:415–420.
32. Caster, W. O., Wade, A. E., Norred, W. P., and Bargman, R. E. (1968): Differential effect of dietary saturated fat on the metabolism of aniline and hexobarbital by the rat liver. *Pharmacology*, 3:117–186.
33. Caster, W. O., Wade, A. E., Greene, F. E., and Meadows, J. S. (1968): Effect of small changes in dietary thiamine or essential fatty acid in altering the rate of drug detoxification in the liver of the rat. *Fed. Proc.*, 27:549.
34. Castro, C. E., Felkner, I. C., and Yang, S. P. (1978): Dietary lipid-dependent activation of the carcinogen N-2-fluoranylacetamide in fats as monitored by *Salmonella typhimurium*. *Cancer Res.*, 38:2836–2841.
35. Catz, C. S., Juchau, M. R., and Yaffe, S. J. (1970): Effects of iron, riboflavin and iodide deficiencies on hepatic drug metabolizing enzyme systems. *J. Pharmacol. Exp. Ther.*, 174:197–205.
36. Cayama, E., Tsuda, H., Sarma, D. S. R., and Farber, E. (1978): Initiation of chemical carcinogenesis requires cell proliferation. *Nature*, 275:60–62.
37. Chandra, R. K. (1974): Rosette-forming T lymphocytes and cell-mediated immunity in malnutrition. *Br. Med. J.*, 545:608–609.
38. Chow, C. K. (1977): Dietary vitamin E and levels of reduced glutathione, glutathione peroxidase, catalase and superoxide dismutase in rat blood. *Int. J. Vitam. Nutr. Res.*, 47:268–273.

39. Clayson, D. B. (1975): Nutrition and experimental carcinogenesis: A review. *Cancer Res.,* 35:3292–3300.
40. Coon, M. J., White, R. E., Nordblom, G. D., Ballon, D. P., and Guengerich, F. P. (1977): Highly purified liver microsomal cytochrome P-450: Properties and catalytic mechanism. *Croatica Chemica Acta.,* 49:163–177.
41. Coon, M. J., and Lu, A. Y. H. (1969): Fatty acid ω-oxidation in a soluble microsomal enzyme system containing P-450. In: *Microsomes and Drug Oxidations,* edited by J. R. Gillette, A. H. Conney, G. J. Cosmides, R. W. Estabrook, J. R. Fouts, and G. J. Mannering, pp. 151–166. Academic Press, New York.
42. Croy, R. G., Essigmann, J. M., Reinhold, V. N., and Wogan, G. N. (1978): Identification of the principal aflatoxin B_1-DNA adduct formed *in vivo* in rat liver. *Proc. Natl. Acad. Sci. USA,* 75:1745–1749.
43. Czygan, P., Greim, H., Garro, A., Schaffner, F., and Popper, H. (1974): The effect of dietary protein deficiency on the ability of isolated hepatic microsomes to alter the mutagenicity of a primary and a secondary carcinogen. *Cancer Res.,* 34:119–123.
44. Degen, G. H., and Neuman, H. -G. (1978): The major metabolite of aflatoxin B_1 in the rat is a glutathione conjugate. *Chem. Biol. Interact.,* 22:239–255.
45. Depiere, J. W., and Dallner, G. (1975): Structural aspects of the membrane of the endoplasmic reticulum. *Biochim. Biophys. Acta,* 415:411–412.
46. Diehl, H., Schadelin, J., and Ullrich, V. (1970): Studies on the kinetics of cytochrome P-450 reduction in rat liver microsomes. *Hoppe Seyler's Z. Physiol. Chem.,* 351:1359–1371.
47. Dietary goals for the United States. (1977): *Nutr. Rev.,* 35:122–127.
48. Diet, Bacteria and the Colon: A Symposium. (1976): *Am. J. Clin. Nutr.,* 29:1409–1484.
49. Dunning, W. F., Curtis, M. R., and Maun, M. E. (1950): The effect of added tryptophane on the occurrences of diethylstilbestrol induced mammary cancer in rats. *Cancer Res.,* 10:319–323.
50. Engel, R. W., and Copeland, D. H. (1952): The influence of dietary casein level on tumor induction with 2-acetylaminofluorene. *Cancer Res.,* 12:905–912.
51. Enig, M. G., Munn, R. J., and Keeney, M. (1978): Dietary fat and cancer trends—a critique. *Fed. Proc.,* 37:2215–2220.
52. Essigman, J. M., Croy, R. G., Nadzan, A. M., Busby, W. F., Jr., Reinhold, V. N., Buchi, G., and Wogan, G. N. (1977): Structural identification of the major DNA adduct formed by aflatoxin B_1 *in vitro. Proc. Natl. Acad. Sci. USA,* 74:1870–1874.
53. Estabrook, R. W., Franklin, M. R., Cohen, B., Shigamatzu, A., and Hildebrandt, A. G. (1971): Influence of hepatic microsomal mixed function oxidation reactions on cellular metabolic control. *Metabolism,* 20:187–199.
54. Franklin, M. R., and Estabrook, R. W. (1971): On the inhibitory action of mersalyl on microsomal drug oxidation: A rigid organization of the electron transport chain. *Arch. Biochem. Biophys.,* 143:318–329.
55. Gammal, E. B., Carroll, K. K., and Plunkett, E. R. (1967): Effects of dietary fat on mammary carcinogenesis by 7,12-dimethyl-benz(a)anthracene in rats. *Cancer Res.,* 27:1737–1742.
56. Garner, R. C., Miller, E. C., and Miller, J. A. (1972): Liver microsomal metabolism of aflatoxin B_1 to a reactive derivative toxic to *Salmonella typhimurium* TA 1530. *Cancer Res.,* 32:2058–2066.
57. Gelboin, H. V. (1969): A microsome-dependent binding of benzo(a)pyrene to DNA. *Cancer Res.,* 29:1272–1276.
58. Gigon, P. L., Gram, T. E., and Gillette, J. R. (1969): Studies on the rate of reduction of hepatic microsomal cytochrome P-450 by reduced nicotinamide adenine dinucleotide phosphate: Effect of drug substrates. *Mol. Pharmacol.,* 5:109–122.
59. Gillette, J. R. (1971): Effect of various inducers on electron transport system associated with drug metabolism. *Metabolism,* 20:215–227.
60. Gortner, W. A. (1975): Nutrition in the United States, 1900 to 1974. *Cancer Res.,* 35:3246–3253.
61. Goth, R., and Rajewsky, M. F. (1974): Persistence of O^6-ethylguanine in rat brain DNA: Correlation with nervous system-specific carcinogenesis by ethylnitrourea. *Proc. Natl. Acad. Sci. USA,* 71:639–643.
62. Gram, T. E., Gigon, P. L., and Gillette, J. R. (1969): Studies on the reduction of hepatic microsomal cytochrome P-450 by NADPH and its role in drug metabolism. *Pharmacologist,* 10:179.

63. Grover, P. L., and Sims, P. (1969): Enzyme catalyzed reactions of polycyclic hydrocarbons with deoxyribonucleic acid and protein *in vitro*. *Biochem. J.,* 110:159–160.

64. Guengerich, F. P. (1977): Separation and purification of multiple forms of cytochrome P-450. Activities of different forms of cytochrome P-450 towards several compounds of environmental interest. *J. Biol. Chem.,* 252:3970–3979.

65. Guengerich, F. P. (1978): Separation and purification of multiple forms of microsomal cytochrome P-450. Partial characterization of three apparently homogeneous cytochromes P-450 prepared from livers of phenobarbital and 3-methylcholanthrene-treated rats. *J. Biol. Chem.,* 253:7931–7939.

66. Gurtoo, H. L., and Campbell, T. C. (1974): Metabolism of aflatoxin B_1 and its metabolism dependent and independent binding to rat hepatic microsomes. *Mol. Pharmacol.,* 10:776–789.

67. Guttenplan, J. B. (1978): Mechanisms of inhibition by ascorbate of microbial mutagenesis induced by N-nitroso compounds. *Cancer Res.,* 38:2018–2022.

68. Habig, W. H., Pabst, M. J., Fleischner, G., Gatmaitan, Z., Arias, I. M., and Jakoby, W. B. (1974): The identity of glutathione S-transferase B with ligandin, a major binding protein of liver. *Proc. Natl. Acad. Sci. USA,* 71:3879–3882.

69. Haenszel, W., Berg, J. W., Segi, M., Kurihara, M., and Locke, F. B. (1973): Large bowel cancer in Hawaiian Japanese. *J. Natl. Cancer Inst.,* 51:1765–1779.

70. Hard, G. C., and Butler, W. H. (1970): Cellular analysis of renal neoplasia: Induction of renal tumors in dietary-conditioned rats by dimethylnitrosamine, with a reappraisal of morphological characteristics. *Cancer Res.,* 30:2796–2805.

71. Haugen, D. A., van der Hoeven, T. A., and Coon, M. J. (1975): Purified liver microsomal cytochrome P-450, separation and characterization of multiple forms. *J. Biol. Chem.,* 250:3567–3570.

72. Hayes, J. R., and Campbell, T. C. (1974): Effect of protein deficiency on the inducibility of the hepatic microsomal drug-metabolizing enzyme system. III. Effect of 3-methylcholanthrene induction on activity and binding kinetics. *Biochem. Pharmacol.,* 23:1721–1731.

73. Hayes, J. R., and Campbell, T. C. (1978): *(Unpublished observations.)*

74. Hayes, J. R., Mgbodile, M. U. K., and Campbell, T. C. (1973): Effect of protein deficiency on the inducibility of the hepatic microsomal drug metabolizing enzyme system: I. Effect on substrate interactions with cytochrome P-450. *Biochem. Pharmacol.,* 22:1005–1014.

75. Hayes, J. R., Mgbodile, M. U. K., Merrill, A. H., Nerurkar, L. S., and Campbell, T. C. (1978): The effect of dietary protein depletion and repletion on rat hepatic mixed function oxidase activity. *J. Nutr.,* 108:1788–1797.

76. Hedegaard, J., and Gunsalus, I. C. (1965): Mixed function oxidation. IV. An induced methylene hydroxylase in camphor oxidation. *J. Biol. Chem.,* 240:4038–4045.

77. Hegsted, D. M. (1975): Summary of the conference on nutrition in the causation of cancer. *Cancer Res.,* 35:3541–3542.

78. Heidelberger, C. (1975): Chemical carcinogenesis. *Annu. Rev. Bioch.* 44:79–121.

79. Hilfrich, J., Haas, H., Kmoch, N., Montesano, R., Mohr, U., and Magee, P. N. (1975): The modifications of the renal carcinogenicity of dimethylnitrosamine by actinomycin D by a protein deficient diet. *Br. J. Cancer,* 32:578–587.

80. Hill, M. J. (1975): Metabolic epidemiology of dietary factors in large bowel cancer. *Cancer Res.,* 35:3398–3402.

81. Hill, M. J., Crowther, J. S., Drasar, B. S., Hasksworth, G., Aries, V., and Williams, R. E. (1971): Bacteria and etiology of cancer of the large bowel. *Lancet,* 1:95–100.

82. Hopkins, G. J., West, C. E., and Hard, G. C. (1976): Effect of dietary fats on the incidence of 7,12-dimethylbenz(a)anthracene induced tumors in rats. *Lipids,* 11:328–333.

83. Irving, C. C., Veazey, R. A., and Hill, J. T. (1969): Reaction of the glucuronide of the carcinogen N-hydroxy-2-acetylaminofluorene with nucleic acids. *Biochem. Biophys. Acta,* 179:189–198.

84. Issenberg, P. (1976): Nitrite, nitrosamines, and cancer. *Fed. Proc.,* 35:1322–1326.

85. Jakoby, W. B., Ketley, J. N., and Habig, W. H. (1976): Rat glutathione S-transferases: Binding and physical properties. In: *Glutathione Metabolism and Function,* edited by I. M. Arias and W. B. Jakoby, pp. 213–223. Raven Press, New York.

86. Jerina, D. M., Lehr, R., Schaefer-Ridder, M., Yagi, H., Karle, J. M., Thakker, D. R., Wood, A. W., Lu, A. Y. H., Ryan, D., West, S., Levin, W., and Conney, A. H. (1977): Bay-region epoxides of dihydrodiols: Concept explaining the mutagenic and carcinogenic activity of benzo(a)pyrene and benzo(a)anthracene. In: *Origins of Human Cancer, Book B. Mechanisms of*

Carcinogenesis, edited by H. H. Hiatt, J. D. Watson, and J. A. Winsten, pp. 639–658. Cold Spring Harbor Laboratory, Cold Spring Harbor, New York.

87. Jose, D. G., and Good, R. A. (1973): Quantitative effects of nutritional essential amino acid deficiency upon immune responses to tumors in mice. *J. Exp. Med.,* 137:1–9.

88. Kasper, C. B. (1971): Biochemical distinctions between the nuclear and microsomal membranes from rat hepatocytes: The effect of phenobarbital administration. *J. Biol. Chem.,* 246:577–581.

89. Kato, R. (1977): Drug metabolism under pathological and abnormal physiological states in animals and man. *Xenobiotica,* 7:25–92.

90. Ketley, J. N., Habig, W. H. and Jakoby, W. B. (1975): Binding of nonsubstrate ligands to the glutathione S-transferases, *J. Biol. Chem.,* 250:8670–8673.

91. Kreis, W., and Goodenow, M. (1978): Methinonine requirement and replacement by homocysteine in tissue cultures of selected rodent and human malignant and normal cells. *Cancer Res.,* 38:2259–2262.

92. Laitinen, M. (1976): Enhancement of hepatic drug metabolism with dietary cholesterol in the rat. *Acta Pharmacol. Toxicol. (Kbh),* 39:241–249.

93. Lang, M. (1976): Depression of drug metabolism in liver microsomes after treating rats with unsaturated fatty acids. *Gen. Pharmacol.,* 7:415–419.

94. Lang, M. (1976): Dietary cholesterol caused modification in the structure and function of rat hepatic microsomes, studied by fluorescent probes. *Biochim. Biophys. Acta,* 455:947–960.

95. Lang, M., Laitinen, M., Hietanen, E., and Vainio, H. (1976): Modification of microsomal membrane components and induction of hepatic drug biotransformation in rats on a high cholesterol diet. *Acta Pharmacol. Toxicol.,* 39:273–288.

96. Lee, D. J., Sinnhuber, R. O., Wales, J. H., and Putnam, G. A. (1978): Effect of dietary protein on the response of rainbow trout *(Salmo gairdneri)* to aflatoxin B_1. *J. Natl. Cancer Inst.,* 60:317–320.

97. Lin, J.-K., Miller, J. A., and Miller, E. C. (1977): 2,3-Dihydro-2-(guan-7-yl)-3-hydroxy-aflatoxin B_1, a major hydrolysis product of aflatoxin B_1-DNA or ribosomal RNA adducts formed in hepatic microsome-mediated reactions and in rat liver *in vivo. Cancer Res.,* 37:4430–4438.

98. Litwak, G., Ketterer, B., and Arias, I. M. (1971): Ligandin: A hepatic protein which binds steroids, bilirubin, carcinogens and a number of exogenous organic anions. *Nature,* 234:466–467.

99. Lotlikar, P. D., Baldy, W. J., Nyce, J., and Dwyer, E. (1976): Phospholipid requirement for dimethylnitrosamine demethylation by hamster hepatic microsomal cytochrome P-450 enzyme system. *Biochem. J.,* 160:401–404.

100. Lotlikar, P. D., Dwyer, E. N., Baldy, W. J., and Nyce, J. (1977): Phospholipid requirement for 2-acetaminofluorene N- and ring-hydroxylation by hamster liver microsomal cytochrome P-450 enzyme system. *Biochem. J.,* 168:571–574.

101. Lu, A. Y. H., and Coon, M. J. (1968): Role of hemoprotein P-450 in fatty acid ω-hydroxylation in a soluble enzyme system from liver microsomes. *J. Biol. Chem.,* 243:1331–1332.

102. Lu, A. Y. H., Kuntzman, R., West, S., Jacobson, M., and Conney, A. H. (1972): Reconstituted liver microsomal enzyme system that hydroxylates drugs, other foreign compounds, and endogenous substrates: II. Role of the cytochrome P-450 and P-448 fractions in drug and steroid hydroxylations. *J. Biol. Chem.,* 247:1727–1734.

103. Lu, A. Y. H., Levin, W., West, S. B., Jacobson, M., Ryan, D., Kuntzman, R., and Conney, A. H. (1973): Reconstituted liver microsomal enzyme system that hydroxylates drugs, other foreign compounds and endogenous substrates: VI. Different substrate specificities of the cytochrome P-450 fractions from control and phenobarbital treated rats. *J. Biol. Chem.,* 248:456–460.

104. Madhavan, T. V., and Gopalan, C. (1965): Effect of dietary protein on aflatoxin liver injury in weanling rats. *Arch. Pathol.,* 80:123–126.

105. Madhavan, T. V., and Gopalan, C. (1968): The effect of dietary protein on carcinogenesis of aflatoxin. *Arch. Pathol.,* 85:133–137.

106. Marshall, W. J., and McLean, A. E. M. (1969): The effect of oral phenobarbitone on hepatic microsomal cytochrome P-450 and demethylation activity in rats fed normal and low protein diets. *Biochem. Pharmacol.,* 18:153–157.

107. Maso, M., Smolin, L., and Campbell, T. C. (1977): *(Unpublished observations).*

108. McLean, A. E. M., and Day, P. A. (1974): The use of new methods to measure the effect

of diet and inducers of microsomal enzyme synthesis on cytochrome P-450 in liver homogenates, and on metabolism of dimethylnitrosamine. *Biochem. Pharmacol.,* 23:1173–1180.

109. McLean, A. E. M., and Magee, P. N. (1970): Increased renal carcinogenesis by dimethylnitrosamine in protein deficient rats. *Br. J. Exp. Pathol.,* 51:587–590.

110. McLean, A. E. M., and McLean, E. K. (1966): The effect of diet and 1,1,1-trichloro-2,2-dis (*p*-chlorophenyl) ethane (DDT) on microsomal hydroxylating enzymes and on sensitivity of rats to carbon tetrachloride poisoning. *Biochem. J.,* 100:564–571.

111. McLean, A. E. M., and McLean, E. K. (1967): Protein depletion and toxic liver injury due to carbon tetrachloride and aflatoxin. *Biochem. Soc. Proc.,* 26:13–14.

112. McPherson, F. J., Markham, A., Bridges, J. W., Hartman, G. C., and Parke, D. V. (1975): A comparison of the properties *in vitro* of biphenyl 2- and 4-hydroxylase in the mesocarp from avocado pear *(Persea americana)* and Syrian hamster hepatic tissue. *Biochem. Soc. Trans.,* 3:281–286.

113. Mgbodile, M. U. K., Hayes, J. R., and Campbell, T. C. (1973): Effect of protein deficiency on the inducibility of the hepatic microsomal drug metabolizing enzyme system. II. Effect on enzyme kinetics and electron transport system. *Biochem. Pharmacol.,* 22:1125–1132.

114. Mgbodile, M. U. K., Holscher, M., and Neal, R. A. (1975): A possible role for reduced glutathione in aflatoxin B_1 toxicity: Effect of pretreatment of rats with phenobarbital and 3-methylcholanthrene on aflatoxin toxicity. *Toxicol. Appl. Pharmacol.,* 34:128–142.

115. Miller, E. C. (1978): Some current perspectives on chemical carcinogenesis in humans and experimental animals: Presidential address. *Cancer Res.,* 38:1479–1496.

116. Miller, J. A. (1970): Carcinogenesis by chemicals: An overview. *Cancer Res.,* 30:559–576.

117. Mirvish, S. S., Cardesa, A., Wallcave, L., and Shubik, P. (1975): Induction of mouse lung adenomas by amines and ureas plus nitrite and by N-nitroso compounds: Effect of nitrite dose and of ascorbate, gallate, thiocyanate, and caffeine. *J. Natl. Cancer Inst.,* 55:633–636.

118. Mitchell, J. R. and Jollow, D. J. (1975): Metabolic activation of drugs to toxic substances. *Gastroenterology,* 68:392–410.

119. Moon, R. G., Grubbs, C. J., and Sporn, M. B. (1976): Inhibition of 7,12-dimethylbenz(a)anthracene-induced mammary carcinogenesis by rentinyl acetate. *Cancer Res.,* 36:2626–2630.

120. Nerurkar, L. S., Hayes, J. R., and Campbell, T. C. (1978): The reconstruction of hepatic microsomal mixed function oxidase activity with fractions derived from weanling rats fed different levels of protein. *J. Nutr.,* 108:678–686.

121. Norred, W. P., and Wade, A. E. (1972): Dietary fatty acid-induced alterations of hepatic microsomal drug metabolism. *Biochem. Pharmacol.,* 21:2887–2897.

122. Paine, A. J., and McLean, A. E. M. (1973): The effect of dietary protein and fat on the activity of aryl hydrocarbon hydroxylase in rat liver, kidney and lung. *Biochem. Pharmacol.,* 22:2875–2880.

123. Pantuck, E. J., Hsiao, K. C., Loub, W. D., Wattenberg, L. W., Kuntzman, R., and Conney, A. H. (1976): Stimulatory effect of vegetables on intestinal drug metabolism in the rat. *J. Pharmacol. Exp. Ther.,* 198:278–283.

124. Patterson, D. S. P., and Roberts, B. A. (1970): The formation of aflatoxin B_{2a} and G_{2a} and their degradation products during the *in vitro* detoxification of aflatoxin by livers of certain avian and mammalian species. *Food Cosmet. Toxicol.,* 8:527–538.

125. Peers, F. G., Gilman, G. A., and Linsell, C. A. (1976): Dietary aflatoxins and human liver cancer. A study in Swaziland. *Int. J. Cancer,* 17:167–176.

126. Peers, F. G., and Linsell, C. A. (1973): Dietary aflatoxins and liver cancer: A population based study in Kenya. *Br. J. Cancer,* 27:473–484.

127. Pozharisski, K. M., Dushkin, V. A., and Podoprigara, G. I. (1974): The role of microbial flora in induction of intestinal tumors in rats. *Bull. Exp. Biol. Med.* (USSR) 78:81–84.

128. Preston, R. S., Hayes, J. R., and Campbell, T. C. (1976): The effect of protein deficiency on the *in vivo* binding of aflatoxin B_1 to rat liver macromolecules. *Life Sci.,* 19:1191–1198.

129. Raj, H. G., Santhanam, K., Gupta, R. P., and Venkitasubramanian, T. A. (1975): Oxidative metabolism of aflatoxin B: observations on the formation of epoxide-glutathione conjugate. *Chem. Biol. Interact.,* 11:301–305.

130. Reddy, B. S., Mastromarino, A., and Wynder, E. L. (1975): Further leads on metabolic epidemiology of large bowel cancer. *Cancer Res.,* 35:3403–3406.

131. Reddy, B. S., Narisawa, T., Maronpot, J. H., Weisburger, J. H., and Wynder, E. L. (1975): Animal models for the study of dietary factors and cancer of the large bowel. *Cancer Res.,* 35:3421–3426.

132. Reddy, B. S., Narisawa, T., Vukusich, D., Weisburger, J. H., and Wynder, E. L. (1976): Effect of quality and quantity of dietary fat and dimethylhydrazine in colon carcinogenesis in rats. *Proc. Soc. Exp. Biol. Med.,* 151:237–239.

133. Reddy, B. S., Narisawa, T., and Weisburger, J. H. (1976): Colon carcinogenesis in germ free rats with intrarectal 1,2-dimethylhydrazine and subcutaneous azoxymethane. *Cancer Res.,* 36:2874–2876.

134. Reddy, B. S., Narisawa, T., Weisburger, J. H., and Wynder, E. L. (1976): Promoting effect of sodium deoxycholate on adenocarcinomas in germ-free rats. *J. Natl. Cancer Inst.,* 56:441–442.

135. Reddy, B. S., and Watanabe, K. (1978): Effect of intestinal microflora on 3,2'-dimethyl-4-aminobiphenyl-induced carcinogenesis in F-344 rats. *J. Natl. Cancer Inst.,* 61:1269–1271.

136. Reddy, B. S., Watanabe, K., Weisburger, J. H., and Wynder, E. L. (1977): Promoting effect of bile acids in colon carcinogenesis in germ-free and conventional F-344 rats. *Cancer Res.,* 37:3238–3242.

137. Reddy, B. S., Weisburger, J. H., and Wynder, E. L. (1974): Effects of dietary fat level and dimethylhydrazine on fecal bile acid and neutral sterol excretion and colon carcinogenesis in rats. *J. Natl. Cancer Inst.,* 52:507–511.

138. Reddy, B. S., Weisburger, J. H., and Wynder, E. L. (1974): Fecal bacterial β-glucuronidase: Control by diet. *Science,* 183:416–417.

139. Reddy, B. S., Weisburger, J. H., and Wynder, E. L. (1975): Effect of high risk and low risk diets for colon carcinogenesis on fecal microflora and steroids in man. *J. Nutr.,* 105:878–884.

140. Reddy, B. S., and Wynder, E. L. (1973): Large bowel carcinogenesis: Fecal constituents of populations with diverse incidence rates of colon cancer. *J. Natl. Cancer Inst.,* 50:1437–1442.

141. Remmer, H., Schenkman, J., and Estabrook, R. W. (1966): Drug interaction with hepatic microsomal cytochrome P-450. *Mol. Pharmacol.,* 2:187–190.

142. Renwick, A. G. (1977): Microbial metabolism of drugs. In: *Drug Metabolism From Microbe to Man,* edited by D. V. Parke and R. L. Smith, pp. 169–189. Taylor & Francis Ltd., London.

143. Reuber, M. D. (1978): Carcinogenicity of saccharin. *Environ. Health Perspect.,* 25:173–200.

144. Rogan, E., Roth, R., Katomski, P., Benderson, J., and Cavalieri, E. (1978): Binding of benzo (a)pyrene at the 1,3,6 positions to nucleic acids *in vivo* on mouse skin and *in vitro* with rat liver microsomes and nuclei. *Chem. Biol. Interact.,* 22:35–51.

145. Rogers, A. E. (1975): Variable effects of a lipotrope deficient, high fat diet on chemical carcinogenesis in rats. *Cancer Res.,* 35:2469–2474.

146. Rogers, A. E., and Newberne, P. M. (1975): Dietary effects on chemical carcinogenesis in animal models for colon and liver tumors. *Cancer Res.,* 35:3427–3431.

147. Ross, M. H., and Bras, G. (1965): Tumor incidence patterns and nutrition in the rat. *J. Nutr.,* 87:245–260.

148. Ross, M. H., and Bras, G. (1973): Influence of protein under- and over-nutrition on spontaneous tumor prevalence in the rat. *J. Nutr.,* 103:944–963.

149. Ross, M. H., Bras, G., and Ragbeer, M. S. (1970): Influence of protein and caloric intake upon spontaneous tumor incidence of the anterior pituitary gland of the rat. *J. Nutr.,* 100:177–189.

150. Schenkman, J. B., Jansson, I., and Robie-Suh, K. M. (1976): The many roles of cytochrome b_5 in hepatic microsomes. *Life Sci.,* 19:611–624.

151. Schenkman, J. B., Remmer, H., and Estabrook, R. W. (1967): Spectral studies of drug interaction with hepatic microsomal cytochrome P-450. *Mol. Pharmacol.,* 3:113–123.

152. Silverstone, H., and Tannenbaum, A. (1949): Influence of thyroid hormone on the formation of induced skin tumors in mice. *Cancer Res.,* 9:684–688.

153. Sligar, S. G., Shastry, B. S., and Gunsalus, I. C. (1977): Oxygen reactions of the P-450 heme protein. In: *Microsomes and Drug Oxidations,* edited by V. Ullrich, I. Roots, A. Hildebrandt, R. W. Estabrook, and A. H. Conney, pp. 192–201. Pergamon Press, New York.

154. Smith, N. J. (1977): Comparative detoxication of invertebrates. In: *Drug Metabolism From Microbe to Man,* edited by D. V. Parke and R. L. Smith, pp. 219–232. Taylor & Francis Ltd., London.

155. Spatz, L., and Strittmatter, P. (1971): A form of cytochrome b_5 that contains an additional hydrophobic sequence of 40 amino acid residues. *Proc. Nat. Acad. Sci. USA,* 68:1042–1046.

156. Sporn, M. B., Dunlop, N. M., Newton, D. L., and Smith, J. M. (1976): Prevention of chemical carcinogenesis by vitamin A and its synthetic analogs (retinoids). *Fed. Proc.,* 35:1332–1338.

157. Stern, K., and Willheim, R. (1943): *The Biochemistry of Malignant Tumors.* Reference Press, Brooklyn, New York.
158. Strobel, H. W., Lu, A. Y. H., Heidema, J., and Coon, M. J. (1970): Phosphatidylcholine requirement in the enzymatic reduction of hemoprotein P-450 and in fatty acid, hydrocarbon, and drug hydroxylation. *J. Biol. Chem.,* 245:4851–4854.
159. Sugimura, T., Nagao, M., Kawachi, T., Honda, M., Yahagi, T., Seino, V., Sato, S. Matsukura, N., Matsushima, T., Shirai, A., Sawamura, M., and Matsumoto, H. (1977): Mutagen-carcinogens highly mutagenic pyrolytic products in broiled foods. In: *Origins of Human Cancer, Book C,* edited by H. H. Hiatt, J. D. Watson, and J. A. Winsten, pp. 1561–1577. Cold Spring Harbor Laboratory, Cold Spring Harbor, New York.
160. Swann, P. F., and McLean, A. E. M. (1968): The effect of diet on the toxic and carcinogenic action of dimethylnitrosamine. *Biochem. J.,* 107:141.
161. Swann, P. F., and McLean, A. E. M. (1971): Cellular injury and carcinogenesis. The effect of a protein-free high-carbohydrate diet on the metabolism of dimethylnitrosamine in the rat. *Biochem. J.,* 124:283–288.
162. Swenson, D. H., Lin, J. K., Miller, E. C., and Miller, J. A. (1977): Aflatoxin B_1 2,3-oxide as a probable intermediate in the covalent binding of aflatoxins B_1 and B_2 to rat liver DNA, and ribosomal RNA *in vivo. Cancer Res.,* 37:172–181.
163. Swenson, D. H., Miller, E. C., and Miller, J. A. (1974): Aflatoxin B_1-2,3-oxide: Evidence for its formation in rat liver *in vivo* and by human liver microsomes *in vitro. Biochem. Biophys. Res. Commun.,* 60:1036–1043.
164. Swenson, D. H., Miller, J. A., and Miller, E. C. (1973): 2,3-Dihydro-2,3-dihydroxy-aflatoxin B_1: An acid hydrolysis product of an RNA-aflatoxin B_1 adduct formed by hamster and rat liver microsomes *in vitro. Biochem. Biophys. Res. Commun.,* 53:1260–1267.
165. Syrotuck, J. A., and Worthington, R. S. (1977): Nutritional effects on syngeneic tumor immunity and carcinogenesis in mice. *Fed. Proc.,* 36:1163.
166. Tannenbaum, A. (1940): Relationship of body weight to cancer incidence. *Arch. Pathol.,* 30:509–517.
167. Tannenbaum, A. (1942): The genesis and growth of tumors. II. Effects of caloric restriction *per se. Cancer Res.,* 2:460–467.
168. Tannenbaum, A. (1942): The genesis and growth of tumors. III. Effects of a high-fat diet. *Cancer Res.,* 2:468–475.
169. Tannenbaum, A. (1944): The dependence of the genesis of induced skin tumors on the caloric intake during different stages of carcinogenesis. *Cancer Res.,* 4:673–677.
170. Tannenbaum, A. (1944): The dependence of the genesis of induced skin tumors on the fat content of the diet during different stages of carcinogenesis. *Cancer Res.,* 4:683–687.
171. Tannenbaum, A. (1945): The dependence of tumor formation on the composition of the calorie restricted diet as well as on the degree of restriction. *Cancer Res.,* 5:616–625.
172. Tannenbaum, A. (1947): The role of nutrition in the origin and growth of tumors. In: *Approaches to Tumor Chemotherapy,* edited by F. R. Moulton, pp. 96–127. Science Press, Lancaster, Pa.
173. Tannenbaum, A. (1959): Nutrition and Cancer. In: *The Physiopathology of Cancer,* edited by F. Humberger, pp. 517–562. Hoeber-Harper, New York.
174. Tannenbaum, A., and Silverstone, H. (1949): The genesis and growth of tumors: IV. Effects of varying the proportion of protein (casein) in the diet. *Cancer Res.,* 9:162–173.
175. Temcharoen, P., Anukarahanonta, T., and Bhamarapravati, N. (1978): Influence of dietary protein and vitamin B_{12} on the toxicity and carcinogenicity of aflatoxins in rat liver. *Cancer Res.,* 38:2185–2190.
176. Thomas, P. E., Lu, A. Y. H., West, S. B., Ryan, D., Miwa, G. T., and Levin, W. (1977): Accessibility of cytochrome P-450 in microsomal membranes: Inhibition of metabolism by antibodies to cytochrome P-450. *Mol. Pharmacol.,* 13:819–831.
177. Ullrich, V. (1977): The mechanism of cytochrome P-450 action. In: *Microsomes and Drug Oxidations,* edited by V. Ullrich, I. Roots, A. Hildebrandt, R. W. Estabrook, and A. H. Conney, pp. 192–201, Pergamon Press, New York.
178. Vessey, D. A., and Zakim, D. (1971): Regulation of microsomal enzymes by phospholipids: II. Activation of hepatic uridine diphosphate-glucuronyltransferase. *J. Biol. Chem.,* 246:4649–4656.
179. Visek, W. J., Clinton, S. K., and Truex, C. R. (1978): Nutrition and experimental carcinogenesis. *Cornell Vet.,* 68:3–39.

180. Vitale, J. J., and Good, R. A. (eds.). (1974): Nutrition and immunology. Symposium on nutrition and immunology. *Am. J. Clin. Nutr.,* 27:623–669.
181. Viviani, A., and Lutz, W. K. (1978): Modulation of the binding of the carcinogen benzo(a)pyrene to rat liver DNA *in vivo* by selective induction of microsomal and nuclear aryl hydrocarbon hydroxylase activity. *Cancer Res.,* 38:4640–4644.
182. Watanabe, K., Reddy, B. S., and Kirtchevsky, D. (1978): Effect of various dietary fibers and food additives on azoxymethane or methylnitroso-urea-induced colon carcinogenesis in rats. *Fed. Proc.,* 37:262.
183. Watanabe, K., Reddy, B. S., Wong, C. Q., and Weisburger, J. H. (1978): Effect of dietary undegraded carrogeenan on colon carcinogenesis in F-344 rats treated with azoxymethane or methylnitrosourea. *Cancer Res.,* 38:4427–4430.
184. Wattenberg, L. W. (1971): Studies of polycyclic hydrocarbon hydroxylases of the intestine possibly related to cancer: Effect of diet on benzpyrene hydroxylase activity. *Cancer,* 20:99–102.
185. Wattenberg, L. W. (1972): Inhibition of carcinogenic and toxic effects of polycyclic hydrocarbons by phenolic antioxidants and ethoxyquin. *J. Natl. Cancer Inst.,* 48:1425–1430.
186. Wattenberg, L. W. (1975): Effects of dietary constituents on the metabolism of carcinogens. *Cancer Res.,* 35:3326–3331.
187. Wattenberg, L. W., Lam, L. K. T., Speier, J. L., Loub, W. D., and Borchert, P. (1977): Inhibitors of chemical carcinogenesis. In: *Origins of Human Cancer, Book B,* edited by H. H. Hiatt, J. D. Watson, and J. A. Winsten, pp. 785–799. Cold Spring Harbor Laboratory, Cold Spring Harbor, New York.
188. Wattenberg, L. W., and Loub, W. D. (1978): Inhibition of polycyclic aromatic hydrocarbon induced neoplasia by naturally occurring indoles. *Cancer Res.,* 38:1410–1413.
189. Wattenberg, L. W., Loub, W. D., Lam, L. K., and Speier, J. L. (1976): Dietary constituents altering the responses to chemical carcinogens. *Fed. Proc.,* 35:1327–1331.
190. Waxler, S. H. (1960): Obesity and cancer susceptibility in mice. *Am. J. Clin. Nutr.,* 8:760–766.
191. Weisburger, E. K., Evarts, R. P., and Wenk, M. L. (1977): Inhibitory effect of butylated hydroxytoluene (BHT) on intestinal carcinogenesis in rats by azoxymethane. *Food Cosmet. Toxicol.,* 15:139–141.
192. Wells, P., Aftergood, L., and Alfin-Slater, R. B. (1976): Effect of varying levels of dietary protein on tumor development and lipid metabolism in rats exposed to aflatoxin. *J. Am. Oil Chem. Soc.,* 53:559–562.
193. White, F. R., and White, J. (1944): Effect of a low lysine diet on mammary tumor formation in strain C3H mice. *J. Natl. Cancer Inst.,* 5:41–42.
194. White, F. R., and White, J. (1944): Effect of diethylstilbestrol on mammary tumor formation in strain C3H mice fed a low cystine diet. *J. Natl. Cancer Inst.,* 4:413–415.
195. White, J., and Andervont, H. B. (1943): Effect of a diet relatively low in cystine on the production of spontaneous mammary-gland tumors in strain C3H female mice. *J. Natl. Cancer Inst.,* 3:449–451.
196. White, J., and Mider, G. B. (1941): The effect of dietary cystine on the reaction of dilute brown mice to methylcholanthrene (preliminary report). *J. Natl. Cancer Inst.,* 2:95–97.
197. Wilson, R. B., Hutcheson, D. P., and Widerman, L. (1977): Dimethylhydrazine induced colon tumors in rats fed beef fat or corn oil with and without wheat bran. *Am. J. Clin. Nutr.,* 30:176–181.
198. Wood, G. C., and Woodcock, B. G. (1970): Effects of dietary protein deficiency on the conjugation of foreign compounds in rat liver. *J. Pharm. Pharmacol.,* 22:605–635.
199. Woodcock, B. G., and Wood, G. C. (1971): Effect of protein-free diet on UDP-glucuronyl transferase and sulfotransferase activities in rat liver. *Biochem. Pharmacol.,* 20:2703–2713.
200. Wynder, E. L. (1975): The epidemiology of large bowel cancer. *Cancer Res.,* 35:3388–3394.
201. Wynder, E. L. (1975): Status of research on nutrition and cancer: concluding remarks. *Cancer Res.,* 35:3548–3550.
202. Wynder, E. L. (1976): Nutrition and cancer. *Fed. Proc.,* 35:1309–1315.
203. Wynder, E. L., and Reddy, B. S. (1974): The epidemiology of cancer of the large bowel. *Am. J. Dig. Dis.,* 19:937–946.
204. Yang, C. S. (1977): The organization and interaction of monooxygenase enzymes in the microsomal membrane. *Life Sci.,* 21:1047–1058.

Carcinogenesis, Vol. 5: Modifiers of Chemical
Carcinogenesis, edited by T. J. Slaga.
Raven Press, New York, 1980.

12

Cancer: Etiology, Mechanisms, and Prevention— A Summary

Thomas J. Slaga

*Cancer and Toxicology Program, Biology Division, Oak Ridge National Laboratory,
Oak Ridge, Tennessee 37830*

Based on knowledge derived from epidemiological studies, it is currently thought that the majority of cancers in humans are caused by environmental factors. Table 1 shows the major environmental factors that are thought to be associated with specific cancers in the human population. Other than skin cancer for which solar ultraviolet light is an important causative factor (14), emphasis has been placed on environmental chemicals as major factors in the cause of cancer in man. Along with the epidemiological data, studies with experimental animals have provided evidence that some chemicals in our environment are responsible for a significant proportion of such cancers. The role of diet as an important environmental factor in the etiology of cancer will be discussed later in this chapter.

Although there are two major classes of chemicals that induce cancer, i.e., direct acting carcinogens and indirect carcinogens requiring metabolic activation by cells, most are related to the latter category. Table 2 summarizes some of the more important direct and indirect carcinogenic compounds. Shown in Table 3 are the chemicals that are generally recognized as carcinogens in the human and the sites where they cause tumors. As can be seen, the majority of chemicals related to cancers in humans have to be metabolized before they are active as described in detail in Chapter 1 *of this volume.* In addition to the chemicals generally recognized as carcinogens in humans as a result of industrial, medical, and societal exposures, a number of other chemicals in the environment, such as aflatoxin B_1 (AFB_1) and certain N-nitrosamines and N-nitrosamides are strongly suspected of causing cancer (21,26). It appears likely that additional chemical carcinogens of both natural and synthetic origin will be identified as cancer causing.

TABLE 1. *Epidemiological studies have implicated certain environmental factors in the development of tumors in humans*

Target	Environmental factors
Skin	Environmental chemicals
	Sunlight
	Occupation
Head and neck	Smoking
	Smoking and alcohol
	Occupation
Stomach	Diet
	Direct and indirect food additives
Liver	Diet
	Occupation
	Prescription drugs
Leukemia	Radiation
	Occupation
Thyroid	Radiation
Bone	Occupation
Lungs	Smoking
	Air pollution
	Smoking and alcohol
	Occupation
Colon	Diet
Bladder	Smoking
	Prescription drugs
	Occupation
Vagina	Prescription drugs
Cervix	Social habits

TABLE 2. *Carcinogenic compounds and metabolic activation*

Substances that do not require metabolic activation
   Biological alkylating agents
      S-mustards, *N*-mustards, epoxides, arizidines, alkyl alkanes, sulfonates, strained ring lactones, nitrosamides
   Inorganic chemicals
      Certain metals and metalloids, asbestos.
   Radiochemicals

Substances that do require metabolic activation
   Polycyclic aromatic hydrocarbons
      Carbocyclic compounds, heterocyclic analogues
   Aromatic amines
      Carbocyclic compounds, heterocyclic amino and nitrocompounds, aminoazo-compounds
   Nitrosamines
   Hydrazines
      Hydrazine, alkyl hydrazines, alkyl azocompounds, alkyl azoxy-compounds
   Hormones and related substances
      Estrogens, goitrogens
   Miscellaneous
      Urethane, carbon tetrachloride, DDT, dieldrin, mycotoxins (aflatoxin), cycasin, vinyl chloride, ethionine, safrole, pyrrolizidine alkaloids, mitomycin C

TABLE 3. *Chemicals considered as carcinogens in the human[a]*

Chemical	Sites of tumor formation
Industrial exposures	
2(or β)-naphthylamine	Urinary bladder
benzidine(4,4'-diaminobiphenyl)	Urinary bladder
4-aminobiphenyl and 4-nitrobiphenyl	Urinary bladder
bis(chloromethyl) ether	Lungs
bis(2-chloroethyl) sulfide	Respiratory tract
vinyl chloride	Liver mesenchyme
certain soots, tars, oils	Skin, lungs
chromium compounds	Lungs
nickel compounds	Lungs, nasal sinuses
asbestos	Pleura, peritoneum
asbestos plus cigarette smoking	Lungs, pleura, peritoneum
benzene	Bone marrow
mustard gas	Respiratory system
Medical exposures	
N,N-bis(2-chloroethyl)-2-naphthylamine	
(chlornapthazine)	Urinary bladder
diethylstilbestrol	Vagina
estrogenic steroids	Breast and uterus
Societal	
cigarette smoke	Lungs, urinary tract, pancreas
betel nut and tobacco quids	Buccal mucosa

[a] See refs. 20 and 27 for details.

TWO-STAGE OR MULTISTAGE CARCINOGENESIS

Current information suggest that chemical carcinogenesis is a multistep process with one of the best studied models in this regard being the two-stage carcinogenesis system using mouse skin. Table 4 summarizes some aspects of carcinogenesis in experimental animals. The initiation phase requires only a single application of either a direct or indirect carcinogen at a subthreshold dose and is essentially irreversible, whereas the promotion phase is brought about by repetitive treatments after initiation and is initially reversible, later becoming irreversible. This system has not only provided an important model for studying carcinogenesis and for bioassaying carcinogenic agents, but it is

TABLE 4. *Carcinogenesis in experimental animals and man*

Complete carcinogenesis
Cocarcinogenesis
Tumor initiation
Tumor promotion
Additive effects of carcinogens, tumor initiators, and promoters
Coinitiating agents
Copromoting agents

TABLE 5. *Two-stage carcinogenesis systems*

Organ system	Tumor initiators	Tumor promoters
Mouse skin	PAH Direct-acting electrophiles	Croton oil, phorbol esters, fatty acids and fatty acid esters, surface-active agents, linear long-chain alkanes, tobacco smoke condensate and extracts of unburned tobacco, certain euphorbia macrocyclic diterpenes, citrus oil, anthralin and other phenols.
Rat and mouse liver	2-Acetylaminofluorene, diethylnitrosamine, 2-methyl-N,N-dimethyl-4-aminoazobenzene	Phenobarbital, DDT, BHT, PCB
Mouse lung	Urethan, PAH	BHT, phorbol
Rat colon	Dimethylhydrazine	Bile acids, high-fat diet, high-cholesterol diet
Rat bladder	N-methyl-N-nitrosourea	Saccharin, cyclamate
Rat and mouse mammary gland	PAH	Hormones, high-fat diet, phorbol
Rat stomach	N-methyl-N'-nitro-N-nitrosoguanidine	Surfactants
Rat esophagus	Diethylnitrosamine	Diet
Mouse cell culture systems	PAH, radiation	Phorbol esters, saccharin
Rat tracheal cell culture system	N-methyl-N'-nitro-N-nitrosoguanidine	Phorbol esters

also one of the best systems for investigating the effects of inhibitors of chemical carcinogenesis.

Recently, the generality of the two-stage system or multistage carcinogenesis has been shown to exist in a number of systems besides the skin such as the liver, lung, bladder, colon, esophagus, stomach, mammary, transplacental, as well as cells in culture (36). The various two-stage systems known and the

TABLE 6. *Possible tumor promoters and/or cocarcinogens in man*

Alcohol
Asbestos
Smoking
High-fat, protein, and caloric content of food
Vitamin deficiencies
Unnatural balance of endogenous hormones
Exogenous hormones, diethylstilbesterol (DES)
Diterpenes from plant sources (tea, etc.)
Environmental chemicals such as hydrocarbons and chlorinated hydrocarbons
Drugs
Radiation
Viruses

initiating and promoting agents involved in each system are shown in Table 5 (36). As is apparent, quite a diversity of promoting agents exists among the various two-stage systems. Table 6 summarizes the possible tumor promoters and cocarcinogens related to cancers in humans (36). This does not mean, however, that some of these agents are not carcinogens. Current information suggests that alcohol, smoking, asbestos, diet, and an imbalance of endogenous hormones are associated with a large percentage of cancer in man (50,51).

GENERAL MODIFIERS OF CHEMICAL CARCINOGENESIS

There are also a number of general factors that have been shown to play a modifying role in chemical carcinogenesis in experimental animals, and, more than likely, these factors play similar roles in cancer in man. These factors are shown in Table 7. As stated in Chapter 6 of this volume, a number of other carcinogens can have an additive, synergistic, or inhibitory effect on the carcinogenic activity of a given carcinogen. Chapters 1, 3, 4, and 8 detail the influence various modifiers have on the metabolism of chemical carcinogens. There are agents that can inhibit chemical carcinogenesis by counteracting the metabolism of the carcinogen as well as by increasing the metabolism of the carcinogen but favoring detoxification. This will be discussed in more detail later in this chapter when some anticarcinogenic agents are discussed.

An important determinant of whether a cell becomes initiated by a chemical carcinogen or not is DNA repair. Inhibition of the excision repair system allows a greater chance that the carcinogenic damage will not be repaired, thus leading to the irreversible initiated carcinogenic state. Likewise, as discussed in Chapter 7, inhibition or induction of error prone DNA repair could lead to a drastic modification of the carcinogenesis process.

Age is known to have quite a modifying influence on carcinogenesis with

TABLE 7. *General factors or modifiers*
of chemical carcinogenesis

Other chemical carcinogens
Metabolism of carcinogen (activation vs. detoxification)
Anticarcinogenic chemicals
DNA repair
Age
Sex
Hormonal
Immunological
Trauma
Radiation
Viral
Cocarcinogenesis and tumor promotion
Diet, nutrition, and life style
Genetic constitution

the noted correlations between the incidence of cancer and aging of a population (31). Likewise, Van Duuren and his associates demonstrated a small but general decrease in the rate of tumor production with an increasing age at the time of tumor promotion (45). On the other hand, when the mouse skin of both young and old animals was treated with several applications of 7,12-dimethyl-benz(a)anthracene (DMBA) and then grafted to young recipients, a higher incidence of carcinoma developed in grafts from old donors than from young (12). These experiments suggest that adult tissue is more prone toward tumor initiation because of either a faulty DNA repair system or a greater DNA error prone system and is less susceptible to tumor promotion whereas the reverse appears to be true in newborn tissue.

Sex and hormones are known to also have a modifying influence on tumor growth. Mammary tumors in rats are essentially always hormone dependent. For example, breast tumors in rats regress following the removal of the ovaries showing the cocarcinogenic effect of female sex hormones (6,19). A similar situation has been observed with prostate cancer and the male sex hormones (6). Besides the sex hormones, the pituitary is decisive in tumor growth. Instead of removing the ovaries, one can extirpate the pituitary in order to stop mammary carcinomas. It is also well known that the sex of the animal is important in carcinogenesis by certain chemicals. 2-Acetylaminofluorene (AAF) is a potent liver carcinogen in male rats but not females (26). If the testes and thyroid are removed from rats, they will not develop liver cancer; however, AAF will induce hepatomas after supplementary dosing with testosterone and thyroxine (19).

It is well known that the immunological status of the animal is also an important factor in chemical carcinogenesis. It has been shown that Baccillus Calmette-Guerin (BCG) vaccination reduces the carcinogenic effect of both carcinogens and promoters (30,32). It is thought that BCG vaccination exerts its effect on neoplasms through the nonspecific enhancement of the immunologic surveillance mechanism of the host (30). It has been suggested that the establishment and proliferation of malignant neoplasms may result from the inability of the host to recognize the tumor immunologically as foreign and thus destroy it (24). Experiments have shown that substances that alone cause cancer and substances that can act only to promote cancer, such as croton oil and phorbol esters, are immunosuppressive agents (5,37,39). It should be pointed out that the potent antipromoting steroids are also potent immunosuppressive agents (33). However, the antipromoting ability of glucocorticoids appears to be related to some early effect on tumor promotion not involving the immune system. In fact, if the glucocorticoids are applied topically to existing carcinomas and papillomas, they appear to enhance their progression (33). The demonstration of tumor-associated transplantation antigens in the majority of the malignancies studied (24,39) and the presence in the tumor-bearing host of concomitant immune reactions against those antigens (24) have led to theories suggesting that the immune system plays a major role as a protection against malignancy (39).

Thus, in all the presentations of the "immune surveillance" theory, the effects of immunodepression (thymectomy and other procedures and drugs) favoring tumor development are quoted as experimental evidence that some sort of control of tumor development is exerted by the intact immune system (39). Such immune surveillance theories would predict a high risk of tumor development in the athymic-nude mice. However, Stutman's results do not support that prediction, since tumor incidence after exposure to 3-methylcholanthrene (MCA) at birth were similar in the immunologically normal nude heterozygotes and the immunologically deficient athymic-nude homozygotes (39).

The relationship of trauma and cancer is also well known. Any long-lasting wound or sore is considered a potential site for cancer and is thus listed as one of the warning signs. It has been shown that wound healing alone can promote the formation of skin tumors initiated by DMBA (20). As pointed out in Chapter 6 of this volume, inflammation and cellular proliferation are related to chemically induced cancer. Chemical carcinogens and tumor promoters induce inflammation and hyperplasia in mouse skin, but it is also known that not all inflammatory-hyperplastic agents cause skin cancer or promote it (35).

The role of radiation alone or in combination with carcinogenic chemicals in the etiology of skin cancer has been known for a long time. A correlation has been noted between the occurrence of skin cancer and ultraviolet light exposure with the incidence notably higher in sunny regions, in outdoor workers, in people with fair complexions as well as in the more exposed skin areas (14). The first report of a suspected interaction between radiation and chemical carcinogens in humans was related to the high incidence of skin cancer among sailors which was thought to be caused by a combination of the high doses of sunlight and coal tar to which they were exposed. More recently, epidemiological studies of uranium miners have indicated an interaction between ionizing radiation and cigarette smoke (3). Both alone and to some extent in combination with chemical carcinogens and tumor promoters, the role of both ultraviolet and ionizing radiation in the induction of skin cancer, as well as other cancers in experimental animals, has been extensively studied (14,38,44). It is quite apparent from these studies that when either ultraviolet or ionizing radiation is combined with chemical carcinogens, the times of tumor appearance are accelerated and/or the tumor incidence are increased. Although both ultraviolet and ionizing radiation have been shown to be either promoting or enhancing agents for chemically initiated tumors and initiating agents for chemically promoted tumors, their primary influence appears to be related to their tumor expression or tumor-promoting activities rather than initiation. Chapter 9 goes into detail concerning the interactions of chemicals and radiation in inducing cancer.

Experiments dealing with the interaction between viruses and chemical carcinogens were carried out soon after the first tumor viruses were isolated (see ref. 9). Such interactions generally result in a higher incidence of tumors in animals exposed to both agents than in animals exposed to either agent alone. Chapter 10 of this volume discusses these interactions in detail. Although studies related to the induction of cancer by a combination of chemicals, viruses, and radiation have not been done, such investigations may indeed reveal a closer relationship among chemical, viral, and radiation carcinogenesis.

Diet and nutrition are important modifying factors of chemical carcinogenesis in experimental animals as well as in cancer in humans (50). These factors, plus cocarcinogenesis and tumor promotion will be discussed in more detail later in this chapter. Suffice it to say, diet appears to be more a cocarcinogen and/or a tumor promoter in carcinogenesis than the causative agent. Epidemiological studies have revealed that there are notable differences in the incidence of specific cancers from country to country and even within countries (2,11). These differences in the geographic incidence of cancer do not appear to be primarily genetically determined since the cancer patterns for migrants from one country to another generally change from those characteristics of the mother country to those of the inhabitants of the new country.

Although the above studies suggest that the genetic makeup of an individual appears not to be primarily important in certain cancer patterns, it is well known that the genetic constitution of a person can make him prone to cancer. Not to be mistaken as a contradiction, the changing patterns of cancer related to migrants appear to be related to the diet and life style of the individual which act more as cocarcinogens and/or tumor promoters (51). If a migrant adopts the cancer-related diet of a country and was genetically prone to cancer, there probably would be a good chance that the migrant would develop the diet-related cancer; however, if the migrant was not genetically prone, he probably would not develop the diet-related cancer. In the above situation the new diet promoted the cancer. Promotion is probably the rate limiting factor in cancer since we are all more than likely initiated because of the large number of initiating agents present in our environment.

It is well known that there are several genetically determined diseases such as xeroderma pigmentosum (XP), Fanconi's anemia, Bloom's syndrome, ataxia-telangiectasia and porokeratosis Mibelli in which individuals have an increased if not invariable incidence of cancer (16,18). These diseases are associated with DNA repair defects, thought to be the cause of the cancer sensitivity (18). In the case of a person with XP, the oversensitivity of the skin to ultraviolet light is inherited and the condition leads to skin cancer.

Furthermore, it is well known that mice can be bred with high and low sensitivity to chemical carcinogens. Boutwell (6) accomplished this by stressing mice with DMBA-promoter two-stage system of tumorigenesis and then selecting for sensitivity and resistance to the carcinogenic treatment for eight generations. The outcome is a remarkable sensitivity and resistance to the chemical induction of cancer. These and other experiments force us to conclude that chemical induction of cancer is also dependent on the genetic constitution of the animal (16). Here, as with spontaneous tumors, genetic constitution can mean many things, among them the loss of the capability to activate carcinogens, faulty DNA repair, and incompetent immune system.

TUMOR INITIATION

As stated earlier, the tumor-initiation phase appears to be an irreversible step which probably involves a somatic cell mutation as evidenced by a good correlation between the carcinogenicity of many chemical carcinogens and their mutagenic activities (1,25). Most tumor-initiating agents either generate or are metabolically converted to electrophilic reactants, that bind covalently to cellular DNA and other macromolecules (19,26). Previous studies have demonstrated a good correlation between the carcinogenicity of several polycyclic aromatic hydrocarbons (PAH) and their ability to bind covalently to DNA (7,34). Recent data suggest that the "bay region" diol epoxide is the ultimate carcinogenic form of PAH carcinogens that react with DNA (22,23). The Millers have proposed a significant general theory to explain the initial event in chemical carcinogenesis which states that all chemical carcinogens that are not electrophilic reactants must be converted metabolically into a chemically reactive electrophilic

TABLE 8. *Millers' unifying theory on chemical carcinogenesis*

All chemical carcinogens that are not themselves chemically reactive must be converted metabolically into a chemically reactive form

The activated metabolite is an electrophilic reagent

This activated metabolite reacts with nucleophilic groups in cellular macromolecules to initiate carcinogenesis

form that then reacts with some critical macromolecule to initiate the carcinogenic process (26,27). This unifying theory on chemical carcinogenesis is depicted in Table 8.

COCARCINOGENESIS AND TUMOR PROMOTION

The term cocarcinogenic action means the augmentation of carcinogenesis by a noncarcinogenic agent applied concomitantly with a carcinogen (36). A promoting agent is one applied repeatedly after a single dose of a tumor-initiating agent that results in tumors (36). Tumor promoters can be either weak carcinogens or noncarcinogens. Some cocarcinogens such as croton oil, phorbol esters, and anthralin are also tumor promoters. A cocarcinogen primarily has an influence on the initiation of the carcinogenic response through an effect on the carcinogen (permeability, metabolism, or repairability of the carcinogenic damage) or the target tissue (for example, hormonal stimulation of mammary gland growth and croton oil stimulation of epidermal growth). A wide variety of agents have been found to be cocarcinogenic in experimental animals such as aliphatic hydrocarbons, aromatic hydrocarbons, phenols, long-chain acids, alcohols, hormones, radiation, viruses, food additives, and diet (36). Table 9 lists some of the more important cocarcinogenic agents that have been tested (36,46). Owing primarily to the ease of determining cocarcinogens as well as promoters in the skin system, most of the cocarcinogens have been discovered using that system.

Refer to Table 5 which summarizes the various two-stage systems used and the various promoting agents associated with them. In many cases, it is difficult to distinguish between a cocarcinogen or a promoter because many of the agents have not been critically tested.

The phorbol ester tumor promoters are the most potent of the known tumor promoters, having been shown to have many cellular and biochemical effects (36). Some of the most important effects which seem to be intimately associated with the phorbol ester tumor promoters' action are as follows: (a) They induce changes in the phenotype of normal cells that mimic features of transformed cells. (b) They induce dedifferentiation of adult epidermal cells to embryonic looking cells. (c) They induce a 200- to 400-fold increase in epidermal ornithine decarboxylase activity which specifically correlates with tumor promotion. (d) They induce protease activity. (e) They stimulate phospholipid synthesis and DNA, RNA, and protein synthesis. (f) They stimulate cellular proliferation.

TABLE 9. *Cocarcinogens in various tissues*

Skin	
catechol	benzo(g,h,i)perylene
pyrogallol	anthralin
lauryl alcohol	croton oil
decane	phorbol esters
undecane	phenols
tetradecane	nicotine
n-dodecane	surfactants
pyrene	radiation
benzo(*e*)pyrene	viruses
fluoranthene	
Lung	
asbestos	ferric oxide
radiation	magnesium oxide
n-dodecane	hypoxia
Mammary gland	
hormones	prolactin
estradiol	
Bladder	
L-tryptophan	cyclamate
saccharin	
Cheek pouch	
X-radiation	croton oil
Liver	
cyclopropenoid fatty acids	alcohol

(g) They inhibit terminal differentiation not only in the skin but in other cellular systems such as Friend erythroleukemic cells, chicken myoblasts, and neuroblastoma cells (36). Chapter 2 discusses the phorbol esters in more detail. Only a limited number of studies have been performed concerning the mechanism by which other tumor promoters act. Both phenobarbitol and BHT (butylated hydroxytoluene) stimulate DNA synthesis followed by cell proliferation in the liver and lung, respectively (29,49).

ANTICARCINOGENESIS BY CHEMICALS

Although prevention of the exposure of man to carcinogens is theoretically the best way to reduce cancer incidence, such an approach is not practical for obvious reasons. Therefore, alternative means of modifying the process of carcinogenesis in man must be found and since carcinogenesis is a prolonged multistage process, a variety of approaches may be considered toward the inhibition of either the initiation or the promotion phases. Table 10 summarizes various chemical agents used to inhibit complete chemical carcinogenesis; however, such a system does not allow one to determine at what stage of carcinogenesis these agents inhibit.

Using the two-stage skin tumorigenesis system, one can specifically study the effects of potential inhibitors on both the initiation and the promotion phases. Studies have been performed on many compounds that have the capacity to inhibit tumor initiation by either (a) alteration of the metabolism of the carcinogen (decreased activation and/or increased detoxification), (b) scavenging of active molecular species of carcinogens to prevent their reaching critical target sites in the cells, or (c) competitive inhibition. In addition, there have been a number of studies on compounds that inhibit promotion or the progression of cancer by altering the state of differentiation, inhibiting the promoter-induced cellular proliferation, or preventing gene activation by the tumor promoters. Table 11 summarizes the potent inhibitors of tumor initiation by various chemical carcinogens. 5,6-Benzoflavone and quercetin have been found to be inhibitory to skin, lung, and mammary carcinogenesis, whereas 7,8-benzoflavone inhibits skin carcinogenesis caused by some PAH and enhances carcinogenesis by others (see Chapter 3). The antioxidants butylated hydroxyanisole (BHA) and butylated hydroxytoluene (BHT) are widely used as food preservatives and have been

TABLE 10. *Inhibitors of complete chemical carcinogenesis*

Retinoids
Protease inhibitors; leupeptin, antipain
Antioxidants: BHT, BHA, ethoxyquin, disulfuran, and selenium
Flavones
Vitamin A, B2, C, and E
Antiinflammatory steroids
Poly 1:C

TABLE 11. *Inhibitors of tumor initiation*

Antioxidants: BHT, BHA, and selenium
Flavones: 7,8-benzoflavone, 5,6-benzoflavone, and quercetin
Vitamins: A, C, and E
Certain noncarcinogenic PAH: dibenz(*a,c*)anthracene, benz(*a*)anthracene, benzo(*e*)pyrene, and pyrene
Environmental contaminants: TCDD and PCB
Sulfur mustard
Poly I:C
Antiinflammatory steroids

---

shown to inhibit skin, lung, mammary, forestomach, colon, and liver cancer in experimental animals induced by a wide range of chemicals (see Chapter 4). BHT has also been shown to act as a tumor promoter in the lung and liver (29,49). Similar inhibitory results have been found for selenium and vitamins C and E. In addition, Vitamin C (ascorbic acid) blocks nitrosamine formation from secondary amines and nitrite in the acid environment of the stomach, by causing breakdown of nitrite (28). Certain chemicals in cruciferous plants (brussel sprouts, cabbage, and cauliflower) and citrus fruits are potent inducers of the mixed-function oxidase system (48). These chemicals have been shown to inhibit carcinogenesis by favoring detoxification of carcinogens. Certain noncarcinogenic PAH are potent inducers of the metabolism (favoring detoxification) of carcinogenic PAH, thus causing a decreased carcinogenic response. This is epitomized by the environmental contaminants 2,3,7,8-tetrachlorodibenzo-*p*-dioxin (TCDD) and polychlorobiphenyls (PCB) which are extremely potent inducers of PAH carcinogen metabolism and potent inhibitors of their carcinogenic effect (see Chapter 8). Although TCDD is one of the most toxic agents known, its inhibitory effect on PAH carcinogenesis is at nontoxic dose levels. Some of the flavones and antioxidants appear to inhibit carcinogenesis by inhibiting the metabolism of the carcinogen to its ultimate carcinogenic form. The noncarcino-

TABLE 12. *Inhibitors of phorbol ester skin tumor promotion*

Antiinflammatory steroids: cortisol, dexamethasone, and fluocinolone acetonide
Vitamin A derivatives
Combination of retinoids and antiinflammatory agents
Protease inhibitors: Tosyl lysine chloromethyl ketone (TLCK); tosyl arginine methyl ester (TAME); tosyl phanylalanine chloromethyl ketone (TPCK); antipain and leupeptin
Cyclic nucleotides
DMSO
Butyrate
BCG
Poly I:C

---

genic PAH and the environmental contaminants appear to inhibit skin carcinogenesis by inducing the metabolism of the carcinogen to detoxified products. Sulfur mustard inhibits tumor initiation by actually killing the initiated cells (10). The polyinosinic:polycytidylic acid (Poly I:C) and anti-inflammatory steroids appear to inhibit tumor initiation by slowing down carcinogen metabolism by their antigrowth effect (17,43). Some of the agents listed in Table 11 have been shown to inhibit carcinogenesis in a number of tissues and against a variety of chemical carcinogens, indicating they may be useful agents in the chemoprevention of cancer in man.

Table 12 summarizes the potent inhibitors of skin tumor promotion in mice by phorbol ester tumor promoters. The anti-inflammatory steroid fluocinolone acetonide has been found to be an extremely potent inhibitor of phorbol ester tumor promotion in mouse skin (see Chapter 6). Repeated applications of as little as 0.01 μg almost completely counteract the skin tumorigenesis. Fluocinolone acetonide also effectively counteracts the tumor promoter-induced cellular proliferation. Certain retinoids have also been found to be potent inhibitors of

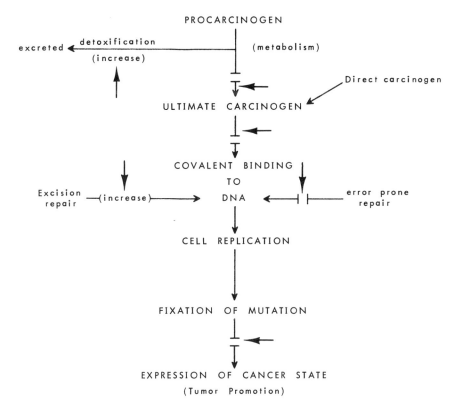

FIG. 1. Illustration of potential sites of action of inhibitors of chemical carcinogenesis. Bold face arrows represent sites where inhibitors may be effective.

mouse skin tumor promotion. In addition, Sporn and co-workers (see Chapter 5) have found that certain retinoids are potent inhibitors of lung, mammary, bladder, and colon carcinogenesis. Verma and co-workers (47) have shown that certain retinoids are potent inhibitors of phorbol ester-induced epidermal ornithine decarboxylase activity. This, plus their effect on epithelial differentiation, appears to be related to their anticarcinogenic effect. Recently it has been found that a combination of fluocinolone acetonide and retinoids produce an inhibitory effect on skin tumor promotion greater than that produced by each separately (see Chapter 6). Belman and Troll (4) have found that protease inhibitors, cyclic nucleotides, DMSO (dimethyl sulfoxide) and butyrate also inhibit mouse skin tumor promotion by phorbol esters. Schinitsky and co-workers (32) reported the inhibitory effect of BCG vaccination on skin tumor promotion. It has been shown that Poly I:C has an inhibitory effect on carcinogenesis and tumor promotion (13,17). This appears to be mediated by its inhibition of promoter and carcinogen induced cell proliferation (47).

In general, Fig. 1 depicts where both the antiinitiators and antipromoters are effective in counteracting chemical carcinogenesis. The bold-face arrows illustrate where these inhibitors are effective.

The results presented here suggest that certain flavones (5,6-benzoflavone and quercetin), antioxidants (BHA, selenium and Vitamins C and E), noncarcinogenic hydrocarbons, antiinflammatory steroids, retinoids, and protease inhibitors may be useful agents in the chemoprevention of cancer in man. Combinations of some of the above agents at very low, nontoxic doses may be a rational approach to the prevention of cancer because of their multiple points of attack.

DIET, NUTRITION, LIFE STYLE, AND CANCER

As stated earlier, there is increasing epidemiological evidence that diet, nutrition, and life style play significant roles in the pathogenesis of several types of human cancer (see also Table 1). Table 3 summarizes the various chemicals known at present to be associated with some occupational cancers, with more and more being added to such a list yearly. The relationship between life style and cancer is illustrated in Table 13, with many of these conclusions supported by results from experimental animal studies. It should be emphasized that smoking is the single most important known cause of cancer in the United States today with some 100,000 Americans dying of cancer each year because of their use of tobacco products (6). Equally alarming, the number of deaths from cardiovascular diseases associated with smoking is even greater. There is considerable epidemiological evidence showing that alcoholism, and the associated nutritional deficiencies, significantly increases the risk of smokers to cancer of the alimentary tract (51). Experimental animal studies have shown that the tumorigenic activity of tobacco smoke condensate depends on a close interaction of tumor initiators, cocarcinogens, and promoters (51). Nevertheless, analysis of the data related

TABLE 13. *Cancer and life style*

Colon cancer: acculturated Hawaiian Japanese whose diet includes beef and legumes
Colon cancer: overrefined carbohydrates, lack of roughage (developed vs. underdeveloped countries)
Esophageal cancer: pickled vegetables with nitrosamines (China)
Buccal cavity, pharynx, esophagus and liver cancer: alcohol
Lung cancer: smoking and asbestos
Oral and esophageal cancer: smoking and drinking alcohol
Skin cancer: drinking well water with arsenic traces (Taiwan)
Skin cancer: agricultural workers
Skin, respiratory system, and bladder cancers: occupational cancer (industry), highest rates of cancer (big cities)
Stomach cancer: more common in countries without refrigeration
Stomach cancer: smoked food
Bladder cancer: coffee and smoking
Breast, uterine, prostate, testis, and kidney cancer: increased fat consumption
Favorable cancer rates for Seventh Day Adventists and Mormons

to the decline of lung cancer in exsmokers suggests more tumor promoting activity of cigarette smoke than that of potent initiating activity (51).

The evidence indicating a relationship between diet and cancer comes from studies showing a wide variation in the incidence of cancer in particular populations or ethnic groups in different geographic areas and change in cancer risk of migrant populations as they assume the dietary habits of either a high or a low risk population (2). Investigations are currently under way to determine the particular dietary factors and regimens that may be responsible for these differences. This is no doubt a complex problem since potential carcinogenic contaminants including pesticides, herbicides, mycotoxins, environmental pollutants, and synthetic hormones may be ingested in food or drink and each component of the diet including proteins, carbohydrates, fats, vitamins, and trace elements may individually or in combination modify carcinogenesis. Furthermore, the extensive use of food additives for purposes of improving food color, flavor, texture, preservation, or nutritive value provides the opportunity for the introduction into foods of potential carcinogens, cocarcinogens, and/or promoters. The magnitude of the role these contaminating agents play in cancer is at present not known.

Nutritional influences may occur in three ways: (a) nutrients, food additive, or contaminants acting as complete carcinogens, tumor initiators, cocarcinogens and/or promoters, (b) dietary deficiencies that influence the initiation or the promotion of the neoplastic process, and (c) nutritional excesses (calories, protein, fats, etc.) inducing a variety of metabolic abnormalities that in turn modify tumor initiation or promote the carcinogenic process. As alluded to above, the nutritional state of an animal can influence carcinogensis by modifying tumor initiation or acting as a tumor promoter (51). One of the major effects of nutrition on tumor initiation appears to be related to its influence on the metabolism of chemical carcinogens. Low-protein levels, and lipotrope-deficient, riboflavin-deficient, iodine-deficient and selenium-deficient diets have been shown to enhance tumor induction by a number of carcinogens in several different tissues (see Chapter 11). These conditions appear to enhance tumor induction by influencing the level of metabolism of the chemical carcinogen. This is described in detail in Chapter 11 of this volume. A high-fat diet has been shown to influence breast and colon cancer induction by acting mainly as an indirect promoter (51). In other words, a high-fat diet causes prolactin and estradiol to be produced in large amounts which act as promoters in mammary carcinogenesis (51). Likewise, a high-fat diet causes bile acids to be produced in excessive amounts which in turn act as promoters in colon carcinogenesis (50,51).

The effect of restricted dietary intake and caloric restriction on the development of spontaneous and induced tumors was first reported by Tannenbaum (41). He found that underfeeding mice and rats not only led to a lower tumor incidence but also increased the life span (41,42). In his studies the amounts of the various dietary components were reduced proportionately to each other. Calorie-restricted diets (reduced amounts of carbohydrate) also were found to reduce the incidence of mammary and skin tumors (6,42). The mechanism by which dietary restriction inhibits tumorigenesis is unknown. Initiation-promotion studies in mouse skin suggest that the dietary and caloric restriction were effective in the promotion stage of tumor formation (6). Tannenbaum and Silverstone (49) concluded that the relevant effect of dietary and caloric restriction was probably mediated through its effect on body weight. They suggested that the inhibition of tumorigenicity is associated with an overall nutritional deficiency at the cellular level. It is known that dietary or caloric restriction brings about an increase in endogenous glucocorticoids that could be responsible for the inhibition of tumorigenesis as described in Chapter 6.

Epidemiological evidence as well as studies using experimental animals suggest that nutritional deficiencies may relate to cancers of the stomach, cervix, and thyroid, whereas overnutrition significantly affects the development of cancers of the colon, pancreas, kidney, breast, ovary, endometrium, and prostate (51). Both epidemiological and experimental data suggest that the etiological factors of overnutrition relate to a high intake of fats and possibly other variables associated with high fat intake (50,51). Another explanation for the increased incidence of colon cancer is the decreased fiber in the diet and the associated

TABLE 14. *Dietary factors related to cancer in man*

High-fat, protein, and caloric intake
Refined carbohydrates; low fiber
Vitamin deficiencies; Vitamin A, riboflavin, and pyridoxine
Inorganic elements; iodine and selenium deficiencies
Certain food additives may be carcinogenic
Vehicle for environmental carcinogens, including PAH, insecticides, herbicides, and mycotoxins
Alcohol and smoking

TABLE 15. *Ways to prevent cancer and possibly cardiovascular diseases*

Decrease the fat (both saturated and unsaturated), protein, and caloric content of diet
Increase the unrefined carbohydrates and roughage content of food
Decrease the food additives used only for cosmetic purposes
Decrease the nitrites as preservatives in food
Decrease the unintentional carcinogens associated with food and water
Decrease the overall level of environmental and occupational carcinogens
Decrease smoking and alcohol consumption
Increase the amount of harmless anticarcinogenic agents to diet

increased intake of refined carbohydrates, protein and fat (50). Fiber-depleted refined diets influence stool consistency and bulk, transit time through the intestine and the nature and number of bacterial flora of the feces (8). There is an inverse relationship between the transit time and bulk of the stools and the fiber content of the food eaten. This could provide more time for bacterial proliferation and for bacterial grading action on bile acids and cholesterol as well as other chemicals associated with the feces (8).

The association between high dietary fat intake and cancer has pointed to high animal fat diet as the culprit. However, Enig and co-workers (15) have recently analyzed the existing data on dietary fat consumption noting that although the total fat consumption per capita has increased, the relative and absolute amount of animal fat consumed per capita has actually decreased. They also found that epidemiological data on various geographic and cultural groups did not support the idea of an association of animal fat consumption with colon or breast cancer. The overall increase in fat consumption is explained by increased use of vegetable fats. Their analyses showed that there was no correlation between animal fat and cancer but a significant positive correlation with vegetable fat (more unsaturated fat). Since vegetable fat has been stated to be more beneficial than animal fat in relationship to cardiovascular diseases, it would seem based on the above data that a decrease in total fat intake, i.e., saturated and unsaturated should be recommended.

Table 14 summarizes the various known dietary factors related to cancer in man. Rational ways to prevent this disease and possibly cardiovascular diseases in man are illustrated in Table 15. As previously discussed, it would be very difficult, if not virtually impossible, to eliminate all carcinogens known to exist in our environment as well as in the food we eat. However, if man would only heed warnings concerning the dangers of smoking, strive to eat a well-balanced and prudent diet, and regulate that to which he is exposed environmentally, certainly the incidence of cancer would decline.

ACKNOWLEDGMENT

This research was supported by NIH Grant CA 20076 and the Division of Biomedical Research, U.S. Department of Energy under contract W-7405-eng-26 with the Union Carbide Corporation.

REFERENCES

1. Ames, B. N., McCann, J., and Yamasaki, E. (1975): Methods for detecting carcinogens and mutagens with the Salmonella/mammalian-microsome mutagenicity test. *Mutat. Res.*, 31:347–364.

2. Armstrong, B., and Doll, R. (1975): Environmental factors and cancer incidence and mortality in different countries, with special reference to dietary practices. *Int. J. Cancer*, 15:617–631.

3. Bair, W. J. (1970): Inhalation of radionuclides and carcinogenesis. In: *Inhalation Carcinogenesis,* edited by P. Nettesheim, M. G. Hanna, Jr., and J. R. Gilbert, pp. 77–97. USAEC, Division of Technical Information, Symposium Series 18, National Technical Information Service, Springfield, Va., Conf-691001.

4. Belman, S., and Troll, W. (1978): Hormones, cyclic nucleotides, and prostaglandins. In: *Mechanisms of Tumor Promotion and Cocarcinogenesis,* Vol. 2, edited by T. J. Slaga, A. Sivak, and R. K. Boutwell, pp. 117–134. Raven Press, New York.

5. Bluestein, H. G., and Green, I. (1970): Croton oil-induced suppression of the immune response of guinea pigs. *Nature*, 228:871–872.

6. Boutwell, R. K. (1964): Some biological aspects of skin carcinogenesis. *Prog. Exp. Tumor Res.,* 4:207–250.

7. Brookes, P., and Lawley, P. D. (1964): Evidence for the binding of polynuclear aromatic hydrocarbons to nucleic acids of mouse skin: Relation between carcinogenic power of hydrocarbons and their binding to DNA. *Nature*, 202:781–784.

8. Burkitt, D. P., Walker, A. R., and Pointer, N. S. (1972): Effect of dietary fiber of stools and transit times and its role in the causation of disease. *Lancet,* 2:1408–1412.

9. Casto, B. C., and DiPaolo, J. A. (1973): Virus, chemicals and cancer. *Prog. Med. Virol.,* 16:1–47.

10. DeYoung, L. M., Mufson, R. A., and Boutwell, R. K. (1977): An apparent inactivation of initiated cells by the potent inhibitor of two-stage mouse skin tumorigenesis, bis(2-chloroethyl) sulfide. *Cancer Res.,* 37:4590–4594.

11. Doll, R. (1969): The geographical distribution of cancer. *Br. J. Cancer*, 23:1–8.

12. Ebbesen, P. (1974): Aging increases susceptibility of mouse skin to DMBA carcinogenesis independent of general immune status. *Science,* 183:217–220.

13. Elgjo, K., and Degre, M. (1975): Polyinosinic·polycytidylic acid: inhibition of cell proliferation in carcinogenesis treated epidermis and in carcinogen-induced skin tumors in mice. *J. Natl. Cancer Inst.,* 54:219–221.

14. Emmett, E. A. (1973): Ultraviolet radiation as a cause of skin tumors. *CRC Critical Rev. Toxicol.,* 2:211–255.

15. Enig, M. G., Munn, R. J., and Keeney, M. (1978): Dietary fat and cancer trends: A critique. *Fed. Proc.,* 37:2215–2200.

16. Frei, J. V. (1976): Some mechanisms operative in carcinogenesis: A review. *Chem. Biol. Interact.,* 13:1–25.

17. Gelboin, H. V., and Levy, H. B. (1970): Polyinosinic-polycytidylic acid inhibits chemically induced tumorigenesis in mouse skin. *Science,* 167:205–207.

18. German, J. (1972): Genes which increase chromosomal instability in somatic cells and predispose to cancer. *Prog. Med. Genet.,* 8:61–78.

19. Heidelberger, C. (1975): Chemical carcinogenesis. *Annu. Rev. Biochem.,* 44:79–121.

20. Hennings, H., and Boutwell, R. K. (1970): Studies on the mechanism of skin tumor promotion. *Cancer Res.,* 30:312–320.

21. International Agency for Research on Cancer (1972–1977): *IARC Monographs on the Evaluation of Carcinogenic Risk of Chemicals to Man,* Vols. 1 to 15. International Agency for Research on Cancer, Lyon, France.

22. Jerina, D. M., and Daly, J. W. (1977): Oxidation at carbon. In: *Drug Metabolism,* edited by D. V. Parke, and R. L. Smith, pp. 15–33. Taylor & Francis, Ltd., London.

23. Jerina, D. M., Lehr, R. E., Yagi, H., Hernandez, O., Dansette, P. M., Wislocki, P. G., Wood, A. W., Chang, R. L., Levin, W. and Conney, A. H. (1976): Mutagenicity of benzo(a)pyrene derivatives and the description of a quantum mechanical model which predicts the ease of carbonium ion formation from diol epoxides. In: *In Vitro Metabolic Activation and Mutagenesis Testing.* edited by F. J. deSerres, J. R. Fouts, J. R. Bend, and R. M. Philpot, pp. 159–177. Elsevier/North Holland Biomedical Press, Amsterdam.

24. Keast, D. (1970): Immunosurveillance and Cancer. *Lancet,* 2:710–712.
25. McCann, J., and Ames, B. N. (1976): Detection of carcinogens as mutagens in Salmonella microsome test: Assay of 300 chemicals: Discussion. *Proc. Natl. Acad. Sci. USA,* 73:950–954.
26. Miller, E. C. (1978): Some current perspectives on chemical carcinogenesis in humans and experimental animals: Presidential address. *Cancer Res.,* 38:1479–1496.
27. Miller, E. C., and Miller, J. A. (1976): The metabolism of chemical carcinogenesis to reactive electrophiles and their possible mechanism of action in carcinogenesis. In: *Chemical Carcinogens,* edited by C. E. Searle p. 732. American Chemical Society, Washington, D.C.
28. Mervish, S. S., Wallcave, L., Eagen, M., and Shubik, P. (1972): Ascorbate-nitrite reaction: Possible means of blocking the formation of carcinogenic N-nitroso compounds. *Science,* 177:65–68.
29. Peraino, C., Fry, R. J. M., and Grube, D. P. (1978): Drug-induced enhancement of hepatic tumorigenesis. In: *Mechanisms of Tumor Promotion and Cocarcinogenesis,* Vol. 2, edited by T. J. Slaga, A. Sivak, and R. K. Boutwell, pp. 421–432. Raven Press, New York.
30. Piessens, W. F., Heimann, R., Legros, N., and Heuson, J. C. (1971): Effect of Bacillus Calmette-Guerin on mammary tumor formation and cellular immunity in dimethylbenz(a)anthracene-treated rats. *Cancer Res.,* 31:1061–1065.
31. Pitot, H. C. (1978): Interactions in the natural history of aging and carcinogenesis. *Fed. Proc.,* 37:2841–2847.
32. Schinitsky, M. R., Hyman, L. R., Blazkovec, A. A., and Burkholder, P. M. (1973): Bacillus Calmette-Guerin vaccination and skin tumor promotion with croton oil in mice. *Cancer Res.,* 33:659–663.
33. Schwarz, J. A., Viaje, A., Slaga, T. J., Yuspa, S. H., Hennings, H., and Lichti, U. (1977): Fluocinolone acetonide: A potent inhibitor of mouse skin tumor promotion and epidermal DNA synthesis. *Chem. Biol. Interact.,* 17:331–347.
34. Slaga, T. J., Buty, S. G., Thompson, S., Bracken, W. M., and Viaje, A. (1977): A kinetic study on the *in vitro* covalent binding of polycyclic hydrocarbons to nucleic acids using epidermal homogenates as the activating system. *Cancer Res.,* 37:3126–3131.
35. Slaga, T. J., Fischer, S. M., Viaje, A., Berry, D. L., Bracken, W. M., LeClerc, S., and Miller, D. L. (1978): Inhibition of tumor promotion by anti-inflammatory agents: An approach to the biochemical mechanism of promotion. In: *Mechanisms of Tumor Promotion and Cocarcinogenesis,* Vol. 2, edited by T. J. Slaga, A. Sivak, and R. K. Boutwell, pp. 173–195. Raven Press, New York.
36. Slaga, T. J., Sivak, A., and Boutwell, R. K., editors (1978): *Mechanism of Tumor Promotion and Carcinogenesis, Vol. 2, Carcinogenesis: A Comprehensive Survey,* 588 pp. Raven Press, New York.
37. Stjernsward, J. (1967): Immunological studies of chemical carcinogenesis. *J. Natl. Cancer Inst.,* 38:515–526.
38. Storer, J. B. (1975): Radiation carcinogenesis. In: *Cancer,* edited by F. F. Becker, Vol. 1. Plenum Press, New York.
39. Stutman, O. (1974): Tumor development after 3-methylcholanthrene in immunologically deficient athymic-nude mice. *Science,* 183:534–536.
40. Stutman, O. (1969): Carcinogen-induced immune depression: Absence in mice resistant to chemical carcinogenesis. *Science,* 166:620–621.
41. Tannenbaum, A. (1940): Relationship of body weight to cancer incidence. *Arch. Pathol.,* 30:509–517.
42. Tannenbaum, A., and Silverstone, H. (1957): Nutrition and genesis of tumors. In: *Cancer,* Vol. 1, edited by R. W. Raven, p. 306. Butterworth & Co., London.
43. Thompson, S., and Slaga, T. J. (1976): The effects of dexamethasone on mouse skin initiation and aryl hydrocarbon hydroxylase. *Eur. J. Cancer,* 12:363–370.
44. Upton, A. C. (1968): Radiation carcinogenesis. In: *Methods in Cancer Research,* Vol. 4, edited by H. Busch. Academic Press, New York.
45. VanDuuren, B. L., Sivak, A., Katy, C., Seidman, I., and Melchionne, S. (1975): The effect of aging and interval between primary and secondary treatment in two-stage carcinogenesis on mouse skin. *Cancer Res.,* 35:502–505.
46. VanDuuren, B. L., Wity, G., and Goldschmidt, B. M. (1978): Structure-activity relationships of tumor promoters and cocarcinogens and interaction of phorbol myristate acetate and related esters with plasma membranes. In: *Mechanisms of Tumor Promotion and Cocarcinogenesis,*

Vol. 2, edited by T. J. Slaga, A. Sivak, and R. K. Boutwell, pp. 491–507. Raven Press, New York.

47. Verma, A. K., Rice, H. M., Shapas, B. G., and Boutwell, R. K. (1978): Inhibition of 12-0-tetradecanoylphorbol-13-acetate-induced ornithine decarboxylase activity in mouse epidermis by vitamin A analogs (Retinoids). *Cancer Res.,* 38:793–801.

48. Wattenberg, L. W. (1978): Inhibition of chemical carcinogenesis. *J. Natl. Cancer Inst.,* 60:11–18.

49. Witschi, H., and Lock, S. (1978): Butylated hydroxytoluene: A possible promoter of adenoma formation in mouse lung. In: *Mechanisms of Tumor Promotion and Cocarcinogenesis,* Vol. 2, edited by T. J. Slaga, A. Sivak, and R. K. Boutwell, pp. 475–490. Raven Press, New York.

50. Wynder, E. L. (1976): Nutrition and Cancer. *Fed. Proc.,* 35:1309–1315.

51. Wynder, E. L., Hoffmann, D., McCoy, G. D., Cohen, L. A., and Reddy, B. S. (1978): Tumor promotion and cocarcinogenesis as related to man and his environment. In: *Mechanisms of Tumor Promotion and Cocarcinogenesis,* Vol. 2, edited by T. J. Slaga, A. Sivak, and R. K. Boutwell, pp. 59–77. Raven Press, New York.

Subject Index

Acetanilide, 62
Acetic acid, 112
N-Acetoxy-acetylaminofluorene (AAF), 229
2-Acetylaminofluorene, 13–16, 58, 63, 73, 91, 92, 158, 210, 219, 248; see also N-Acetylaminofluorene
N-Acetylaminofluorene-N-hydroxylase, 63, 230
N-α-Acetyl-L-lysine methyl ester [(^{3}H)ALME], 131
Actinomycetes, 129
Actinomycin D, 132
Activation of carcinogen, 6, 24, 253
  nutrition and, 209–211
Adenine, 6
Adenoma (s), pulmonary, 87, 179
Adenylate cyclase, activation of, 137
Adipocyte, induction of, 37
β-Adrenergic response, 42
Adrenohypophyseal system, 133
Aflatoxicol (AFOL), 223
  action of, 22
Aflatoxin(s), 2, 20, 21, 145, 158, 207, 225–227
Aflatoxin B_1 (AFB$_1$), 21–23, 219, 221, 223–227
Aflatoxin B_1-2,3-dichloride 23
Aflatoxin B_{2a}, 21, 223, 224
Aflatoxin M, 22, 223
  action of, 21, 22
Aflatoxin P_1, 22, 23
Aflatoxin Q_1, 23
Age, influence on carcinogenesis, 209, 247, 248
AKR cells, 197, 198
L-Alanine-L-phenyl-D-lysine-CH$_2$Cl, 135
Alcohol(s), 60, 252
Alcoholism, 256
Aldehyde, 17, 129
Aldrin, 60, 157
Aliphatic hydrocarbons, 252
Alkene, 2

Alkylate sulfhydryl, 129
Alkylation, 13, 229
Allylisopropylacetamide, 60
Ames system, 68
Amine (s), 19, 254
  see also Aromatic amines
Amino acid(s), 218
6-Aminochrysene, 75
Amphotropic virus, features of, 186
Anchorage-independent growth, 35, 36, 38, 39
Androgenic steroid hormones, 101
Antabuse, 93
Anthralin, 133, 251
Anticarcinogenesis, 99
  compounds for, 247–251, 253, 254 256
Antigen(s), 248
Antiinflammatory steroids, 256
  effects of, 117, 118, 121, 122
  inhibition of tumor promotion by, 45, 47, 113, 114–117, 122, 133, 255
Antimetabolites, 1
Antioxidant(s), 146, 253, 256
  inhibition of chemical carcinogenesis by, 61, 86–96
    by BHA, BHT, and ethoxyquin, 87 90–93, 95
    by cysteamine-HCl, 95
    by disulfiram and related compounds, 93–95
    of PAH, 151–153, 163
    by selenium and selenium salts, 94, 95
Antipain, 138
Antipyrene, 68
Apigenin, 65
Aromatic amine(s), 2, 12–16, 73, 145
Aroclor 1254, inhibition of PAH carcinogenesis by, 158–160, 162
Aryl epoxide(s), 212
Aryl hydrocarbon hydroxylase (AHH), 150–152, 155